T0122463

Smart Innovation, Systems and Technologies

357

Series Editors

Robert J. Howlett, *KES International Research, Shoreham-by-Sea, UK*
Lakhmi C. Jain, *KES International, Shoreham-by-Sea, UK*

The Smart Innovation, Systems and Technologies book series encompasses the topics of knowledge, intelligence, innovation and sustainability. The aim of the series is to make available a platform for the publication of books on all aspects of single and multi-disciplinary research on these themes in order to make the latest results available in a readily-accessible form. Volumes on interdisciplinary research combining two or more of these areas is particularly sought.

The series covers systems and paradigms that employ knowledge and intelligence in a broad sense. Its scope is systems having embedded knowledge and intelligence, which may be applied to the solution of world problems in industry, the environment and the community. It also focusses on the knowledge-transfer methodologies and innovation strategies employed to make this happen effectively. The combination of intelligent systems tools and a broad range of applications introduces a need for a synergy of disciplines from science, technology, business and the humanities. The series will include conference proceedings, edited collections, monographs, handbooks, reference books, and other relevant types of book in areas of science and technology where smart systems and technologies can offer innovative solutions.

High quality content is an essential feature for all book proposals accepted for the series. It is expected that editors of all accepted volumes will ensure that contributions are subjected to an appropriate level of reviewing process and adhere to KES quality principles.

Indexed by SCOPUS, EI Compendex, INSPEC, WTI Frankfurt eG, zbMATH, Japanese Science and Technology Agency (JST), SCImago, DBLP.

All books published in the series are submitted for consideration in Web of Science.

Yen-Wei Chen · Satoshi Tanaka · R. J. Howlett · Lakhmi C. Jain

Editors

Innovation in Medicine and Healthcare

Proceedings of 11th KES-InMed 2023

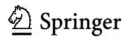
Springer

Editors
Yen-Wei Chen
Ritsumeikan University
Kyoto, Japan

R. J. Howlett
KES International Research
Shoreham-by-Sea, UK

Satoshi Tanaka
Ritsumeikan University
Kyoto, Japan

Lakhmi C. Jain
KES International
Selby, UK

ISSN 2190-3018   ISSN 2190-3026 (electronic)
Smart Innovation, Systems and Technologies
ISBN 978-981-99-3313-6   ISBN 978-981-99-3311-2 (eBook)
https://doi.org/10.1007/978-981-99-3311-2

This Springer imprint is published by the registered company Springer Nature Singapore Pte Ltd.
The registered company address is: 152 Beach Road, #21-01/04 Gateway East, Singapore 189721, Singapore

Preface

The 11th KES International Conference on Innovation in Medicine and Healthcare (InMed-23) was held in Rome, Italy, on June 14–16, 2023.

The InMed-23 is the 11th edition of the InMed series of conferences. The conference focuses on major trends and innovations in modern intelligent systems applied to medicine, surgery, health care and the issues of an aging population including recent hot topics on artificial intelligence for medicine and health care. The purpose of the conference is to exchange the new ideas, new technologies and current research results in these research fields.

We received submissions from many countries around the world. All submissions were carefully reviewed by at least two reviewers of the International Program Committee. Finally, 35 papers were accepted to be presented in this proceeding, which covers a number of key areas in smart medicine and health care including: (1) innovations in assessment, education and interventions for children with developmental disorders; (2) data-driven models for healthcare systems; (3) projects, systems and applications for smart medicine/health care; (4) medical image processing; (5) machine/deep learning for medicine and health care; and (6) deep learning in medical imaging. In addition to the accepted research papers, a number of keynote speeches by leading researchers were presented at the conference.

We would like to thank Ms. Yuka Sato of Ritsumeikan University for their valuable assistance in editing this volume. We are also grateful to the authors and reviewers for their contributions.

June 2023

Yen-Wei Chen
Satoshi Tanaka
Robert J. Howlett
Lakhmi C. Jain

InMed 2023 Organization

Honorary Chair

Lakhmi C. Jain — University of Canberra, Australia, and Bournemouth University, UK

Executive Chair

Robert J. Howlett — Bournemouth University, UK

General Chair

Yen-Wei Chen — Ritsumeikan University, Japan

Program Chair

Satoshi Tanaka — Ritsumeikan University, Japan

International Program Committee Members

Alanis Arnulfo G. — Instituto Tecnológico de Tijuana, Mexico
Ahmad Taher Azar — Prince Sultan University, Saudi Arabia
Adrian S. Barb — Penn State University, USA
Smaranda Belciug — University of Craiova, Romania
Alvaro Bertelsen — VICOMTECH, Spain
Isabelle Bichindaritz — State University of New York, Oswego, USA
Brenda Bogaert — University Jean Moulin Lyon 3, France
Christopher Buckingham — Aston University, UK
Jose Manuel Fonseca — NOVA University of Lisbon, Portugal
Yoshiaki Fukami — Keio University/Gakushuin University, Japan
Oana Geman — University Stefan cel Mare of Suceava, Romania
Maria Jesus Garcia-Gonzalez — VICOMTECH, Spain
Kyoko Hasegawa — Ritsumeikan University, Japan
Maria Iacob — University of Twente, Netherlands

Anca Ignat	University "Alexandru Ioan Cuza" of Iasi, Romania
Rahul Kumar Jain	Ritsumeikan University, Japan
Rashmi Jain	Montclair State University, USA
Bill Kapralos	Ontario Tech University, Canada
Dalia Kriksciuniene	Vilnius University, Lithuania
Jingbing Li	Hainan University, China
Liang Li	Ritsumeikan University, Japan
Jing Liu	Zhejiang Lab, China
Yinhao Li	Ritsumeikan University, Japan
Karen Lopez-Linares	VICOMTECH, Spain
Jiaqing Liu	Ritsumeikan University, Japan
Michaela Luca	Institute of Computer Science, Romanian Academy
Daniela López De Luise	CI2S Labs
Yoshimasa Masuda	Keio University, Japan
Kazuyuki Matsumoto	Tokushima University, Japan
Rashid Mehmood	King Abdul Aziz University, Saudi Arabia
Mayuri Mehta	Sarvajanik College of Engineering and Technology, India
Polina Mihova	New Bulgarian University, Bulgaria
Victor Mitrana	Polytechnic University of Madrid, Spain
Marek R. Ogiela	AGH University of Science and Technology, Krakow, Poland
Ivan Macia Oliver	VICOMTECH, Spain
Liying Peng	Zhejiang University, China
Vijayalakshmi Ramasamy	University of Wisconsin, Parkside, USA
Joel J. P. C. Rodrigues	China University of Petroleum, China
Virgilijus Sakalauskas	Vilnius University, Lithuania
Donald Shepard	Brandeis University, USA
Margarita Stankova	New Bulgarian University, Bulgaria
Maialen Stephens	VICOMTECH, Spain
Ruxandra Stoean	University of Craiova, Romania
Kazuyoshi Tagawa	Aichi University, Japan
Tomoko Tateyama	Fujita Health University, Japan
Eiji Uchino	Yamaguchi University, Japan
Athanasios V. Vasilakos	University of Agder, Norway
Didier Vinot	University Jean Moulin Lyon 3, France
Hongyi Wang	Zhejiang University, China
Weibin Wang	Zhejiang Lab, China
Junzo Watada	University Teknologi Petronas, Malaysia
Rui Xu	Dalian University of Technology, China

Yingying Xu	Zhejiang Lab, China
Yoshiyuki Yabuuchi	Shimonoseki City University, Japan
Shuichiro Yamamoto	Nagoya University, Japan
Yulin Yang	Ritsumeikan University, Japan
Hiroyuki Yoshida	Harvard Medical School/Massachusetts General Hospital, USA
Gan Zhan	Ritsumeikan University, Japan
Chujie Zhao	Zhejiang Lab, China

Organization and Management

KES International (www.kesinternational.org)
in partnership with
the Institute of Knowledge Transfer (www.ikt.org.uk).

Contents

Medical Image Processing

About the Authors

Prof. Yen-Wei Chen received his B.E. degree in 1985 from Kobe University, Kobe, Japan. He received his M.E. degree in 1987 and his D.E. degree in 1990, both from Osaka University, Osaka, Japan. He was a research fellow at the Institute of Laser Technology, Osaka, from 1991 to 1994. From October 1994 to March 2004, he was an associate professor and a professor at the Department of Electrical and Electronic Engineering, University of the Ryukyus, Okinawa, Japan. He is currently a professor at the College of Information Science and Engineering, Ritsumeikan University, Kyoto, Japan. He is also a visiting professor at the College of Computer Science and Technology, Zhejiang University, Hangzhou, China. He was a visiting scholar at Oxford University, Oxford, UK, in 2003 and at Pennsylvania State University, Pennsylvania, USA, in 2010. His research interests include medical image analysis and computer vision. He has published more than 300 research papers. He has received many distinguished awards including Best Scientific Paper Award of ICPR2013. He is the principal investigator of many projects in biomedical engineering and image analysis, funded by the Japanese Government.

Prof. Satoshi Tanaka got his Ph.D. in theoretical physics at Waseda University, Japan, in 1987. After experiencing assistant professors, a senior lecturer, and an associate professor at Waseda University and Fukui University, he became a professor at Ritsumeikan University in 2002. His current research target is computer visualization of complex 3D shapes such as 3D scanned cultural heritage objects, inside structures of a human body, and fluid simulation results. He was the vice president of Visualization Society of Japan (VSJ), the president of Japan Society for Simulation Technology (JSST), and the president of ASIASIM (Federation of Asia Simulation Societies). Currently, he works as a cooperation member of Japan Science Council. He received best paper awards at Asia Simulation Conference (2012 and 2022), Journal of Advanced Simulation in Science and Engineering in 2014, and many others.

R. J. Howlett is the Academic Chair of KES International a non-profit organisation which facilitates knowledge transfer and the dissemination of research results in areas including Intelligent Systems, Sustainability, and Knowledge Transfer. He is Visiting Professor at 'Aurel Vlaicu' University of Arad, Romania, and has also been Visiting Professor at Bournemouth University, UK. His technical expertise is in the use of artificial intelligence and machine learning for the solution of industrial problems. His current interests centre on the application of intelligent systems to sustainability, particularly renewable energy, smart/micro grids and applications in housing and glasshouse horticulture. He previously developed a national profile in knowledge and technology transfer, and the commercialisation of research. He works with a number of universities and international research groups on the supervision teams of PhD students, and the provision of technical support for projects.

Professor Lakhmi C. Jain , PhD, Dr H.C., ME, BE(Hons), Fellow (Engineers Australia), is with the University of Arad. He was formerly with the University of Technology Sydney, the University of Canberra and Bournemouth University.

Professor Jain founded the KES International for providing a professional community the opportunities for publications, knowledge exchange, cooperation and teaming. Involving around 5,000 researchers drawn from universities and companies world-wide, KES facilitates international cooperation and generate synergy in teaching and research. KES regularly provides networking opportunities for professional community through one of the largest conferences of its kind in the area of KES.

His interests focus on the artificial intelligence paradigms and their applications in complex systems, security, e-education, e-healthcare, unmanned air vehicles and intelligent agents.

Innovations in Assessment, Education, and Interventions for Children with Developmental Disorders

Online Platforms and Applications for the Development and Treatment of Reading Skills in Children - A Comparison Between Three Countries

Polina Mihova[1]([✉]) [iD], Maria Mavrothanasi[1] [iD], Haneen Alshawesh[1] [iD], and Tsveta Stoyanova[2] [iD]

[1] Department of Health Care and Social Work, New Bulgarian University, 1618 Sofia, Bulgaria
pmihova@nbu.bg
[2] Bocconi University, Milan, Italy

Abstract. After schools were closed due to the COVID-19 pandemic, children were left with distance learning as their only option for a considerable amount of time. The impact on students with special education needs, especially those who have reading difficulties, is still not completely clear. Children with reading comprehension difficulties may be more vulnerable to negative learning outcomes following the COVID-19 lockdown. This is because they require constant, focused, and deliberate care in order to meet their educational goals. The purpose of this article is to examine three nations' free, online tools geared towards improving and rehabilitating the reading skills of preschool and elementary school-aged students. For children who have trouble while learning to read, it has been found that enrichment reading online treatment tools and programs can be helpful in developing their reading ability.

Keywords: Online platform · Therapeutic tools · Reading skills · Special educational needs

1 Introduction

Text comprehension has become increasingly dependent - in recent years, as a result of the proliferation of technology in many aspects of day-to-day life - on an increasing number of digital reading devices (computers and laptops, e-books, and tablet devices). These devices have the potential to become fundamental support to improving traditional reading, learning, and understanding skills. This pattern can be observed in schools, at home when doing homework, and at the workplace (e.g., inference generation). Since most children are exposed to technology well before they enter kindergarten, parents make use of the various smart devices in their homes to give their children a head start on their reading abilities.

The formation of solid reading skills and good reading habits begins with learning the fundamental abilities related to perception, sound detection, word recognition, word

Y.-W. Chen et al. (Eds.): KES InMed 2023, SIST 357, pp. 3–12, 2023.
https://doi.org/10.1007/978-981-99-3311-2_1

discrimination, semantics, syntax, linguistic processes, and comprehension. Creating conducive reading settings that take these needs into account might help those, who have trouble reading, succeed. The early identification of kids who have trouble reading and the implementation of accessible and affordable therapeutic programs for reading challenges are also crucial. One approach that might be adopted is the use of open-access online reading platforms, designed as enrichment reading programs that serve as therapeutic instruments.

Most countries have temporarily closed their educational institutions in 2020, including Bulgaria, Greece, and Libya. Because of the lengthy disruption in traditional classroom settings, many parents have put their faith into online education. Online education for young children, however, requires a substantial investment of time and effort from busy parents, especially when it comes to youngsters with special educational needs (SEN). Different online and app solutions were created and used by governments and NGOs to support children with special needs.

Many educators, parents, and kids were caught off guard by this unexpected shift, and they are now facing new issues as a result of the growing role that parents play in supporting their children's education at home.

The article presents an overview of online platforms for training and therapeutic support of children with SEN and their parents in three countries – Bulgaria, Greece, and Libya.

2   Reading Skills

In international scientific literature on the topic of computerized training programs for reading comprehension, a variety of strategies and skills have been identified as being important. In particular, various studies include activities that promote cognitive (such as vocabulary and inference-making) and metacognitive (such as the use of strategies, comprehension monitoring, and identification of relevant parts in a text) components of reading comprehension. For example, vocabulary is one cognitive component, and inference-making is another. Capodieci et al. (2020) evaluate papers on computerized training systems and summarize the results. Most participants are middle and high school students of various ages and academic levels. Training program participants outperformed comparison group peers and sustained their progress, contributing to the good outcomes of the investigations. The training program improved comprehension abilities, which lasted during the follow-up.

The ability to read and write may benefit from new technology in a meaningful way. Reading refers to the process by which printed texts are converted into speech (often while pupils are reading the printed materials themselves). Literacy requires a wide range of mental operations, including, but not limited to, letter and word recognition [2]. Interaction with multimedia also extends and improves learning and reading abilities in productive ways, which may expand educational opportunities for students who are not currently achieving their potential to become strong readers [3]. In addition, the use of technology is appreciated by children and their parents, and both groups have a positive attitude towards the use of additional means in learning and therapy of cognitive disorders [4–6].

2.1 Aetiology for Reading Difficulties

Given that a quite large portion of the student population is on the learning difficulties spectrum, which is related to functional, social, emotional, and behavioural difficulties with poorer long-term social and vocational outcomes, early detection of and intervention in those deficits is a high priority.

Literature review suggests that students with reading disabilities, show significant deficits in decoding, fluency, slow or/and inaccurate reading, and difficulties in overall text comprehension [7]. A neurobiological background seems to be involved [8], which affects specific domains of cognitive processes, rather than causing an overall intellectual disability [9]. Finally, environmental factors also determine the characteristics of individuals with Specific Learning Disabilities (SLD). The effects of instructional practices, family literacy, and peer influences can moderate or magnify reading difficulties, alongside the genetic basis.

The necessity of early intervention [10] is grounded on findings, according to which it can be cautionary supported that neural processes may normalize if the intervention is successful [11]. Therefore, intervention goals should aim at developing the mediate neural systems that compose the reading comprehension procedure. For instance, vocabulary and visual sequential memory enhancement, phonological awareness, and development of the semantical network are significant requirements for immediate access to word meaning and decoding.

Other adjustments of the educational environment such as individualization, increment instructional time, and reduction of group size, are crucial factors to improve reading skills.

Assistive technology meets all these requirements, as educational software could promote individual learning. In addition, there are findings that suggest that even high-quality intensive intervention could be inadequate for many students on the SLD spectrum. However, they "may profit from assistive technology (e.g., computer programs that convert text-to-speech;) [12].

As discussed, students with reading disabilities face difficulties in decoding. Studies have shown that word recognition plays a key role in decoding and, consequently, in comprehension [13]. Intervention orientated at presenting reading material orally [12], facilitates students' access to the meaning of the text [14].

In this paper, some educational tools developed in the Greek, Libyan, and Bulgarian languages, addressed to teachers, logotherapists, and other experts will be presented, in light of the encouraging data research [15] regarding the effectiveness of the technology-assisted intervention, in all areas of developmental disorders [16–18].

3   Types of Online Educational and Therapeutics Tools

An online learning tool is a piece of software that gives students the option to participate in classroom activities in a virtual capacity. This category of software can have a wide variety of features and functions that can help analyse the performance of students and determine which instructional methods work best. If you have a working knowledge of what an online learning tool is, you will be better able to engage with your students and create an inclusive learning environment for them. This article will provide an explanation of what an online learning tool is, a list of the benefits of using one, and a few online learning tools for you to consider using in your own therapy sessions and practice.

3.1 Online Learning Tools

Online learning tools are software platforms that provide multiple educational functions such as collaborative communication, digital education materials, and immediate feedback to students. Some of these functions include access to a variety of educational tools developed by a number of different software providers via the internet. A platform that can deliver either broad or narrowly focused functionality is what we mean when we refer to an online learning tool. Some of the instructional tools available online, for instance, may place an emphasis on communication, while others may keep students' attention through educational games. Below, we have provided a list of some of the most common settings you can find in an online learning tool.

3.2 Learning Management Systems

A learning management system, sometimes known as an LMS, is a piece of software that may be used for online instruction and contains various methods to evaluate the performance of students. An LMS is often the most comprehensive online learning tool because of its ability to record assessment results, personalize online classes, and select certain learning content. Students of all ages, from elementary school up through college, could benefit from the use of such online tools.

3.3 Communication Tools

Communication tools are online forums where one can participate in conversations with other individuals, such as students or co-workers. The educational functions of communication tools, such as the creation of tests and the recording of the results, are not always included. Communication tools often focus on facilitating group conversations. Utilizing these technologies in conjunction with many other virtual learning tools may prove to be effective. When compared to other educational tools, communication tools typically offer more facilities for creating forums and engaging in topical discussion.

3.4 Internet-Based Educational Resources

Online learning resources are commonly understood as a platform that has a variety of learning materials, such as research articles, pre-set tests, quizzes, and interactive activities. Students can access a wide variety of learning materials if their educator uses an online learning resource. Students can benefit from this by becoming more interested in learning, which may inspire them to grow their skills and expand their knowledge.

3.5 Video Games with an Educational Component

Students have access to a variety of fun and educational online activities using digital educational games, which are hosted on internet platforms. These interactive learning activities are often better suited for pupils in elementary school and younger pupils difficult and provide more information could be beneficial to students in high school. Young children can benefit greatly from playing digital games since it can help them feel more interested in their education and more motivated to come to school.

4 Materials and Method

This study considered all ethical research standards in accordance with the General Data Protection Requirements (GDPR) and complied with the ethical recommendations of the Department of Health care and Social Services, NBU. The authors conducted a literature search of available materials and identified the issue, which is the use of mobile applications in enhancing reading comprehension in first language acquisition.

We searched those four major online databases, using the search terms ("online" OR "web") AND "platforms" AND ("serious games" OR "computer games" OR "computer-based" OR "mobile app" OR "portable" OR "software") AND "reading skills". The search and selection of the results were conducted in November-December 2022. Eleven of the twenty platforms were selected as they present original technologies and thera-peutics tools by the authors. A brief summary of each of these publications is presented below.

5 Results

5.1 Bulgarian Platforms

Digital Backpack
In 2023, students, instructors and parents will use a free unified e-education platform with 5 modules. It will be installed on the MES cloud and will be accessible via electronic profiles at https://edu.mon.bg/. Students shall carry "digital backpacks". The school's distant learning platform won't affect the work interface. Teachers may construct lessons, exercises, and examinations using the new platform. Texts, photos, interactive presenta-tions, 3D models, video and audio clips, virtual and augmented reality, and more will be available development. The projects purpose is to build a "bank" of high-quality interac-tive lessons, exercises, and examinations prepared by teachers for all general education disciplines. The EU's structural and investment funds co-finance the "Education for Tomorrow" initiative of the Operational Program "Science and Education for Intelligent Growth" 2014–2020.

eProsveta
On February 15, 1945, the Regents of Bulgaria decreed that Prosveta Publishing House would "produce textbooks, teaching aids, notebooks, and drawing pads for all academic disciplines in all sorts of schools and academic institutions" within the Ministry and

Education and Science. Prosveta has published more than 50,000 writers and 28,000 titles in 788 series in over two billion copies, according to statistics.

FlipBooks are ePosvetas' interactive electronic textbooks (digital versions of traditional paper volumes that have additional educational exercises, video lessons, brief e-lessons, and tests).

Quick online tutorials in basic English can aid self-education, and the platform has an assessments section with interactive exams that grade students after each lesson. There are e-books and textbooks for pre-K tin the last school year and instructional videos, so all Bulgarian kids may acquire high-quality online education from professional teachers through video courses. The platform reads the textbook's task conditions to the youngest and visually impaired pupils on a computer. Almost 40,000 interactive items make information visible and easy to learn (videos, animations, 360-degree panoramas, 3D animations, etc.).

Shkolo

Shkolo, founded in 2016 by Lyubomir Vanyov (CTO), Miroslav Dzhokanov (CEO), Simeon Predov (CCO), and Alexander Stoyanov (Chief Mobile Division), is Bulgaria's premier digital education platform. Bulgaria joins the UK, Estonia, and the US in using school administration software with the team's e-diary.

The tech startup's key aims are reducing bureaucracy, involving parents in their children's education, and engaging students in class. Shkolo's solution optimizes schools' back-end and administrative procedures by automating reports, alerts, student and parent reminders, online payments, and asset monitoring.

5.2   Libyan Platforms

The Libyan Platform for Training and Distance[1]

The platform in numbers is as follows: 16,506 active users for a total of 913 courses with 21,619 resources in the form of assignments, links and references, images, and videos. The platform also has a mobile version.

Alef Ba Ta Educational Games[2]

- **Games Section** - 200 games ranked and numbered by difficulty. Each game genre is themed. Pupils are taught the Arabic alphabet, the Harakat, and appropriate pronunciation.
- **Texts Section** - short stories and longer instructional essays. Discusses various political and ethical problems to enrich the reader's experience. Interactive, vocabulary-building exercises. Targeted towards 8–10-year-olds.
- **Sights Section** - the top 100 sight words in children's literature. Each set of five sight words has a review component. Each sight word's introduction is followed by exercises to help students understand and remember it. This section teaches sight words and helps kids remember them, improving their reading abilities. Presents and certificates inspire and reward kids for completing tasks.

---

[1] https://school-ly.com/school.

[2] https://www.alefbata.com/lessons.

- Educational Activities - over 1,000 interactive exercises. Over 100 educational activities are intriguing. Interactive courses and PDFs provide exercises. From learning Arabic letters through grammar and comprehension, the tasks are grouped by difficulty.

3asafeer[3]

3asafeer's online digital library makes high-quality Arabic reading materials affordable and easy to find for schools and public libraries. In addition to a variety of instructional aids, tools, and worksheets. Providing material organized by level based on the latest research on teaching Arabic to youngsters. Partnering with KHDA to offer levelled reading and 3asafeer's ICT education innovation to Dubai schools. Pilot initiatives in many schools will do this.

They are working with The Breteau Foundation (BF) to give refugee camp students in Jordan and Lebanon free access to the entire digital library. The charity provides online teaching materials to help disadvantaged kids reach their potential. In the past month, children spent 367,250 h reading 2,602,360 stories on the platform. It is available also as an app, both for Play Store and Apple Store.

Nafham[4]

Nafham is a free online K-12 educational platform that relies on crowdsourcing for its content and adheres to the public curriculum. The five to twenty-minute crowdsourced videos on Nafham are edited by professionals. Students are provided a variety of learning strategies to choose from when watching instructional videos. By doing so, according to grade, subject, term, and academic schedule, they will have a much easier time locating the courses they require. The platform contains 3000 videos that have been seen more than 120 million times by one million viewers.

The "Free Education" section provides several general education courses, unrelated to formal education, on the fundamentals and principles of various fields to enrich and develop the skills and knowledge of society. These courses are offered in addition to the schools' curricula. The platform is available also as an app, on both Play Store and Apple Store.

5.3 Greek Platforms

"Text Detective"

"Text Detective" is an educational software where students play the role of real detectives. Based on the clues they are given in the text and the strategies taught, they are asked to "solve their guesses" by finding the meaning of the text. The strategies concern the active use of prior knowledge, finding text difficulties, and summarizing narrative or factual texts to understand them. Finally, students are asked to use the reading comprehension strategies without external reinforcement through the self-regulation strategy. It is a conversion of a successful reading enhancement program that has been applied over

---

[3] https://3asafeer.com.

[4] https://www.nafham.com/courses/subject/16064.

4 months to 286 students, with 76 among whom had reading comprehension difficulties (Antoniou 2006). It aimed at developing self-regulation strategies for students to use when trying to find a text's meaning.

"Write Simple. Read Fast"[5]

This company has developed a software for students with learning disabilities. It is aimed at primary school students, focusing on the cultivation of skills in which students show significant deficits.

The "Write Simple. Read Fast" software interactively and playfully cultivates basic reading skills, such as phonological awareness, and vocabulary development, through pictures, sequencing, sentence structure, categorization etc.

Development and Weighting of the 12 Tools[6]

The University of Patras' department of Primary school education undertook the "Construction and weighting of 12 exploratory-detection tools (criteria) of learning difficulties", aiming at the early detection and diagnostic evaluation of students' learning difficulties. Furthermore, this program wishes to set the psycho-pedagogical diagnostic framework in order to organize and implement personalized educational intervention programs both for the prevention and treatment of learning difficulties.

Tool 1 and 8 focus on the investigation of the cognitive-linguistic factors that make up the reading function and the identification of those parameters that show deficient development or function, in order to diagnose and interpret the nature of the difficulty and, therefore, to draw up an individualized educational intervention program for prevention (according to preschool age) or its treatment (during school age).

6 Conclusions

In general, all three nations have devised programs and resources to help students improve their reading abilities. This indicates that reading is a priority in each of the three societies, as well as for each of the three languages; for state institutions as well as for non-governmental groups, whose mission is to promote children's literacy. Reading abilities should not be pushed to the background in the process of obtaining visual information, and the policies towards children's literacy are obviously also geared at introducing the technologies that are increasingly demanded by current young people.

At the same time, however, our research has shown that there are not enough therapeutic tools available to provide children who struggle with reading and writing with activities that are expressly aimed at overcoming these types of difficulties. This is related, on the one hand, to the fact that the symptoms of the diseases are frequently extremely specific to the individual, and, on the other hand, to the fact that the treatment of these disorders is very specialized and challenging.

The findings lead to the conclusion that efforts in the creation of assistive technologies should also be aimed towards children and people, who suffer from reading and writing impairments, making use of the resources for the successful adoption of technology by

---

[5] https://www.d-all.gr.

[6] http://www.elemedu.upatras.gr/tests-madyskolies/content-1.htm.

youngsters. Reading problems may be treated with the use of technology, which can increase the effectiveness of the treatment for reading disorders, assist professionals in their work, and assist parents who wish to work with their children at home.

References

1. Capodieci, A., Cornoldi, C., Doerr, E., Bertolo, L., Carretti, B.: The use of new technologies for improving reading comprehension. Front. Psychol. **11**, 751 (2020). https://doi.org/10.3389/fpsyg.2020.00751
2. Nicolielo-Carrilho, A.P., Crenitte, P.A.P., Lopes-Herrera, S.A., Hage, S.R.V.: Relationship between phonological working memory, metacognitive skills and reading comprehension in children with learning disabilities. J. Appl. Oral Sci. Revista FOB **26**, e20170414 (2018). https://doi.org/10.1590/1678-7757-2017-0414
3. Ahmad, N.A., Khoo, Y.Y.: Using interactive media to support reading skills among underachieving children **8**, 81–88 (2019)
4. Mihova, P., et al.: Parental attitudes towards online learning - data from four countries. In: Uskov, V.L., Howlett, R.J., Jain, L.C. (eds.) SEEL-22 2022. Smart Innovation, Systems and Technologies, vol. 305, pp. 508–517. Springer, Singapore (2022). https://doi.org/10.1007/978-981-19-3112-3_47
5. Stankova, M., Tuparova, D., Mihova, P., Kamenski, T., Tuparov, G., Mehandzhiyska, K.: Educational computer games and social skills training. In: Ivanović, M., Klašnja-Milićević, A., Jain, L.C. (eds.) Handbook on Intelligent Techniques in the Educational Process. LAIS, vol. 29, pp. 361–392. Springer, Cham (2022). https://doi.org/10.1007/978-3-031-04662-9_17
6. Stankova, M., Ivanova, V., Kamenski, T.: Use of educational computer games in the initial assessment and therapy of children with special educational needs in Bulgaria. TEM J. **7**(3), 488–494 (2018)
7. Cain, K., Oakhill, J., Bryant, P.: Children's reading comprehension ability: concurrent prediction by working memory, verbal ability, and component skills. J. Educ. Psychol. **96**(1), 31–42 (2004). https://doi.org/10.1037/0022-0663.96.1.31
8. Morris, R.D., et al.: Subtypes of reading disability: a phonological core. J. Educ. Psychol. **90**, 347–373 (1998)
9. Grigorenko, E.L., Compton, D.L., Fuchs, L.S., Wagner, R.K., Willcutt, E.G., Fletcher, J.M.: Understanding, educating, and supporting children with specific learning disabilities: 50 years of science and practice. Am. Psychol. **75**(1), 37–51 (2020). https://doi.org/10.1037/amp0000452. Epub 2019 May 13. PMID: 31081650; PMCID: PMC6851403
10. Lovett, M.W., Frijters, J.C., Wolf, M.A., Steinbach, K.A., Sevcik, R.A., Morris, R.D.: Early intervention for children at risk for reading disabilities: the impact of grade at intervention and individual differences on intervention outcomes. J. Educ. Psychol. **109**, 889–914 (2017)
11. Barquero, L.A., Davis, N., Cutting, L.E.: Neuroimaging of reading intervention: a systematic review and activation likelihood estimate meta-analysis. PLoS ONE **9**, e83668 (2014)
12. Wood, S.G., Moxley, J.H., Tighe, E.L., Wagner, R.K.: Does use of text-to-speech and related read-aloud tools improve reading comprehension for students with reading disabilities? A meta-analysis. J. Learn. Disabil. **51**, 73–84 (2018)
13. Perfetti, C.A.: Reading Ability. Oxford University Press, New York (1985)
14. Olson, R.K.: Individual differences in gains from computer-assisted remedial reading. J. Exp. Child Psychol. **77**(3), 197–235 (2000). https://doi.org/10.1006/jecp.1999.2559
15. Stetter, M.E., Hughes, M.T.: Computer-assisted instruction to enhance the reading comprehension of struggling readers: a review of the literature. J. Spec. Educ. Technol. **25**(4), 1–16 (2010)

16. Iordanova, N.: Mobile application prototype of Pumpelina training and therapeutic system (PTES). In: Uskov, V.L., Howlett, R.J., Jain, L.C. (eds.) SEEL-22 2022. Smart Innovation, Systems and Technologies, vol. 305, pp. 498–507. Springer, Singapore (2022). https://doi.org/10.1007/978-981-19-3112-3_46

17. Kamenski, T.: Application of online fidelity assessment of caregivers skills in the implementation of home-administered parent-mediated program for children with ASD. In: Uskov, V.L., Howlett, R.J., Jain, L.C. (eds) SEEL-22 2022. SIST, vol. 305, pp. 518–523. Springer, Singapore (2022). https://doi.org/10.1007/978-981-19-3112-3_48

18. Stankova, M., Mihova, P., Kamenski, T., Mehandjiiska, K.: Emotional understanding skills training using educational computer game in children with autism spectrum disorder (ASD) – case study. In: 2021 44th International Convention on Information, Communication and Electronic Technology, MIPRO, pp. 724–729 (2021). ISSN 1847-3946

19. Stankova, M., Kamenski, T., Mihova, P., Datchev, T.: Online application of a home-administered parent-mediated program for children with ASD. In: Lim, C.-P., Chen, Y.-W., Vaidya, A., Mahorkar, C., Jain, L.C. (eds.) Handbook of Artificial Intelligence in Healthcare. ISRL, vol. 212, pp. 149–167. Springer, Cham (2022). https://doi.org/10.1007/978-3-030-836 20-7_6

Development of Three Language Digital Platform for Early Childhood Development Screening PTES – Preliminary Parents Self-check Results

Nina Iordanova[1,2(✉)] ⓘ, Kornilia Tsoukka[2] ⓘ, and Maria Mavrothanasi[2] ⓘ

[1] Pumpelina, 1113 Sofia, Bulgaria
nina@pumpelina.eu
[2] New Bulgarian University, 1309 Sofia, Bulgaria

Abstract. It is of the utmost importance to address the lack of scalable cognitive assessment tools for preschool-aged children to facilitate the identification of children who may be at risk of developing below their full potential and to assist in the timely referral of these children to appropriate interventions. Since digitalization can be utilized in the diagnosis and treatment of language disorders, reading, and writing disorders, the upgrade of counting abilities, the development of social skills, communication development, help with anxiety disorders, as well as counselling and collaborating with parents, it can be utilized in all of these areas. The results of 113 children, filled out by their parents on the digital platform for early childhood development screening PTES, are provided in this research. PTES is intended as an observation tool for the child's behaviour while they are engaged in play.

Keywords: Online platform · Child assessment · Child development

1 Introduction

The evaluation of a child's growth is a difficult task. It encompasses their entire development since any disturbance that manifests itself throughout this process will invariably have an effect on other functions. In addition, every developmental illness is unique because it reflects the effect of the kid's upbringing and the settings in which the child is raised. Consideration of developmental phases, expectations for mastery of certain abilities at specific age periods, and simultaneous examination of a great deal of information, are all necessary steps in the process of formulating a technique for assessing developmental progress. This is especially important for children who are still in preschool. During this phase of the process, technology would be of tremendous assistance to both experts and parents in organizing the information, constructing it appropriately, and making it uniform for all children of a given age. The development of technology has made it feasible to rapidly compare the evaluations provided by professionals and parents and to examine the degree to which they are consistent with one another for the same child.

© The Author(s), under exclusive license to Springer Nature Singapore Pte Ltd. 2023
Y.-W. Chen et al. (Eds.): KES InMed 2023, SIST 357, pp. 13–20, 2023.
https://doi.org/10.1007/978-981-99-3311-2_2

As digitalization can be used in the assessment of emotional and social development, cognitive assessment [1, 2], the therapy of language disorders, reading and writing disorders, and upgrading counting abilities [3–8], the development of social skills [4–8], communication development [9], help with anxiety disorders [10], as well as in counselling and working with parents [11, 12], it can be utilized in all of these areas.

In recent years, a great number of platforms have been developed for the purposes of digitizing and automating assessment data, matching data on the same person from various sources, performing comparisons and quick calculations, as well as facilitating the collection of research data in a quick and efficient manner. A few of them also have particular objectives that are focused on specific information [13], or at a specific infraction [14, 15], in addition to providing specialized assistance for a certain group [16].

While we are in the process of digitizing the collection and processing of information on child development, it is important to keep in mind the perspective that both parents and professionals have on the application of technology. This attitude is typically favourable [17–20], and children are particularly responsive to the inclusion of technology in the evaluation and therapy [21].

2   Digital Platform for Early Childhood Development Screening PTES

2.1   Theoretical Model

The digital platform for early childhood development screening PTES is constructed as an observation of child behaviour through play. It is protected under the trademark Pumpelina [22].

A lot of screenings are based on play observation because play is one of the most important activities during the first 3 years of life. The Munich Functional Developmental Diagnostic [23] is constructed over movement, perceptive, social, speech and language development and the observation material is presented through play.

Denver Development screening test (DDST) [24] - is constructed as a screening tool for motor, social, language, and perceptive. Observation is introduced through play.

Bayley Scales of Infant and Toddler Development Screening Test [25] is presented as well at the same areas – cognitive, communication (receptive and expressive), fine motor skills, and gross motor skills. The test materials are presented as well during the play.

All that facts have directed us to look for similar theories, based on the child's abilities to play, such as Piaget. So, we have focused on the Penelope Leach child game theory. Her theory is presented on the appearance and disappearance of particular game types through different ages [26].

We have organized the questions according to the following game types – child's solitary play, child's play with the parent; partnership games; imitation games; child's play with the objects and their variations, communications games, and their variations; child's play during feeding. PTES consists of 159 items. All the items are created by Nina Iordanova and verified through MFED. The verification process is still open.

2.2 Platform for Observers – Specialist SLT of Psychologists

The platform is constructed on WordPress with the usage of a specially developed add-on. The data collection is protected with special tools and requirements. User entrance is supervised via user name and password. Parents have no access to this platform. All 159 items are organized in four questionnaires - first age with thirty-four items, second age with 47 items, third age with 39 items: fourth age with 39 items. The starting point is the child's age according to the birth date, the specialist does the check following the instruction.

2.3 Platform for Parent's Self-check – Independent Users

The platform is constructed on WordPress with the usage of a specially developed add-on. The data collection is protected with special tools and requirements. User entrance is supervised via user name and password.

The platform was made available for trial and feedback on June 1, 2022. Eighty-nine parents and professionals evaluated it. Following several important recommendations, the platform was rebuilt. All parent questionnaires were rearranged for optimal reality-based outcomes. Currently, four questionnaires are available for the second test period: 0–3 months with 23 items, 3–6 months with 28 items, 6–9 months with 36 items, and 9–12 months with 33 items. There are a total of 120 items for the age of one, which are sub-questions for the 34 things from the questionnaire for experts that pertain to the age of one. The portal is available to parents for unsupervised use. Specialists and users who use the platform to observe do not have access to the results of the parents. In the feature, the link might be established via the platform administrator in response to a special request from the parents to transmit the findings to a certain specialist. All of the platform's users (in our example - the parents) are provided with results, explanations, and instructions for extra activities. The parents are allowed to use the knowledge and send it to any home that may be affected.

3 Preliminary Results from the Parents' Self-check Platform and Feedback

The platform was reopened on 01.09.2022 after the correction and reorganization of the questionnaires.

3.1 Data Collection Age 0–3 Months

Total Submissions: 28. Average point – 17.95 from all 23 No focus on child gender.
Average Results: 20 personal answers show normal development with a profile over 80% coverage of the items; 5 personal answers show a developmental profile within 60% coverage of the items; 3 personal answers show a developmental profile under 50% coverage of the items.
Conclusions. No negative feedback has been received through the site email. Three families have used the site email to consult specialists for further recommendations, and to express their concerns.

3.2   Data Collection Age 3–6 Months

Total Submissions: nineteen individual answers. Average point – 22.53 from all twenty-eight. No focus on child gender.

Average Results: 12 personal answers show normal development with a profile over 80% coverage of the items; 2 personal answers show a developmental profile in 80 to 60% coverage of the items; 2 personal answers show a developmental profile within 60% coverage of the items; 3 personal answers show developmental profile under 50% coverage of the items.

It is interesting to look at the items from different game types – child's play with the objects and mealtime games. Both are connected to movement development and to communication development. This is the reason why we could have a variety of different results within 80% of normal development, but with a deviation either on communication given, incl. Meal time; or at the child's play with the objects.

Conclusions. No negative feedback has been received through site email. Three families have used the site email to consult specialists for further recommendations, and to express their concerns.

3.3   Data Collection Age 6–9 Months

Total Submissions: twenty-one. Average point from 28.55 from all 36 No focus on child gender.

Average Results: 15 personal answers show normal development with a profile over 80% coverage of the items; 2 personal answers show a developmental profile in 80 to 60% coverage of the items; 1 personal answer shows a developmental profile within 60% coverage of the items 2 personal answers shows developmental profile under 50% coverage the items.

The same difference with the answers was found among the results: there are deviations found among the result of 80% of the items connected to the movement and communication development, including mealtime games.

Conclusions. No negative feedback has been received through site email. One family has received email to consult specialists for further recommendations, and to express their concerns.

3.4   Data Collection Age 9–12 Months

Total Submissions: forty-five. Average point – 23.86 from all 33 No focus on child gender.

Average Results: 30 personal answers show normal development with a profile over 80% coverage of the items; 10 personal answers show a developmental profile within 60% coverage of the items 5 personal answers show a developmental profile under 50% coverage of the items.

Because of the huge influence of social communication and the child's ability for shared attention, we could have interesting deviations in the area of imitation games, communication games with a focus on speech and language development and partnership games. All those games' abilities relate to the social rules within the particular family, as well as with the reflection of mother-child interaction and the willingness of the family members to play with the child.

Conclusions. No negative feedback has been received through the site email. 17 families have contacted via site email with concerns for further recommendations and consultations with specialists. Figure 1 provides a graphical representation of an overview of the findings.

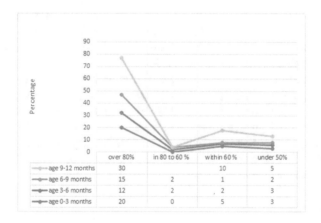

Fig. 1. 118 Parents' responses and their results according to PTES

4 Translation of the Questionnaire for Specialists in Different Regions

Translating questionnaires into all local languages in the study region is an essential part of any survey. Incomplete or inaccurate translations may lose the meaning that the impact research team intended, or at worst, completely change it. As a result, the questionnaire may become invalid. Our research team allows for extra time to perform tasks like translation, reverse translation, reconciliation, and enumerator validation. Due to version control, information is preserved even when translated.

We translated the PTES into 2 languages, following the actions listed below:

1. "Forward translation" – translation from the research team's language uses to the language spoken where the study is being conducted. The time required for this step was less than a week.
2. "Second translation" – the returned document was retranslated again to the original language using the local language version only.

3. "Reconciliation" – is used to describe the process of comparing the original question-naire to the back-translated questionnaire. Any differences found at this point should be highlighted by researchers and sorted into two categories: minor (such as phrasing errors) and major (like changes in the meaning of a question).

5   Future Directions

The use of technology in the process of evaluating a child's progress is both practical and uncomplicated. Its inclusion in professionals' daily work is unavoidable. In order to make use of digital forms for the gathering of information, those forms must fulfill certain requirements. Namely, they must be simple to fill out, brief, and the questions must be articulated in an understandable manner. In this instance, the scale needs to fulfil the criterion that the completion is parent-friendly, which is especially important when taking into account the fact that the parents' levels of general knowledge would vary. The data shall be able to be processed quickly and easily, and it should be easy to compare the information gathered from the various respondents.

One of the most difficult aspects of creating a tool is doing it in several languages. This is because the terminology that is typically used does not have a straight translation, or the word that is used in common speech does not correlate to the phrase. It is necessary to put translations into other languages through a series of phases that focus on how precisely the obtained information can be compared. The following step for the researchers will involve gathering data from respondents located in a variety of nations and analysing the results to draw conclusions about child development.

6   Conclusions

Helping children who have development difficulties is a concern shared by all pro-fessionals working in the therapeutic field. In recent years, when speech therapy was unavailable, therapists began to explore and assess applications that make use of infor-mation and communication technology (ICT) to aid developmentally delayed children in meeting their learning goals. The COVID-19 pandemic has resulted in an increased need for telepractice, which necessitates the urgent digitalization of PTES.

The treatment team, as well as the parents, receive additional resources and feedback on the progress that their kid makes in therapy thanks to the prototype of a mobile version of the PTES systems and the therapist scale.

This study considered all ethical research standards in accordance with the General Data Protection Requirements (GDPR) and complied with the ethical recommendations of the Department of Health care and Social Services, NBU. The authors conducted a literature search of available materials and identified the issue, which is the use of mobile applications in enhancing reading comprehension in first language acquisition.

References

1. Bhavnani, S., et al.: The association of a novel digital tool for assessment of early childhood cognitive development, "DEvelopmental assessment on an E-Platform (DEEP)", with growth in rural India: a proof of concept study. EClinicalMedicine **37**, 100964 (2021). https://doi.org/10.1016/j.eclinm.2021.100964

2. Stankova, M., Ivanova, V., Kamenski, T.: Use of educational computer games in the initial assessment and therapy of children with special educational needs in Bulgaria. TEM J. **7**, 488–494 (2018)
3. Sudarmilah, E., Ferdiana, R., Nugroho, L.E., Susanto, A., Ramdhani, N.: Tech review: game platform for upgrading counting ability on preschool children. In: International Conference on Information Technology and Electrical Engineering (ICITEE), Yogyakarta, Indonesia, pp. 226–231 (2013). https://doi.org/10.1109/ICITEED.2013.6676243
4. Stankova, M., Tuparova, D., Mihova, P., Kamenski, T., Tuparov, G., Mehandzhiyska, K.: Educational computer games and social skills training. In: Ivanović, M., Klašnja-Milićević, A., Jain, L.C. (eds.) Handbook on Intelligent Techniques in the Educational Process. LAIS, vol. 29, pp. 361–392. Springer, Cham (2022). https://doi.org/10.1007/978-3-031-04662-9_17
5. Levy, J., Dunsmuir, S.: Lego therapy: building social skills for adolescents with an autism spectrum disorder. Educ. Child Psychol. **37**(1), 58–83 (2020). ISSN 0267-1611
6. Mihova, P., Stankova, M., Andonov, F., Stoyanov, S.: The use of serious games for developing social and communication skills in children with autism spectrum disorders—review. In: Lim, C.P., Vaidya, A., Chen, YW., Jain, V., Jain, L.C. (eds.) Artificial Intelligence and Machine Learning for Healthcare. ISRL, vol. 229, pp. 181–196. Springer, Cham (2023). https://doi.org/10.1007/978-3-031-11170-9_7
7. Grossard, C., Grynspan, O., Serret, S., Jouen, A. L., Bailly, K., Cohen, D.: Serious games to teach social interactions and emotions to individuals with autism spectrum disorders (ASD). Comput. Educ. **113**, 195–211 (2017). ISSN 0360-1315 https://doi.org/10.1016/j.compedu.2017.05.002
8. Stankova M., Mihova, P., Kamenski, T., Mehandjiiska, K.: Emotional understanding skills training using educational computer game in children with autism spectrum disorder (ASD) – case study. In: 2021 44th International Convention on Information, Communication and Electronic Technology, MIPRO 2021, pp. 724–729 (2021). ISSN 1847-3946
9. Bernardini, S., Porayska-Pomsta, K., Smith, T.J.: ECHOES: an intelligent serious game for fostering social communication in children with autism. Inf. Sci. **264**, 41–60 (2014)
10. Simon, E., de Hullu, E., Bögels, S., et al.: Development of 'learn to dare!': an online assessment and intervention platform for anxious children. BMC Psychiatry **20**, 60 (2020). https://doi.org/10.1186/s12888-020-2462-3
11. Stankova, M., Kamenski, T., Mihova, P., Datchev, T.: Online application of a home-administered parent-mediated program for children with ASD. In: Lim, C.-P., Chen, Y.-W., Vaidya, A., Mahorkar, C., Jain, L.C. (eds.) Handbook of Artificial Intelligence in Healthcare. ISRL, vol. 212, pp. 149–167. Springer, Cham (2022). https://doi.org/10.1007/978-3-030-836 20-7_6
12. Kamenski, T.: Application of online fidelity assessment of caregivers skills in the implementation of home-administered parent-mediated program for children with ASD. In: Uskov, V.L., Howlett, R.J., Jain, L.C. (eds.) SEEL-22 2022. Smart Innovation, Systems and Technologies, vol. 305, pp. 518–523. Springer, Singapore (2022). https://doi.org/10.1007/978-981-19-3112-3_48
13. Richter, L.M., Naicker, S.N.: A data-free digital platform to reach families with young children during the COVID-19 pandemic: online survey study. JMIR Pediatr. Parent. **4**(2), e26571 (2021). https://doi.org/10.2196/26571
14. Guxin, L., Qiufang, L.: Construction of website-based platform on development assessment of children with autism. In: 2013 3rd International Conference on Consumer Electronics, Communications and Networks, Xianning, China, pp. 199–202 (2013). https://doi.org/10.1109/CECNet.2013.6703306
15. Armas, J., Pedreschi, V., Gonzalez, P., Díaz, D.: A technological platform using serious game for children with Autism Spectrum Disorder (ASD) in Peru (2019). https://doi.org/10.18687/LACCEI2019.1.1.278

16. Trilevic, I.: KidExplore: a new online platform to support child development during a pandemic. In: Hovestadt, C., Recker, J., Richter, J., Werder, K. (eds.) Digital Responses to Covid-19. SpringerBriefs in Information Systems, pp. 55–61. Springer, Cham (2021). https://doi.org/10.1007/978-3-030-66611-8_4

17. Smith, S.J., Burdette, P.J., Cheatham, G.A., Harvey, S.P.: Parental role and support for online learning of students with disabilities: a paradigm shift. J. Spec. Educ. Leadersh. **29**(2), 101–112 (2016)

18. Stankova, M., et al.: Barriers to the use of serious computer games in the practical work with children with educational difficulties.TEM J. **10**(3), 1175–1183 (2021) https://www.temjournal.com/archives/vol10no3.html

19. Garbe, A., Ogurlu, U., Logan, N., Cook, P.: COVID-19 and remote learning: experiences of parents with children during the pandemic. Am. J. Qual. Res. **4**(3), 45–65 (2020). https://doi.org/10.29333/ajqr/8471

20. Mihova, P., et al.: Parental attitudes towards online learning - data from four countries. In: Uskov, V.L., Howlett, R.J., Jain, L.C. (eds.) SEEL-22 2022. Smart Innovation, Systems and Technologies, vol. 305, pp. 508–517. Springer, Singapore (2022). https://doi.org/10.1007/978-981-19-3112-3_47

21. Stankova, M., Ivanova, V., Kamenski, T.: Use of educational computer games in the initial assessment and therapy of children with special educational needs in Bulgaria. TEM J. **7**(3), 488–494 (2018)

22. Iordanova, N.: Mobile application prototype of Pumpelina training and therapeutic system (PTES). In: Uskov, V.L., Howlett, R.J., Jain, L.C. (eds.) SEEL-22 2022. SIST, vol. 305, pp. 498–507. Springer, Singapore (2022). https://doi.org/10.1007/978-981-19-3112-3_46

23. Munich functional developmental diagnosis for the first, second, and third year of life, Hellbruegge, Theodor. Theodor Hellbruegge International Institute (1995). ISBN 10: 8186312110 ISBN 13: 9788186312117

24. Hansen, R.: Denver development screening test (DDST). In: Volkmar, F.R. (eds.) Encyclopedia of Autism Spectrum Disorders. Springer, New York (2013). https://doi.org/10.1007/978-1-4419-1698-3_613

25. Leach, P.: Your baby and child, NY (2010). ISBN 9780375712036

26. Balasundaram, P., Avulakunta, I.D.: Bayley scales of infant and toddler development. In: StatPearls [Internet]. Treasure Island (FL). StatPearls (2022). https://www.ncbi.nlm.nih.gov/books/NBK567715/. Accessed 21 Nov 2022

27. Leach, P., Gerber, E., Peters, D.R.: Die Ersten Jahre dines Kindes, Hallwag Ag, Bern (1990). Lech P. Babyhood, NY (2001). ISBN 0374714369

Online Parent Counselling in Speech and Language Therapy - The View of the Professionals

Margarita Stankova(✉) ⓘ, Tsveta Kamenski ⓘ, Kornilia Tsoukka ⓘ,
Haneen Alshawesh ⓘ, and Alexandros Proedrou ⓘ

Department of Health Care and Social Work, New Bulgarian University, 1618 Sofia, Bulgaria
mstankova@nbu.bg

Abstract. Families and caregivers of children with speech and language disorders, as well as with developmental delays, face considerable challenges, such as lack of reliable information and support or of regular access to therapy. This is particularly true when they are in remote places, or with limited resources, while trying to best support the development of their children. One solution to such challenge is the provision of online consultations and therapeutic sessions, which became quite popular during the COVID-19 pandemic as a replacement for conventional speech and language therapy.

Our objective is to shed a light on various aspects of online counselling and to analyse the impact on professionals, parents, and children in terms of engagement and involvement, as well as the effectiveness and perceived value of the process itself through collecting and studying views and opinions from professionals' experience.

Through the work of a focus group (participants N = 8) of speech and language therapists, aged between 30 and 50, with various degrees of experience, some positive and negative aspects of online counselling were identified, including possible barriers, challenges, and future implications were outlined and discussed.

Keywords: Online Counselling · Speech and Language Therapy · Parental Involvement

1 Introduction

1.1 Speech and Language Therapy, Parental Involvement

When discussing speech and language therapy and processes, we should take into consideration several key factors. One basic, but crucial, aspect of the SLT's work with the child is consulting parents on setting the goals and tasks of the therapy. This is a key factor to ensure a positive effect of the intervention for children with speech and language disorders. Often, speech and language therapists (SLTs) set the following goals in the consultation: to provide information about the therapy process; to engage parents in strategies that can be used as home-based interventions; to reduce parents' anxiety regarding the child's development. Therapists can follow three steps that are necessary to prepare for parent training and coaching, such as identifying a target skill, identifying a targeted strategy, and creating parent-friendly procedures [1]. Effective communication with caregivers can contribute to successful therapy outcomes [2]. SLTs must have the skills to engage with parents by focusing on mutual understanding, creating constructive relationships, empowering them, and overcoming barriers [3, 4]. Those barriers often include parental uncertainty about the nature of the intervention and scepticism about the intervention's approach and strategy [5]. Parents' investment in home interventions through the establishment of a good relationship between family and SLTs is highly valued [6, 7].

1.2   Online Interventions for Parents of Children with Speech and Language Disorders

In addition to the conventional therapeutic approaches, and with help of Internet and Information and Communication Technology (ICT) health professionals from various fields exchange clinical information easier and can provide remote health care, thus allowing patients to have health services in their homes [8]. The results of the application of telepractices suggest that their use is promising when it comes to reducing the demands on available resources for families [9]. Teletherapy can improve the quality of service delivery by addressing the challenges in terms of distance in intervening and evaluating people with problems in accessing the services. Several studies showed that telecommuting can address some obstacles to intervention such as time, money, and distance, and it can provide education for children with ASD [10]. In addition, evaluation through means of technology has facilitated the counselling process for parents. Parent education is considered to result into a better situation at home and helps to reduce the stress level in the family [11].

Online work with parents of children with speech and language disorders has many advantages: saving time travelling to the specialist's office, the possibility of participation of both parents, the possibility of organizing a convenient meeting time and the feeling of anonymity during the conversation. Moreover, speech and language pathology online therapy services may be more effective if, before the start of a child's online speech therapy sessions, there is a thorough involvement of parents in the negotiation of meaningful intervention goals, a family member attendance of sessions, and the nature of the home activities likely to be required for progress [12]. Thus, training parents is very important as it gives them the opportunity to understand and acquire the strategies they will be implementing with their child before mastering a specific skill [1].

Preliminary research suggests that telehealth can support parent education and, as a result, improve children's behaviour in some families [13]. Parents reported that they perceived telepractice sessions to be as valuable as those conducted directly by the physician, felt comfortable using the technology, and were willing to continue the intervention with their children at home [9]. Parents consider that the application of online interventions improves their relationship with their children and shows high levels of satisfaction [14].

Telehealth training has increased the use of evidence-based strategies for parents of children with autism. For instance, training parents to implement communication strategies in order to teach communication skills to their children. Such training is also applicable in extraordinary circumstances, e.g., a global pandemic [15]. The telepractice coaching model has a positive impact on therapy outcomes in many targeted communicative behaviours. Furthermore, the telepractice parent training model contributes to children maintaining skills acquired over a month past suspension of intervention and generalization data appears to track the pattern of the targeted behaviour. Telepractice has proven to be effective also with families of children with autism in low-resource countries [16].

1.3   Parental Views of Online Interventions

Parents' views of teletherapy in school settings are that it promotes greater engagement of school staff in the therapeutic process and its understanding [17, 18]. Meanwhile, teletherapy in a home setting gives parents the opportunity to be involved, but it also lets their children take control and ownership of their own therapy, leading to more independence [17]. Parents reported that the teletherapy services were more practical, convenient, and efficient in the transfer of therapy techniques and activities with more frequent verbal parent instruction and feedback, in contrast to conventional speech therapy methods [12]. On the other hand, some disadvantages of teletherapy are reported in the literature. For example, not being in the same environment to physically prompt or comfort the children was reported as a disadvantage to building a trusting relationship via telepractice [19] or building a successful relationship with the families [20]. There are other issues, such as regulatory ones including licensure, reimbursement, and threats to privacy and confidentiality hinder the routine implementation of the telerehab services in the clinical setting [21]. In order to overcome some of these challenges, speech and language therapists indicate that staying connected with children and families outside of the therapy sessions is very important for building a rapport via telepractice [20].

The aim of the present paper is to identify, according to SLP professionals, the positives and the negatives of online consulting of parents of children with developmental disorders. The method that we used consists of open answers to questions and a focus group discussion. A definite strength of it is that the participants can answer questions freely and express opinions. On the other hand, the participants could be influenced by the answers of the other professionals in the group, and they express views with no anonymity of answers granted, which could be considered a weakness of the method. Nevertheless, we believe that through free discussion and focus groups we were able to access information that is impossible to gather by administering a questionnaire. Our expectations were that the professionals would single out mainly the positive experiences they have had with online practice with the parents of children with speech and language disorders.

2   Methods

We formed a focus group of eight speech and language therapists /SLTs/ to check whether the online counselling of parents of children with speech and language disorders can replace face-to-face meetings, and to list the advantages and disadvantages of online counselling as a new form of working with parents, as well as to find out the unwritten rules that professionals follow when using online counselling.

The reason we selected this method is that it gives the participants in the group the opportunity to freely express their opinion in an open format, rather than pick pre-defined answers. In this manner, it is possible to gather new information, out of the presumption of the research team. The discussion follows a strict protocol and is audio-recorded. The answers have been transcribed after the focus group took place.

Focus groups usually consist of 6–8 participants and the method is recommended for investigation of problems, related to communication [22].

The SLTs were selected according to the following criteria: **they work with children with speech and language disorders; they use both face-to-face and online sessions when meeting parents; they include parents in counselling regarding children's disorders and their speech and language therapy; they have more than 5 years of experience as speech and language therapists.**

The participants in the focus group included 7 women and 1 man. Three participants were between 30 and 40 years age-old, four were between 40 and 50 years age-old, and one was over 50.

We assumed that online counselling would support the inclusion of parents in the work of the SLT, as it saves time for both parties, gives the opportunity to arrange a meeting outside of working hours, and allows both parents to be present. However, we believed that professionals were still unsure of the effects of the use of online consultations due to the lack of sufficient information and possibilities to analyse the behaviour/incl. nonverbal/of the parents during the meeting, as well as the uncertainty regarding confidentiality.

An experienced researcher was appointed as a moderator of the focus group.

The following script was agreed upon in advance, containing the following parts:

– **Opening** – introduction of the moderator, introduction of the topic and explanation of the aims of the focus group; explanation of the protocol and the option to have questions asked on behalf of the participants. The following rules were introduced as well: Participants do not interrupt each other; they wait for their turn, follow the protocol, and do not use mobile phones. The participants were assured that their answers will be subject to strict anonymity and confidentiality.
– **Questions and answers of the participants.** We selected the following questions to find out the attitudes of the professionals towards online counselling:

1. *Do you think that online counselling for parents in speech and language therapy is more appropriate than face-to-face and why?*
2. *Do you think that parents participate more eagerly in online counselling than in face-to-face counselling?*
3. *Do you follow certain rules when consulting online that are different from the ones you follow in face-to-face meetings?*
4. *What are the disadvantages of online counselling of parents of children with speech and language disorders compared to face-to-face counselling?*

– **Closure** – end of the discussion and appreciation for the information provided.

Participants confirmed their consent to participate in the focus group. Although the results would be presented anonymously, they also confirmed their consent for information about their gender, age, and years of professional experience to be used and provided to the researchers.

3 Results

Participants' answers to question N1 (*Do you think that online counselling for parents in speech and language therapy is more appropriate than face-to-face and why?*)

Participant 1 shares that she has a lot of experience and a positive attitude towards consulting parents of children with speech and language disorders. When conducting online meetings, Participant 1 states that she manages to give the parents adequate guidance. She concentrates on the conversation and can talk about what happened in the sessions with the child.

Participant 2 supports the first participant and shares that it is very convenient for parents. When they do not travel specifically for the meeting, both parties have time to concentrate on the conversation and discussion. Payment is also easily adjusted.

Participant 3 agrees with participants 1 and 2. Online counselling is much more structured and shorter; time is well-controlled, and everyone is able to follow the structure of the session. But, if it is a first meeting, Participant 3 prefers to have it in person, as she gets more information, which is missing in online meetings, although she is not able to specify the actual disadvantage. Seems that the impression is half done.

Participant 4 points out that trust is probably built more slowly and the relationship between the professional and the patient suffers, if the very first meeting is online.

Participant 5 - believes that online consultations have their place in working with parents, but they cannot replace a face-to-face meeting, which has many more advantages.

Participant 6 says that she uses online consultations only for parents of children with speech and language disorders, who live outside the country, but these online meetings are usually one-time, and their effect is very good.

Participant 7 says that she tries to organize the meetings in person because parents value the meetings in person more and then they get full information about how the work with the child is going. Online counselling works only with parents outside the country.

Participant 8 believes that the fact that the professional uses the time to prepare, dress and go to another place, outside their home, has a more positive effect on working with parents.

Participants' answers to question N2 (*Do you think that parents participate more eagerly in online counselling than in face-to-face counselling?*)

Participant 3 – shares that parents are more regular in their participation; they stick to schedule and do not miss meetings when working online.

Participant 1 – believes that the parents avoid missing participation and manage to exchange more information in online meetings.

Participant 8 – shared that it depends on the family and the capacity of the parents.

Participant 2 – believes that even the first meeting can be done online. However, there are some situations in which we need face-to-face meetings. Online meetings are more affordable and for some parents, they can be their only option.

Participants' answers to question N3 (*Do you follow certain rules when consulting online that are different from the ones you follow in face-to-face meetings?*)

Participant 7 - believes that both online and live counselling should have a structure and framework in terms of time, start, end, approach, information to be collected, and payment. Counselling should be distinguished from ordinary conversation.

Facilitator's clarification: explains that the question is about some specific conditions that are different from face-to-face meetings, e.g., participants turn on cameras.

Participant 7 – shares that the place where the patients are located - their home - is special and gives her a lot of additional information. Sometimes she can see parts of the house, and the furniture, and she can interpret what it means when the patients "show" specific parts of their surroundings.

Participant 3 – thinks that it is necessary to have a quiet place and no other people around, no distractors. Very often there are other people in the room and they are doing things, which is detrimental to the session and its quality.

Participant 8 – agrees that the child should not be present in the room where the conversation with the parents takes place.

Participant 3 – shares that this worries her too because she can't see if the child is really in another room.

Participant 2 – shares that she doesn't impose strict rules, instead, she tries to interpret what the parents do. Recordings are also a problem: she doesn't know what others do in such situations, but she thinks some patients record the meetings.

Participant 5 – says that we usually don't know if the patients are recording our sessions.

Participant 2 – shares that she has had a school principal asking her if they can record the session and play the recording to all the teachers.

Participant 8 – agrees – she was also asked if the parents could record the conversation and play the recording to other family members.

Participant 6 – wonders if the patients realize that the content in question may not fit to the situation if used in a different context.

Participant 1 – thinks that we can warn the parents that if they record it may be irrelevant to other people.

Participant 4 – summarizes that the SLT can introduce a rule - if the parents want to record the session, they must ask for permission.

Participants' answers to question N4 (*What are the disadvantages of online counselling of parents of children with speech and language disorders compared to face-to-face counselling?*)

Participant 7 – shares that one can easily cancel the online meeting because it is probably perceived to be less important than a face-to-face meeting. This has a negative effect on the work with the child in general, as well as on the relationship between the therapist and the parent.

Participant 2 – thinks that meetings are easily cancelled when online, but it is also easier to re-schedule. There is much more flexibility when managing meetings online.

Participant 1 – considers the control over time online to be much more difficult.

Participant 3 – thinks that it is easier to control the time online because the therapist can see it on the computer, otherwise it is necessary to look at the watch.

Participant 4 – shares that when working online, she refrains from checking the time.

The advantages of online counselling for parents of children with speech and language disorders, according to the professionals in our group were the following: no time is wasted in travel, all participants concentrate more on the conversation, time is easier to control; for parents who live abroad this is often the only possible way to receive a consultation.

The disadvantages, in turn, are as follows: some of the information that the therapist receives in the live meetings is missing, especially in the first meeting; trust is more difficult to build; the professional remains undervalued; the professional and the parents might not be fully involved in the meeting.

In terms of trust, communicating entirely online probably gives the feeling of unreality to both parties, with the professional remaining abstract to the patient, who perceives him/her more as information obtained from the Internet than as a real person, and the patient remains somewhat unknown to the professional. Thus, it is likely that some of the effects that come from the presence of another person and their positive impact remain untapped in full when counselling online.

In terms of participation, experts believe that parents are more likely to stick to a schedule with online appointments and are less likely to miss sessions. This is probably due to the fact that the organization of time at home is easier, parents do not waste time travelling, especially in busy traffic after working hours, and it is easier to plan their participation in meetings.

Regarding the rules for online sessions, the following conditions were outlined – they should take place somewhere quiet, the child should not listen to the conversation with the parents, and there should be no distractors in the room where the conversation takes place. An important condition would be to record the conversation only after a special request and permission. The discussion regarding the recording of the sessions was longer, and this leads us to the conclusion that online sessions do not give the participants assurance of confidentiality - in what the environment is, who is listening to the conversation and who would be interested in recording the conversation appears a serious drawback of internet counselling.

As a major disadvantage of online counselling, the participants share the feeling on both sides - therapist and patient - that the consultation online is perceived as less important than the one "in person". In our focus group, participants seemed to pay particular attention to their relationship with parents of children with speech and language disorders, and shared concerns that this relationship suffers when communicating online.

An interesting fact mentioned in our focus group is that age did not appear to be a factor in the positive attitude towards online counselling, as the oldest participants had the most positive experiences in this regard.

4 Discussion

Our preliminary hypothesis that the professionals are completely satisfied with the online work with parents of children with speech and language disorders did not prove completely justified. All participants used remote techniques for work with patients, mainly because they were the only option during the pandemic. Although some patients were willing to continue working remotely after the lockdown period, the SLPs expressed some concerns and possible restrictions in this regard.

In the views of the SLPs, similar to what was reported by other research [14], parents were happy and satisfied with online communication and remote therapeutic work. Due to the nature of the therapy of children with speech and language disorders, SLPs often have to consult families living abroad. In this case, remote work has proven a satisfactory solution and professionals would use it in any conditions. In accordance to our preliminary hypothesis, the participants expressed the opinion that online consulting gives a good structure and clear frame to parents and improves their level of participation. Other authors point out the increased motivation of parents because of the implementation of the telepractices [23].

Our professionals, as well as others in similar studies [19, 20], express concerns about building a trusted relationship with their patients. Some of them prefer to start work with the patient in person, and then continue working online. The long-term outcome from such relationship, built solely on the basis of telepractice, is also unclear [24].

As a possible restriction of this study, we consider the possibility that the answers of the participants could be influenced by the answers of the other professionals in the group, and in turn, affect their opinion. In addition, SLTs have their identity revealed and thus have the opportunity to hear everyone's answers, although they were granted confidentiality by the research team.

5 Conclusion

Online consultations and speech and language therapy are contemporary and quite new methods of conducting therapeutic sessions and counselling. They have their advantages, as well as challenges. Some SLTs would use this new technological solution in their practice, others are more reserved towards using it.

In conclusion, we believe that by managing some aspects of online consultations and sessions, imposing strict rules on the deliverables and relevant permissions, and considering some limitations and restrictions, this telepractice, supporting SLT's work with children and their families, can be an effective replacement of the conventional speech and language therapy.

References

1. Snodgrass, M.R., Chung, M.Y., Biller, M.F., Appel, K.E., Meadan, H., Halle, J.W.: Telepractice in speech–language therapy: the use of online technologies for parent training and coaching. Commun. Disord. Q. **38**(4), 242–254 (2017)

2. Cates, J., Paone, T.R., Packman, J., Margolis, D.: Effective parent consultation in play therapy. Int. J. Play Ther. **15**(1), 87–100 (2006)
3. Klatte, I.S., Harding, S., Roulstone, S.: Speech and language therapists' views on parents' engagement in parent-child interaction therapy (PCIT). Int. J. Lang. Commun. Disord. **54**, 553–564 (2019)
4. Stankova, M., et al.: Cultural and linguistic practice with children with developmental language disorder: findings from an international practitioner survey. Folia Phoniatr. Logop., 1–13 (2020)
5. Levickis, P., McKean, C., Wiles, A., Law, J.: Expectations and experiences of parents taking part in parent–child interaction programmes to promote child language: a qualitative interview study. Int. J. Lang. Commun. Disord. **55**, 603–617 (2020)
6. Melvin, K., Meyer, C., Scarinci, N.: What does a family who is "engaged" in early intervention look like? Perspectives of Australian speech-language pathologists. Int. J. Speech Lang. Pathol. **23**(3), 236–246 (2021)
7. Law, J., Levickis, P., Rodríguez Ortiz, I.R., Matić, A., Lyons, R., Messarra, C., et al.: Working with the parents and families of children with developmental language disorders: an international perspective. J. Commun. Disord. **82**, 105922 (2019)
8. Plantak Vukovac, D., Novosel-Herceg, T., Orehovački, T.: Users' needs in telehealth speech-language pathology services. In: Proceedings of the 24th International Conference on Information Systems Development. Department of Information, Systems, Harbin, Hong Kong, SAR, pp. 1–12 (2015)
9. Baharav, E., Reiser, C.: Using telepractice in parent training in early autism. Telemed. J. E Health **16**(6), 727–31 (2010)
10. Lindgren, S., Wacker, D., Suess, A., Schieltz, K., Pelzel, K., Kopelman, T., et al.: Telehealth and autism: treating challenging behavior at lower cost. Paediatrics **137**(Supply 2), S167–S175 (2016)
11. Barton, E.E., Fettig, A.: Parent-implemented interventions for young children with disabilities: a review of fidelity features. J. Early Interv. **35**(2), 194–219 (2013)
12. Fairweather, G.C., Lincoln, M.A., Ramsden, R.: Speech-language pathology teletherapy in rural and remote educational settings: decreasing service inequities. Int. J. Speech Lang. Pathol. **18**(6), 592–602 (2016)
13. Vismara, L.A., McCormick, C., Young, G.S., Nadhan, A., Monlux, K.: Preliminary findings of a telehealth approach to parent training in autism. J. Autism Dev. Disord. **43**(12), 2953–2969 (2013). https://doi.org/10.1007/s10803-013-1841-8
14. Hicks, B., Baggerly, J.: The effectiveness of child parent relationship therapy in an online format. Int. J. Play Ther. **26**(3), 138–150 (2017)
15. Wattanawongwan, S., Ganz, J.B., Pierson, L., Yllades, V., Liao, C.-Y., Ura, S.K.: Communication intervention implementation via telepractice parent coaching: parent implementation outcomes. J. Spec. Educ. Technol. **37**(1), 35–48 (2022)
16. Samadi, S.A., Bakhshalizadeh-Moradi, S., Khandani, F., Foladgar, M., Poursaid-Mohammad, M., McConkey, R.: Using hybrid telepractice for supporting parents of children with ASD during the COVID-19 lockdown: a feasibility study in Iran. Brain Sci. **10**(11), 892 (2020)
17. Pennington, L., et al.: Internet delivery of intensive speech and language therapy for children with cerebral palsy: a pilot randomised controlled trial. BMJ Open **9**(1), e024233 (2019)
18. Mihova, P., et al.: Parental attitudes towards online learning - data from four countries. In: Uskov, V.L., Howlett, R.J., Jain, L.C. (eds.) SEEL-22 2022. SIST, vol. 305, pp. 508–517. Springer, Singapore (2022). https://doi.org/10.1007/978-981-19-3112-3_47
19. Anderson, K., Balandin, S., Stancliffe, R.J., Layfield, C.: Parents' perspectives on tele-AAC support for families with a new speech generating device: results from an Australian pilot study. Perspect. Telepract. **4**(2), 39–70 (2014)

20. Akamoglu, Y., Meadan, H., Pearson, J.N., Cummings, K.: Getting connected: speech and language pathologists' perceptions of building rapport via telepractice. J. Dev. Phys. Disabil. **30**(4), 569–585 (2018)
21. Cherney, L.R., Van Vuuren, S.: Telerehabilitation, virtual therapists, and acquired neurologic speech and language disorders. In: Seminars in Speech and Language, vol. 33, no. 03, pp. 243–258. Thieme Medical Publishers, August 2012
22. Allen, M. (ed.): The Sage Encyclopedia of Communication Research Methods, vols. 1–4. SAGE Publications, Inc. (2017). https://doi.org/10.4135/9781483381411
23. Sikka, K.: Parent's perspective on teletherapy of pediatric population with speech and language disorder during Covid-19 lockdown in India. Indian J. Otolaryngol. Head Neck Surg. (2022)
24. Murphy, E., Rodríguez-Manzanares, M.A.: Rapport in distance education. Int. Rev. Res. Open Distrib. Learn. **13**(1), 167–190 (2012)

Data Driven Models for Health Care Systems

Modelling Competing Risk for Stroke Survival Data

Virgilijus Sakalauskas[(✉)] and Dalia Kriksciuniene

Vilnius University, Universiteto St. 3, 01513 Vilnius, Lithuania
{virgilijus.sakalauskas,dalia.kriksciuniene}@knf.vu.lt

Abstract. The concept of competing risk explores occurrence of events which prevent or affect observation of the main event. The paper focuses on modelling competing risk from stroke survival data, which enables to identify several types of events over the follow-up time for each patient affected by stroke. We explore the possibilities of recovery or death from stroke complications by exploring medical data of the neurology department. Our main interest is to estimate the probability of recovery event, whereas death from stroke is considered as a competing risk event, and the discharge of the patients from the hospital without completing the follow-up are identified as censored events. The effect of numerous variables from the patient database are analyzed by applying the open-source software R. The results of the research show, that the type of the diagnosed stroke has high influence to the estimated cumulative incidence function (CIF). The influence of the types of medications, rehabilitation procedures and demographics characteristics of the patient in the competing risks settings are explored by the regression model, which enables to confirm the hypothesis of significance of all regression covariates.

Keywords: competing risk · stroke · survival data · cumulative incidence function

1 Introduction

It is a common practice of medical research to assess the probability of survival after some kind of illness or accident. In the scientific literature, this approach is called survival analysis. All subjects who can potentially experience the observed event are considered as a risk group. The risk group for each time period is composed of the individuals who have not yet experienced the event of interest, and the subjects of this group who have not experience the event of interest during the entire observation period form the so-called censored group [1].

In the presence of censored cases the evaluation of probability to survive up until the fixed time point t, usually is done by using non-parametric Kaplan–Meier method from the observed survival time data [2].

To check the statistical differences for survival time of two or more risk groups the Log-Rank test can be applied. The null hypothesis for a Log-Rank test asserts that the explored groups have the same survival probability. The Log-Rank test is based on a

© The Author(s), under exclusive license to Springer Nature Singapore Pte Ltd. 2023
Y.-W. Chen et al. (Eds.): KES InMed 2023, SIST 357, pp. 33–43, 2023.
https://doi.org/10.1007/978-981-99-3311-2_4

Chi-squared statistics which checks if the observed number of events in each group is significantly different from the expected [3].

The Kaplan–Meier method and Log-Rank tests are commonly used for the categorical predictor variables. In order to find the quantitative predictor, the survival regression is applied for exploring covariates of independent variables (e.g. age, illness type, treatment methods, etc.) against the survival or failure times. Most common approach is application of the Proportional Hazard (Cox) model, which aims to represent the hazard rate as a function of t and several covariates [4].

The competing risk analysis complements the traditional survival analysis with the possibility of analyzing time-to-event data in the presence of several mutually exclusive causes of failure events. When just one of several competing events can occur, we understand the probabilities of these events as a *competing risk*. For example, if we are interested in cancer-related mortality, the other causes of death can precede its occurrence. So, the death from other reasons is a typical example of competing risk.

In order to describe the rate of failure from one event type in the presence of others the cause-specific hazard function may be used. The cumulative incidence function measures the probability of failure from event of interest when there are competing risks [5, 7].

In case of competing risk, the use of Kaplan–Meier method generally overestimates the probability of the event of interest. This happens because patients who experienced the competing risk will no longer experience the event of interest and the probability of such an event is equal to 0. According to the traditional Kaplan-Meier method, the probability of such an event is equated to the probability of censored events, which is greater than zero. To overcome these problems, we will use the cumulative incidence competing risk method. According to this method, the CIF is estimated not only for event of interest but also for all competing events, and their estimates depend on each other [8].

The application of the Log-Rank test and the Cox regression methods in the presence of the competing risk require some changes as well. The Log-Rank test should be changed to Gray's test [9] for equality of CIF (cumulative incidence function) across the groups. The method of Fine and Gray [6, 10] extends the Cox regression and models the cumulative incidence function for the competing risks data. Sometimes Fine-Gray model is called subdistribution hazards model, as the statistics derived from Fine-Gray model is sub distribution of the hazard ratio. An important feature of this method is that patients who experience a competing event remain in the risk group (instead of being censored), although they are in fact no longer at risk of the event of interest [1].

Competing risk models described in this section are used for analysis of stroke survival data records, provided by the neurology department of Clinical Center of Montenegro. The following section of this paper describes the database structure and its main statistical characteristics. The Sect. 3 presents the estimates of cumulative incidence function from the competing risk data and investigate the difference between the CIF's across the groups experiencing different stroke types. The Fine-Grey regression model on the effect of covariates on the cumulative incidence function (CIF) for competing risks data is explored in Sect. 4. The article is summarized by a discussion of the most important results and conclusions.

2   Main Statistical Characteristics of the Stroke Clinical Data

The experimental research data is provided by the neurology department of Clinical Centre of Montenegro, located in Podgorica, Montenegro. The original database consists of the clinical data records collected between 02/25/2017 and 12/18/2019. The medical data of patients who have experienced stroke, consists of 944 records, structured in 58 variables, where 50 of them are coded by scale values of {1, 2, 3} corresponding to "Yes, No, Unspecified", and 8 variables consisting of the demographic data, and dates of admission and discharge from the hospital [3]. For applying the approach of competing risk modelling we have cleansed the initial stroke database, recoded some of the variables and selected 8 variables for further research. The brief fragment of the prepared database and its structure is presented in Table 1.

Table 1. The fragment of the prepared Stroke database

TimeH	Status	Disease	Age	Gender	Smoke	Medications	Rehabilitation
8	2	1	17	0	0	Other	Physical
23	0	1	16	1	0	Other	Working
12	1	1	13	0	0	Other	Physical
13	1	0	96	1	0	ANTIKOAG	NoRehab
3	1	0	95	0	0	ANTIKOAG	NoRehab
3	1	1	93	0	0	Other	NoRehab
3	1	0	94	1	0	ANTIAGREGAC	NoRehab
14	1	0	94	0	0	ANTIKOAG	Physical
6	0	0	92	1	0	ANTIAGREGAC	Physical
16	1	1	92	1	1	Other	Physical
16	2	0	91	1	0	ANTIAGREGAC	NoRehab
7	1	1	91	0	0	Other	Physical
18	0	1	93	1	0	Other	Working
21	0	0	91	0	0	ANTIAGREGAC	Physical
12	1	0	91	0	0	ANTIKOAG	NoRehab
1	1	0	92	0	0	ANTIKOAG	Physical

The values of the variables presented in Table 1 are coded for modeling the competing risk. The explanation of coding is provided in Table 2.

Table 2. The definition of stroke clinical database variables

Variable name	Meaning and coding of data
TimeH	The number of days spent in hospital after stroke
Status	2: Recovery after stroke with good health (event of interest), 1: death (competing event), 0: discharge from hospital (censored event)
Disease	0: Ischemic stroke, 1: Hemorag or SAH stroke
Age	Patient age, years
Gender	0: Female, 1: Male
Smoke	0: No, 1: Yes
Medications	Medications received: *ANTIKOAG*-Anticoagulant drugs; *ANTIAGREGAC*-Antiplatelet drugs, *TROMOLIZA*-Thrombolysis, *Other*
Rehabilitation	Procedures assigned during hospitalization: *Physical*-Physical therapy, *Working*-Working therapy, *NoRehab*-No therapy

In general, stroke is diagnosed for the patients whose blood supply to the brain is blocked or when a brain blood vessel bursts. Usually, the stroke is classified into two types: a hemorrhagic stroke and an ischemic stroke. Ischemic strokes (Ishemic) happen when the blood vessels carrying blood to the brain become clogged. The generally observed statistics for his type of stroke reports about 87% of all stroke cases [11]. A hemorrhagic stroke is caused by bleeding which can happen within the brain or in the area between the brain and skull. This is the cause of about 20% of all strokes [12]. Depending on the place where the bleeding occurs, the Hemorrhagic strokes are split to two categories: Intracerebral hemorrhage (Hemorag) and Subarachnoid hemorrhages (SAH). Intracerebral hemorrhages (Hemorag) are caused by a broken blood vessel located in the brain. The SAH stroke occurs when a blood vessel gets damaged, leading to bleeding in the area between the brain and the thin tissues that cover it. SAH is a less common type of hemorrhagic stroke, approximately 5–6% of all strokes [3]. The survival of the patient and health status after stroke and the recovery period may depend not only on the differences of the medical conditions defined by stroke types but also to the severity of damage experienced.

The presented research analyses the recovery conditions after stroke and its dependence from the characteristics of the patient, such as age, the modifiable life-style factors, medications received during hospital stay and additional procedures prescribed and processed for rehabilitation. The main statistical characteristics of our dataset describe the variety of the patient cases and value distribution of the variables. The demographic data of stroke patients varies by age (from 13 to 96 years), gender (485-male, 459-female) and smoking (379 of 944). These data show similar risk and prevalence of stroke among people of different age and gender. In order to characterize data distribution and suitability for applying survival modelling, we calculated the mortality and recovery percentage for different types of strokes (Table 3). In Table 3 the percental distribution of stroke types in the patient database corresponds to the generally observed statistics of stroke cases distribution. The percentage of occurrence of the competing events is very similar as well: the general statistics of recovery from Ischemic stroke is more than 33%, and from Hemorrhagic or SAH – 26%.

Table 3. Event distribution by stroke types: multiple response frequency table

N = 944	Ischemic stroke	Hemorag or SAH stroke	Percent
0 - Censored event	268 (76,1%)	84 (23,9%)	**37.3%**
1 - Death	166 (55,1%)	135 (44,9%)	**31.9%**
2 - Recovered	214 (73,5%)	77 (26,5%)	**30.8%**
All Grps %	**68.6%**	**31.4%**	

The age factor is assumed to have the greatest impact on stroke patients, their recovery status and risk of fatal outcome. Although the occurrence of stroke for younger patients is increasing recently, the stroke complications are significantly more dangerous for elder people.

This trend is well reflected from the analysis in Fig. 1, where the highest risk of having a stroke is observed among people between 60 and 75 years old. There were 401 (42.5%) such records in the database. The risk of stroke is also very high at the age between 75 and 90. The probability to recover from stroke differs significantly across the age groups. Up to the age of 75 years, the probability to recover from a stroke complication is greater than 50%. Unfortunately, at the elder age, this probability decreases sharply.

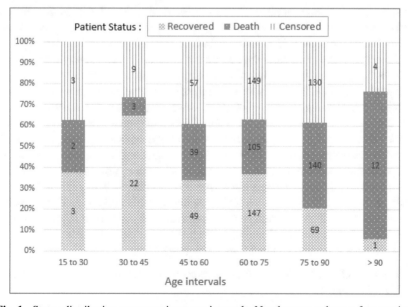

Fig. 1. Status distribution across patients age intervals. Numbers on columns-frequencies.

It is worth paying attention to the relatively high number of censored events between the ages of 45 and 90, as this significantly reduces the reliability of the observed results.

Some interesting findings are observed while exploring the variable of average of days spent in hospital (Table 4).

Table 4. The average days spent in hospital

Stroke_Type	Health_Status		
	Censored	Death (Competing)	Recovered (Event of interest)
Stroke ISHEM	12.4	6.8	9.4
Stroke HEMORAG or SAH	15.7	7.0	10.8

We see that the patients who withdraw from the further investigation, stay in the hospital the longest time. Improvement usually happens around 9–11 days of hospitalization. A fatal outcome follows on average after 7 days. Thus, in the case of a stroke, the first 10 days after the illness are the most dangerous.

In the next section this effect is researched in more details by calculating the cumulative incidence function of the variable "Status".

3   Estimates of Cumulative Incidence Function

In order to evaluate the cumulative incidence function, the cumulative incidence competing risk method (CICR) is applied. CICR is the generalization of Kaplan–Meier method used for the case if we have only one event of interest and no competing event. According to the CICR method, the CIF is estimated at the selected point of time for every competing event, and their estimates depend on each other [8]. Moreover, we need to apply Gray's test [10] to test the equality of cumulative incidence functions across groups.

To implement the CIF calculation for competing risk events and check the Grays' test the statistical software may be applied. Unfortunately, there are few statistical packages which could perform calculations for medical problem domain area. The most suitable tool for competing risk analysis was selected as the add-on package of R. R is an open-source software freely available at www.r-project.org. It can be applied to many statistical problems: linear and non-linear statistical models, time series, parametric and non-parametric hypothesis testing, clustering and survival analysis [13].

We performed CIF calculations for our *Status* variable and checked the hypothesis about equality of CIF across different stroke illnesses by applying R programing language. The program code in R language is attached in Appendix. For CIF calculation we use standard R function, called *CumIncidence()*:

CumIncidence (TimeH, Status, Disease, cencode = 0, xlab = "Days", t = c(0, 1, 3, 6, 10, 15, 21, 28, 36))

The function *CumIncidence()* requires setting of the following arguments: the follow-up time (*TimeH* in our example); the variable containing the competing events (*Status*);

the grouping variable of disease (*Disease*). The argument *cencode* indicates the code for censored observations, and it is set to 0 (default). In addition, we include the argument xlab for the x-axis label, and argument t, which define a vector of user-defined time points [13]. As the first days after the stroke are generally stated as the most important factor of recovery, we emphasized the smaller time values.

The results of CIF calculation are in Table 5.

Table 5. Cumulative incidence function estimates from the competing risk data

Stroke Type	Status	Time intervals								
		0	1	3	6	10	15	21	28	36
0	1	0.008	0.041	0.086	0.154	0.227	0.284	0.313	0.323	0.350
1	1	0.030	0.088	0.201	0.313	0.399	0.438	0.471	0.493	0.564
0	2	0.012	0.014	0.036	0.133	0.287	0.372	0.434	0.451	0.464
1	2	0.014	0.024	0.052	0.086	0.156	0.233	0.289	0.337	0.349

The probability of recovery is higher after experiencing Ischemic stroke (Table 4) at the end of the entire observation period, but for the period of the initial three days this probability is lower, as compared to the Hemorrhagic stroke or SAH. This fact is further supported by the estimated high possibility of the fatal outcome from Hemorrhagic stroke or SAH. The probability of death from Hemorrhagic stroke or SAH at the end of the observation interval is higher than *0.56*, whereas for Ischemic stroke, this outcome does not exceed 0.35.

In order to explore how recovery and death (variable Status) depend on the stroke type, we visualize CIF estimates by the linear graph (Fig. 2).

We check Gray's test for equality of CIFs across groups of Ischemic, Hemorrhagic or SAH stroke by applying R function *CumIncidence()* (Table 6).

The cumulative incidence curves for Ischemic, Hemorrhagic or SAH stroke types are significantly differ for recovery and death, especially for the case of fatal outcome.

The reliability of the results is explored by calculating the standard errors and 95% pointwise confidence intervals of the CIF estimates. This can also be done by applying *CumIncidence()*.

4   Fine-Grey Regression Model of Competing Risk

In this section we explore the effect of treatment procedures processed during hospitalization and disease or patient covariates by applying research of Fine-Grey regression model of competing risk [9]. We estimate cumulative incidence of recovery in the presence of the competing event, defined as death from stroke. As predictive factors and covariates for CIF regression we will use the variables defined and explained in Table 2: Disease, Age, Gender, Smoke, Medications, Rehabilitation.

Fine-Grey regression model is implemented as R function *crr()* contained in crr-addson.R and described in [14]. In order to apply the *crr()* function, the variables were

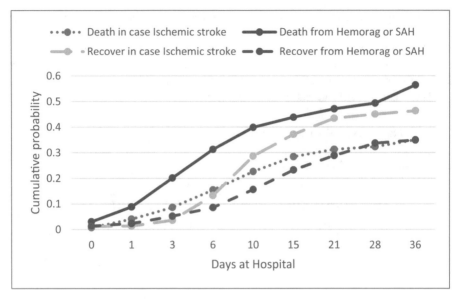

Fig. 2. CIF estimates for Status variable

Table 6. Gray's test for equality of CIFs

Status	Statistics	df	p-value
Death	*31.02*	*1*	*2.5484e−08*
Recovery	*14.60*	*1*	*0.00013294*

recoded accordingly. The numerical variables did not need any change, but the categorical variables had to be recoded by using the so-called 'baseline' codification [14]. If the categorical variable acquires only 2 different values (which in our case applies for *Age, Smoke, Gender, Disease)*, it is sufficient to code values as 0 and 1. However, if the variable acquires more than 2 values (variables *Medications* and *Rehabilitation*) we have to create supplementary indicator variables - variables coded as 1 in the presence of a given category and 0 otherwise. This task is automated by using the R function *factor2ind()*. The arguments for applying this function are the categorical variable name and selected baseline value [14]. The baseline values for *Medications* and *Rehabilitation* were selected "Other" and "NoRehab" respectively.

The R program code for competing risk regression is provided in Appendix. The program execution result sheet is in Fig. 3.

The first part of Fig. 3 lists the estimated regression coefficients, the relative risk as exp (coef), the standard error, the z-value and the corresponding p-value. The p-value indicates the high significance of *Age, Disease* and *Smoke* covariates, *Rehabilitation*, and only marginal significance of *Medications*, whereas we don't see the influence of *Gender*. An overall p-value for *Medications* and *Rehabilitation* can be obtained through

```
> summary(regr)
Competing Risks Regression

Call:
crr(ftime = TimeH, fstatus = Status, cov1 = x)

                          coef exp(coef) se(coef)        z p-value
Age                     0.0287     1.029  0.00548    5.237 1.6e-07
Gender                 -0.0312     0.969  0.12245   -0.255 8.0e-01
Smoke                  -0.2697     0.764  0.13015   -2.072 3.8e-02
Disease                 0.5842     1.794  0.15625    3.739 1.8e-04
Medications:ANTIAGREGAC -0.7809    0.458  0.18262   -4.276 1.9e-05
Medications:ANTIKOAG    0.0215     1.022  0.16312    0.132 9.0e-01
Medications:TROMOLIZA  -0.2720     0.762  0.44525   -0.611 5.4e-01
Rehabilitation:Physical -1.4413    0.237  0.12571  -11.465 0.0e+00
Rehabilitation:working -1.5068     0.222  0.32921   -4.577 4.7e-06

                        exp(coef) exp(-coef)  2.5% 97.5%
Age                         1.029      0.972 1.018 1.040
Gender                      0.969      1.032 0.762 1.232
Smoke                       0.764      1.310 0.592 0.986
Disease                     1.794      0.558 1.320 2.436
Medications:ANTIAGREGAC     0.458      2.183 0.320 0.655
Medications:ANTIKOAG        1.022      0.979 0.742 1.407
Medications:TROMOLIZA       0.762      1.313 0.318 1.823
Rehabilitation:Physical     0.237      4.226 0.185 0.303
Rehabilitation:working      0.222      4.512 0.116 0.423
```

Fig. 3. CIF estimates for Status variable.

the Wald test by using the *aod* library of R. The calculated p-values for *Medications* and *Rehabilitation* is very close to 0, so we can conclude the high significance of those factors for competing risk evaluation.

The second part of the output in Fig. 3 presents the relative risk for all covariates, and 95% confidence interval. For the continuous covariate the relative risk refers to the effect of one unit increase in the covariate, with all other covariates being equal. As an example, if age increases by 1 year, the relative risk increases by 1.029. The relative risk for a categorical variable is interpreted as the relative risk for the actual group with respect to the baseline, with all other covariates being equal. As example, 0.969 is the relative risk of a male with respect to a female.

5 Conclusion

The research of modelling Competing Risk is performed for the dataset of clinical trial records of the neurology department of Clinical Centre in Montenegro. The original database was cleansed and prepared for the time-to-event stroke analysis by selecting 944 records of the medical data of patients who have experience stroke, characterized by 8 variables. The explored event of interest is defined as a chance of recovery after stroke with the status of good health, and death as competing event. The results of the research revealed significant influence of the stroke type (ischemic, haemorrhagic or subarachnoid hemorrhage (SAH)) to the patient's level of recovery or death. The probability to recover from a stroke for the patients younger than 75 years is greater than 50%. Unfortunately, at an older age, this probability decreases to 20%.

CIF calculation for competing risk events, confirms the insight that the probability of recovery is higher after experiencing the Ischemic stroke, and the events of death from Hemorrhagic stroke or SAH by the end of the observation interval is greater than *0.56*. This mean that the cumulative incidence curves for each type of stroke (Ischemic, haemorrhagic or SAH) are significantly different for the recovery and death events.

Application of Fine-Grey model for CIF regression enables us to evaluate the influence of the selected predictive factors and covariates, such as Disease, Age, Gender, Smoke, Medications and Rehabilitation. The calculated p-value confirms the significance of *Age, Disease* and *Smoke* covariates, *Rehabilitation, Medications,* whereas the significance of *Gender* factor is not confirmed.

Appendix

#CIF estimates	#Competing risk regression
install.packages("cmprsk") medicina=read.csv(file.choose()) medicina str(medicina) attach(medicina) table(Disease, Status) tapply(TimeH, list(Disease, Status), mean) source (file.choose()) fit=CumIncidence (TimeH, Status, Disease, cencode = 0, xlab="Days", t=c(0,1,3,6,10,15,21,28,36), level=0.95)	install.packages("cmprsk") regresija=read.csv(file.choose()) regresija str(regresija) attach(regresija) source (file.choose()) x=cbind(Age, Gender, Smoke, Disease, factor2ind(Medications, "Other"), factor2ind(Rehabilitation, "NoRehab")) regr=crr(TimeH, Status, x) summary(regr) install.packages("aod") library(aod) wald.test(regr$var, regr$coef, Terms = 4:6) wald.test(regr$var, regr$coef, Terms = 7:8)

References

1. Noordzij, M., Leffondré, K., van Stralen, K.J., Zoccali, C., Dekker, F.W., Jager, K.J.: When do we need competing risks methods for survival analysis in nephrology? Nephrol. Dial. Transplant. **28**(11), 2670–2677 (2013). https://doi.org/10.1093/ndt/gft355(2013)
2. Kaplan, E.L., Meier, P.: Nonparametric estimation from incomplete observations. J. Am. Stat. Assoc. **53**, 457–481 (1958)
3. Kriksciuniene, D., Sakalauskas, V., Ognjanovic, I., Sendelj, R.: Time-to-event modelling for survival and hazard analysis of stroke clinical case. In: Abramowicz, W., Auer, S., Stróżyna, M. (eds.) BIS 2021. LNBIP, vol. 444, pp. 14–26. Springer, Cham (2022). https://doi.org/10.1007/978-3-031-04216-4_2

4. Cox, D.R.: Regression models and life-tables. J. R. Stat. Soc. Ser. B (Meth.) **34**, 187–202 (1972)
5. Gooley, T.A., Leisenring, W., Crowley, J., Storer, B.E.: Estimation of failure probabilities in the presence of competing risks: new representations of old estimators. Stat. Med. **18**, 695–706 (1999)
6. Freidlin, B., Korn, E.L.: Testing treatment effects in the presence of competing risks. Stat. Med. **24**, 1703–1712 (2005)
7. Guo, C.: Cause-specific analysis of competing risks using the PHREG procedure (2018)
8. Logan, B.R., Zhang, M.-J., Klein, J.P.: Regression models for hazard rates versus cumulative incidence probabilities in hematopoietic cell transplantation data. Biol. Blood Marrow Transplant **12**, 107–112 (2006)
9. Gray, R.J.: A class of K-sample tests for comparing the cumulative incidence of a competing risk. Ann. Stat. **16**, 1141–1154 (1988)
10. Fine, J.P., Gray, R.J.: A proportional hazards model for the subdistribution of a competing risk. J. Am. Stat. Assoc. **94**, 496–509 (1999)
11. Deljavan, R., Farhoudi, M., Sadeghi-Bazargani, H.: Stroke in-hospital survival and its predictors: the first results from Tabriz Stroke Registry of Iran. Int. J. Gen. Med. **11**, 233–240 (2018)
12. Homepage. https://www.world-stroke.org/assets/downloads/WSO_2019_Annual_Report_online.pdf. Accessed 24 Oct 2022
13. Scrucca, L., Santucci, A., Aversa, F.: Competing risk analysis using R: an easy guide for clinicians. Bone Marrow Transplant **40**(4), 381–387 (2007). https://doi.org/10.1038/sj.bmt.1705727. Epub 2007 Jun 11. PMID: 17563735 (2007)
14. Scrucca, L., Santucci, A., Aversa, F.: Regression modeling of competing risk using R: an in depth guide for clinicians. Bone Marrow Transplant **45**(1388–1395) (2010). https://doi.org/10.1038/bmt.2009.359

Artificial Intelligence Chatbots and Conversational Agents – An Overview of Clinical Studies in Health Care

I. Stević[1(✉)], D. Vukmirović[2], V. Vujović[3], and V. Marinković[1,3]

[1] Department of Social Pharmacy and Pharmaceutical Legislation, Faculty of Pharmacy, University of Belgrade, Belgrade, Serbia
ivana.stevic@pharmacy.bg.ac.rs
[2] Faculty of Pharmacy, University of Belgrade, Belgrade, Serbia
[3] United Association in Serbia on Quality – JUSK, Belgrade, Serbia

Abstract. One of the forms of digital health with increasing presence in Health Care are Chatbots or Conversational Agents – computer programs driven by artificial intelligence intended to support different activities in the health care sector. The goal of this research is to present the latest cross section of available trials using chatbots and provide overview of research and development directions in this section of digital health. For our research, we reviewed registered clinical studies related to chatbot or conversational agent at ClinicalTrials.gov database, WHO International Clinical Trials Registry Platform and EU Clinical Trials Register with the cutoff date 31 December 2022. Results were reviewed and cross-checked by authors to confirm eligibility of chatbot/conversational agent presence and their intended use in the study. From 373 results, in final analysis 168 studies were included. Analyzed variables were: Research area, Chatbot support category, Study design, Study funded by, Gender, Age, Country. Behavioral therapy was shown to be the most researched chatbot support category, followed by Disease Management and Disease/Health Risks Training/Education/Prevention. Further research is needed to expand results to include additional sources in conjunction with additional efforts to harmonize chatbot classification in healthcare.

Keywords: Artificial Intelligence · Chatbot · Conversational Agent · Clinical studies · Healthcare

1   Introduction

Digital health is a term that is including wide area of fast evolving technology solutions in healthcare and per the World Health Organization (WHO) can be defined as "field of knowledge and practice related to the development and use of digital technologies intended to improve health" [1].

The speed of digital health development can be illustrated by the growing number of digital health apps, as the most available and used products in this area. Only in 2020 there were more than 90.000 new health related apps added in the market which contributed to a total of more than 350.000 apps available [2].

© The Author(s), under exclusive license to Springer Nature Singapore Pte Ltd. 2023
Y.-W. Chen et al. (Eds.): KES InMed 2023, SIST 357, pp. 44–52, 2023.
https://doi.org/10.1007/978-981-99-3311-2_5

Additionally, it is important to notice that main categories of digital health apps can be defined as wellness management and health condition management. While the initial focus of development was on the first category with intention to facilitate tracking and modification of fitness behaviors, lifestyle, stress and diet, since 2015 the shift towards focus on second category is noticed with the goal to supply information on diseases and conditions, enable access to care, and aid treatment such as through medication reminders [2].

Artificial intelligence (AI) has important place in development of digital health products and can be explained as simulation of human intelligence processes by machines. Focus is on the computer systems that can work and react like human beings. Examples of AI application include expert systems, natural language processing (NLP), speech recognition and machine vision [3].

Digital health products can have different applications, including to diagnose or treat a condition, to inform users about health-related topics or to drive a health assistance. As number of available products and intended uses is constantly increasing, they can be categorized in different ways. One of the possible categorizations include following 4 sections of digital health, where the focus of our research will be on the last section [4]:

- Connected devices (wearable and non-wearable devices)
- Digital patient information collection tools (web portals, smartphone apps, electronic surveys)
- Telehealth (Long distance clinical healthcare)
- Digital assistants (Chatbots/Conversational agents/AI driven software)

Digital assistants are widely used across different industries and their presence in healthcare is increasingly evident [5].

The aim of this review is to present the latest cross section of available clinical studies using chatbots/conversational agents reported in public registries and provide overview of research and development directions in this section of digital health.

2 AI Driven Chatbots/conversational Agents

Chatbots, or conversational agents, are computer programs, driven by artificial intelligence, which interact with humans via speech, text, or other inputs and outputs on different devices/platforms with the intent to simulate conversation with users [6].

Artificial intelligence techniques enable the program to recognize, analyze and process information provided by users, and consequently generate complex replies which mimic human interaction [5].

This makes AI Chatbots attractive for application in supporting different activities in the healthcare sector.

AI chatbots have been used in various ways, with outcomes being improvement of self-management of chronic diseases, disease management personalization, therapy management and behavioral/lifestyle changes, early screening and diagnostics, education/training services and compliance measurements [5, 7, 8].

As chatbots are digital technologies independent of external human maintenance, they provide 24/7 availability to users, regardless of user's access to the traditional healthcare system services (e.g., in-site visits, with available healthcare provider) [5, 8]. AI chatbots may provide relevant support to patients and healthcare providers alike. Utilization of AI chatbots go beyond disease control and management. Through behavioral interventions, in mental status (e.g., stress management), promotion of healthy lifestyle and physical activities (e.g., smoke cessation, healthy diet and calories intake, toothbrushing techniques, etc.), AI chatbots may serve as a platform for disease prevention efforts. This means that AI Chatbot utilization can be applied to support general healthcare topics, and potentially reduce burden of healthcare (e.g., related with lack of physicians, or disease management related costs). As such, AI chatbots became even more important in post-COVID-19 period as potential tool which would address health related challenges during pandemic [8].

Research on artificial intelligence application in the field of health care is increasing. We analyzed publication trend of articles related to healthcare and chatbot or conversational agents (Fig. 1) which is showing rapid increase of publications of such solutions in last 4 years, both in manner of original papers, results of conducted studies, and systematic reviews [9].

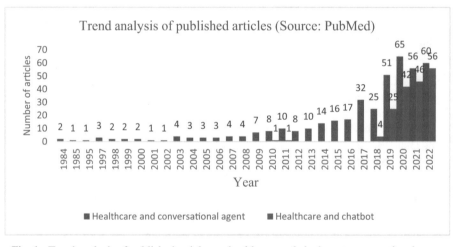

Fig. 1. Trend analysis of published articles on healthcare and chatbot or conversational agent

This is in line with the fact that technological advancements facilitate increasing usage of AI based chatbots [10]. Multi-stakeholder working groups have already been addressing topics about standardization of clinical research involving AI [11].

Providing AI Chatbot performance and safety evaluations in well-regulated and standardized clinical research setting is critical to address in a timely manner ethical, regulatory, and data privacy questions for expanding their future usage in the real world.

3   Clinical Studies Involving Chatbots/Conversational Agents

Chatbots or conversational agents may be integrated as part of the software, and since regulation on software as medical device is different among countries as well as requirement to conduct clinical studies based on software categorization, we did a review of the registered clinical studies related to chatbot or conversational agent [12].

As relevant registries for this review we selected ClinicalTrials.gov database (CT.gov), WHO International Clinical Trials Registry Platform (WHO ICTRP) and EU Clinical Trials Register (EU CTR) with the cutoff date 31 December 2022 [13–15].

Results from these sources were reviewed and crosschecked by authors to confirm eligibility of chatbot/conversational agent presence and their intended use in the study. Total of 373 results were found across all three registries (CT.gov 285, WHO ICTRP 86 and EU CTR 2). It was determined that there were 168 unique eligible studies present in relevant registries that were further analyzed (CT.Gov 122 (including 39 overlapping studies with WHO ICTRP search), 46 unique results from WHO ICTRP search and 0 eligible studies from EU CTR search). Data for eligible studies were extracted, synthesized and database for the purpose of analysis was created.

Based on different level of information, we created variables for which we had information in all of 3 sources. Variables we analyzed were: Research area, Chatbot support category, Study design, Study funded by, Gender, Age, Country.

Conditions category data from registries were used to create Research area, where we divided all studies into the 14 categories: Cardiovascular, Diagnostic, Gastrointestinal, Infectious Disease, Mental Health, Metabolic Disease, Musculoskeletal, Oncology, Pain, Renal, Respiratory, Sense Organs, Substance Abuse and Other (for studies that could not be categorized). Among these categories % of studies varied from 1,19% (Diagnostic) to Mental Health (33,33%). In order to conduct cross-variable analysis, all categories that had less than 5% of the total studies were transferred into category Other, and final number of categories was 6. Most of the studies was in the category Other (60; 35,71%), followed by Mental Health (56; 33,33%), Substance Abuse (16; 9,52%) and Oncology (15; 8,93%), and Infectious Disease and Metabolic Disease with the same frequency (11; 6,55%).

Based on the review of the Interventions, eligible studies were arbitrary divided, as per the type of support that is provided by chatbot/conversational agent, into following 6 categories:

- Behavioral Therapy (45,24%) - addressing items such as wellbeing, lifestyle changes, habits adjustments contributing to improvement of health
- Decision Making - Informed Consents (4,17%) - supporting patients with informed consent process
- Disease/Health Risks Training/Education/Prevention (17,26%)
- Disease Management (19,64%)
- Disease Screening / Tracking / Monitoring (7,74%)
- Medication Therapy Management (5,95%) - including treatment or dosage compliance or dosage modification and adverse event management

Study design types were Observational (13; 7,74%) and Interventional (155; 92,26%). Interventional studies were reviewed by the authors and subcategorized into randomized-clinical trial (118; 76,13%) and non-randomized clinical trial (37; 23,87%). Dominantly studies involving chatbot or conversational agents were interventional, which is in line with data on all clinical studies [13], but is opposite to the current literature [5, 6] which is expected since for the most of research that can be found in literature it is not mandatory to be registered as clinical studies.

Studies were reviewed also according to who was their sponsor i.e., who funded them, and by the Industry 5,95% of the studies were funded, compared to the 86,90% funded by Other, and 7,50% by Other and Industry together. Category "Other" refers to Academia, Public Health Institution, Hospitals etc.

According to Gender, we found almost 90% of studies included all genders, 9,52% only Female and 1,19% only Male participants.

Study analysis per participants age was conducted according to 6 categories:

- Child (7,14%) – participants less than 18 years old
- Adult (9,52%) – participants that were between 18 and 65 years old
- Older adult (2,98%) – participants that were 65 and more years old
- Child, Adult (5,36%) – participants that were less than 65 years old
- Adult, Older Adult (67,86%) – participants that were 18 and more years old
- Child, Adult, Older Adult (6,55%) – no year limitation

From the results above, we can see that almost 20% included Children (of which 53,13% interventional).

Most of the studies were conducted in one country (163; 97,02%), more than one third in the United States of America. If we analyze them based on the Regions, 38,89% were in the North America, followed by EMEA (33,89%) and APAC (26,67%) with only one study in LATAM.

In Table 1 we provide cross-variable overview for each Chatbot support category.

Table 1. Chatbot support category distribution per variables

	Behavioral Therapy	Decision Making - Informed Consents	Disease/ Health Risks Training/Education/Prevention	Disease Management	Disease Screening/Tracking/ Monitoring	Medication Therapy Management
N	**76**	**7**	**29**	**33**	**13**	**10**
%	**45,24**	**4,17**	**17,26**	**19,64**	**7,74**	**5,95**
RESEARCH AREA						
INFECTIOUS DISEASE	1 1,32%	0 0%	9 31,03%	0 0%	1 7,69%	0 0%
MENTAL HEALTH	40 52,63%	2 28,57%	3 10,34%	8 24,24%	3 23,08%	0 0%
METABOLIC DISEASE	3 3,95%	0 0%	0 0%	7 21,21%	1 7,69%	0 0%
ONCOLOGY	1 1,32%	0 0%	4 13,79%	1 3,03%	4 30,77%	5 50,00%
SUBSTANCE ABUSE	15 19,74%	0 0%	1 3,45%	0 0%	3 23,08%	0 0%
OTHER	16 21,05%	5 71,43%	12 41,38%	17 51,52%	1 7,69%	5 50,00%
STUDY DESIGN						
OBSERVATIONAL	2 2,63%	0 0%	2 6,90%	2 6,06%	6 46,15%	1 10,00%

(continued)

Table 1. (continued)

	Behavioral Therapy	Decision Making - Informed Consents	Disease/ Health Risks Training/Education/Prevention	Disease Management	Disease Screening/Tracking/ Monitoring	Medication Therapy Management
INTERVENTIONAL	74 97,37%	7 100%	27 93,10%	31 93,94%	7 53,85%	9 90,00%
RCT	59 77,63%	6 85,71%	18 62,07%	25 75,76%	6 46,15%	4 40,00%
NON-RCT	15 19,74%	1 14,29%	9 31,03%	6 18,18%	1 7,69%	5 50,00%
FUNDED BY						
INDUSTRY	7 9,21%	0 0%	0 0%	0 0%	1 7,69%	2 20,00%
OTHER	60 78,95%	7 100%	28 96,55%	33 100%	11 84,62%	7 70,00%
INDUSTRYI OTHER	9 11,84%	0 0%	1 3,45%	0 0%	1 7,69%	1 10,00%
GENDER						
FEMALE	5 6,58%	0 0%	7 24,14%	2 6,06%	1 7,69%	1 10,00%
MALE	0 0%	0 0%	2 6,90%	0 0%	0 0%	0 0%

(continued)

Table 1. (*continued*)

	Behavioral Therapy	Decision Making - Informed Consents	Disease/ Health Risks Training/Education/Prevention	Disease Management	Disease Screening/Tracking/ Monitoring	Medication Therapy Management
ALL	71 93,42%	7 100%	20 68,97%	31 93,94%	12 92,31%	9 90,00%
AGE[a]						
CHILD	9 11,84%	0 0%	1 3,45%	1 3,03%	1 7,69%	0 0%
ADULT	9 11,84%	1 14,29%	5 17,24%	0 0%	1 7,69%	0 0%
OLDER, ADULT	2 2,63%	0 0%	0 0%	1 3,03%	1 7,69%	1 10,00%
CHILD, ADULT	3 3,95%	0 0%	2 6,90%	2 6,06%	2 15,38%	0 0%
ADULT, OLDER ADULT	45 59,21%	6 85,71%	21 72,41%	27 81,82%	8 61,54%	7 70,00%
CHILD, ADULT, OLDER ADULT	8 10,53%	0 0%	0 0%	2 6,06%	0 0%	1 10,00%

[a] missing data for one study in the category Medication Therapy Management.
RCT - Randomized Clinical Trial.
NON-RCT - Non-Randomized Clinical Trial.

4 Conclusions

Based on our review there is an evident trend in increasing the number of clinical trials investigating AI Chatbots/Conversational agents.

Main research focus of reviewed studies based on the research area was related to non-specific disease, mental health and substance abuse.

Behavioral therapy was shown to be the most researched chatbot support category, followed by Disease Management and Disease/Health Risks Training/Education/Prevention.

This review included data collected from three most significant public clinical studies registries. Further research is needed to expand results to include additional sources, such as local registries. This should be done in conjunction with additional efforts to harmonize chatbot classification in healthcare based on their nature and intended use.

References

1. World Health Organization, Global strategy on digital health 2020–2025 (electronic version) (2021). ISBN 978-92-4-002092-4
2. IQVIA Institute for Human Data Science, Digital Health Trends 2021 (2021)
3. International Pharmaceutical Federation (FIP): Digital health in pharmacy education, developing a digitally enabled pharmaceutical workforce (2021)
4. Garg, S., Williams, N.L., Ip, A., Dicker, A.P.: Clinical integration of digital solutions in health care: an overview of the current landscape of digital technologies in cancer care. JCO Clin. Cancer Inform. **2**, 1–9 (2018)
5. Milne-Ives, M., et al.: The effectiveness of artificial intelligence conversational agents in health care: systematic review. J. Med. Internet Res. **22**(10), e20346 (2020)
6. Tudor Car, L., et al.: Conversational agents in health care: scoping review and conceptual analysis. J. Med. Internet Res. **22**(8), e17158 (2020)
7. Griffin, A.C., et al.: Conversational agents for chronic disease self-management: a systematic review. AMIA Annu. Symp. Proc. **25**(2020), 504–513 (2021)
8. Oh, Y.J., Zhang, J., Fang, M.L., Fukuoka, Y.: A systematic review of artificial intelligence chatbots for promoting physical activity, healthy diet, and weight loss. Int. J. Behav. Nutr. Phys. Act. **18**(1), 160 (2021)
9. Healthcare and Chatbot or Concersational Agent articles trend analysis. https://pubmed.ncbi.nlm.nih.gov. Accessed 08 Jan 2023
10. Schachner, T., Keller, R., V Wangenheim, F.: Artificial intelligence-based conversational agents for chronic conditions: systematic literature review. J. Med. Internet Res. **22**(9), e20701 (2020)
11. Cruz Rivera, S., Liu, X., Chan, A.-W., Denniston, A., Calvert, M.: Guidelines for clinical trial protocols for interventions involving artificial intelligence: the SPIRIT-AI extension. Nat. Med. **26**, 1351–1363 (2020). https://doi.org/10.1038/s41591-020-1037-7
12. Vukmirović, D., Stević, I., Odalović, M., Krajnović, D.: Review of regulatory requirements in the US, EU and Serbia on software: mobile application as a medical device: state of the art. Arhiv za farmaciju **72**(4), 413–427 (2022)
13. ClinicalTrials.gov. https://clinicaltrials.gov/ct2/home. Accessed 31 Dec 2022
14. International Clinical Trials Registry Platform Search Portal. https://trialsearch.who.int/Default.aspx. Accessed 31 Dec 2022
15. EU Clinical Trials Register/EudraCT (Europe). https://www.clinicaltrialsregister.eu/ctr-search/search/. Accessed 31 Dec 2022

Challenges and Solutions for Artificial Intelligence Adoption in Healthcare – A Literature Review

Uldis Donins[(✉)] [iD] and Daiga Behmane [iD]

Riga Stradins University, 16 Dzirciema, Riga 1007, Latvia
`{uldis.donins,daiga.behmane}@rsu.lv`

Abstract. Even though Artificial Intelligence (AI) solutions are already used and have additional potential to revolutionize healthcare (HC), its application in practice tends to face limitations. Objectives of this research are to identify and summarize knowledge on the challenges and solutions for the adoption of AI in HC by a literature review of articles (N = 19) published between 2018 and 2022 in Scopus, Science Direct and BMC Health Services Research using the key terms "challenges", "solutions", "artificial intelligence", "AI", "adoption", and "healthcare". The study reveals several limitations of AI implementation: the lack of transparency in AI decision making, difficulty to trust and use the results; obtaining high-quality properly labeled medical data; concerns about data privacy, regulation and security and hesitancy of HC professionals and patients to trust and use AI-powered systems. To overcome these challenges, studies suggest to apply the solutions: justify the application of AI-powered systems in the context of digital transformation of HC - value-based HC and change management strategies with the aim to benefit patients and improve overall health outcomes; educate stakeholders and involve them in the implementation process to overcome black-box decision making; teaching AI fundamentals and applications to ensure HC professionals can effectively use and understand AI systems; address the challenge of data availability by federated learning and secondary use of health data enabling researchers to discover new knowledge and breakthroughs in medical science. Proper regulation is also essential to ensure the safe and ethical development, testing, and use of AI in HC.

Keywords: Artificial Intelligence · Challenges · Solutions · Healthcare

1 Introduction

In recent years Artificial intelligence (AI) has become a disruptive technology in many sectors, including healthcare (HC) [10]. This has happened due to several factors. One reason is the increasing amount of data available in HC, including electronic health records, imaging, and genomics data. The amount of data that is generated and collected is increasing exponentially every year and collection of HC data from various sources is still emerging. To get maximum out of HC data, the data needs to be analyzed,

Y.-W. Chen et al. (Eds.): KES InMed 2023, SIST 357, pp. 53–62, 2023.
https://doi.org/10.1007/978-981-99-3311-2_6

interpreted, and acted upon. AI and especially its subfields Machine Learning (ML) and Deep Learning (DL) allow extracting valuable information and knowledge from the collected data and can help to reduce the costs of operation, prediction, and diagnosis in HC as HC data can be used to train AI models using different AI algorithms to make predictions and automate tasks. Another reason is the advancements in AI algorithms, which have made it possible to analyze large and complex datasets. Additionally, the cost of computing power and storage has decreased, making it more feasible to run large AI models. These factors have led to the development of a range of AI-powered HC solutions that have the potential to improve patient outcomes, reduce costs, and increase efficiency in the HC system [4].

Even though AI solutions are already used and have additional potential to revolutionize HC, its application in practice tends to face limitations. Objectives of this research are to identify and summarize knowledge on the challenges and solutions for the adoption of AI in HC. This paper is organized as follows. Section 2 describes the applied research method of this paper – a literature review. Section 3 outlines the identified challenges, while Sect. 4 summarizes the identified solutions for AI adoption in HC. Section 5 concludes this article by providing conclusions of the research. This study aims to be useful to both scholars and practitioners.

2   Review Methodology

The review methodology used in this paper is based on the Preferred Reporting Items for Systematic reviews and Meta-Analyses (PRISMA) 2020 statement approach [19]. The review proceeds in the following three steps: 1) identification of articles, 2) screening and inclusion of articles, and 3) data extraction and analysis.

The subsequent sections give a detailed explanation of each step in the process, covering important aspects of the applied review methodology. This provides a better understanding of the procedure, making it easier to replicate or adapt in future.

2.1   Identification of Articles

The process of selecting articles for this review was carried out through a comprehensive search of three different databases: Scopus, Science direct, and BMC Health Services Research. These databases were chosen for their wide coverage of the relevant literature and the high quality of the articles they contain. To identify the most relevant articles for this review, a set of key terms were used for the article selection process. These key terms include: "challenges", "solutions", "artificial intelligence", "AI", "adoption", and "healthcare". The use of these terms ensures that the articles selected for the review are directly related to the topic of interest.

To focus on more recent research papers, additional criteria were applied to include articles that were published in the last four years, specifically between the years 2018 and 2022. This was done to ensure that the review would be based on the most current and up-to-date research available, providing a comprehensive and accurate representation of the current state of the field. By applying these criteria, the review was able to select the

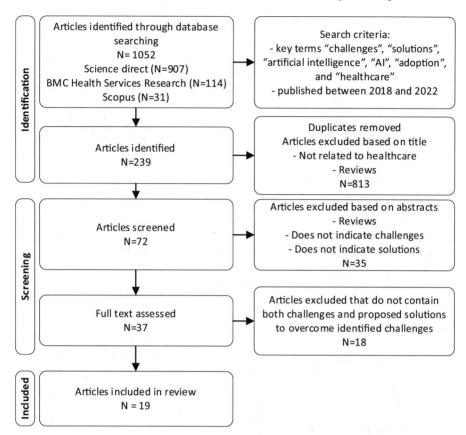

Fig. 1. Article identification, screening, and selection for review

most relevant and current articles, providing a thorough and up-to-date analysis of the challenges, solutions and adoption of AI in HC.

By following the search criteria, 1052 articles were identified. By removing the duplicates and excluding articles that were not related to the HC and that were reviews, 239 articles were selected for further analysis. See Fig. 1 for more details.

2.2 Screening and Inclusion of Articles

Screening and inclusion procedures were carefully implemented to select articles for the main analysis. The first step involved retrieving and analyzing the abstracts of the identified articles. After reviewing the abstracts, a total of 35 articles were excluded from further analysis due to various exclusion criteria. These criteria included articles that were reviews or abstracts that did not indicate challenges or proposed solutions. The remaining 37 articles had their full texts retrieved for detailed analysis.

During the detailed analysis of the full texts, an additional 18 articles were excluded because they did not contain both challenges and proposed solutions to overcome identified challenges. This was done to ensure that the review was based on articles that provided a comprehensive understanding of the challenges and proposed solutions to overcome them.

The final number of articles included in this review was N = 19, consisting of research articles that identified challenges in adopting AI in HC and proposed solutions to overcome those challenges. The selection process was rigorous and meticulous, ensuring that only the most relevant and current articles were included in the analysis. This provided a thorough and accurate representation of the current state of the field, providing valuable insights into challenges and solutions for adoption of AI in HC.

2.3   Data Extraction and Analysis

By reviewing the selected N = 19 articles, the following key challenges for the adoption of AI in HC were identified: 1) black-box decision making, 2) data availability, 3) data privacy, 4) perception and acceptance of AI, and 5) lack of regulation.

To address these challenges, a number of solutions are proposed: 1) value-based HC, 2) change management, 3) explainable AI, 4) teaching AI fundamentals and applications, 5) data availability, 6) federated learning, and 7) regulation.

3   Challenges

Five challenges of adopting AI in HC were identified from the selected and reviewed articles. The contribution of the reviewed articles to each of the challenges are described following subsections.

3.1   Black-Box Decision Making

Black-box decision making in AI solutions relates to the process in which a machine learning model makes predictions or decisions without providing any insight into how the model made it – the working of the model is not transparent or interpretable to the user. Trusting a black box model includes trusting both the algorithm for the model and the entire database that was used for model training. Thus, the black-box models can hide potential mistakes and even a data leakage through its predictions. The opposite of black box is transparent decision-making [24].

Black-box decision making as a challenge is outlined in a number of reviewed articles: [1–3, 5, 6, 11, 12, 15, 16, 20, 21], and [26], pointing to the following problems:

- Difficult or impossible to explain and interpret the results and lack of trust if it is not possible to explain how the AI models make decisions.
- Difficulty in identifying and addressing errors – the root cause can be hidden any-where, starting with the selection of algorithm, and ending with data preparation for the training of selected algorithm.
- Bias might be introduced into the decision-making process if the data used to train the system is biased or the algorithms used are not designed to account for bias.

3.2 Data Availability

AI requires large amounts of high-quality data to be trained on and tested for best results. HC data is often siloed and difficult to access, making it challenging to collect and use the necessary data for training AI models. Additionally, HC data is often sensitive and personal, and strict regulations such as "General Data Protection Regulation" (GDPR) in European Union (EU) and "Health Insurance Portability and Accountability Act" (HIPAA) in USA must be followed to ensure patient privacy and security.

Data availability as a challenge is outlined in a number of reviewed articles: [2, 3, 6, 7, 9, 11, 12, 15, 17], and [20], pointing to the following problems:

- Limited availability of high-quality properly labeled medical data.
- Very expensive to label the medical data.
- Data quality can vary widely and may not be suitable for training AI models.
- Limited diversity as the data may not be representative of the entire population, limiting the generalization and applicability of AI models.

3.3 Data Privacy

HC data is often sensitive and personal with strict regulations that has to be applied, like GDPR and HIPAA. Additionally, AI systems can analyze large amounts of data quickly, making it important to ensure that the data is protected and used in an ethical and responsible manner.

Data privacy as a challenge is outlined in a number of reviewed articles: [3, 6, 9, 11, 13, 16, 17, 20], and [22], pointing to the following problems:

- Data sharing for training AI models raises privacy and security concerns.
- Data security to protect patients from identity theft and other security breaches.
- Compliance with regulations like GDRP and HIPAA to ensure patient privacy and security when collecting, storing, and using HC data.
- Important to ensure that data is protected and used in ethical and responsible way.
- Explainability to ensure that patients understand how their data is being used.

3.4 Perception and Acceptance of AI

Perception and acceptance of AI is related to the fact that people may not fully understand the capabilities and limitations of AI. People may have misconceptions about AI, as it is widely depicted in fiction books, TV shows and movies. Finally, some people may be resistant to using AI systems and applications due to concerns about job displacement, bias, or lack of transparency.

Perception and acceptance of AI as a challenge is outlined in a number of reviewed articles: [5, 17, 22], and [27], pointing to the following problems:

- Resistance to change due to concerns about job displacement, bias, lack of transparency, or fear of the unknown creating mistrust to AI application.
- Ethical concerns like how AI might be used to make decisions about patient care or how AI might impact the doctor and patient relationship.

3.5 Lack of Regulation

As final challenge in our research we have identified lack of regulation related to development, application, and certification of AI solutions. Since the training of AI models involves usage of a large amount of data, data privacy and HC data availability and sharing regulations has to be improved or even created. Without clear guidelines and regulations in place, it can be difficult to ensure that AI systems are tested and validated for safety and effectiveness before they are applied in HC. Lack of regulation can also negatively impact innovation by creating uncertainty about what is and is not allowed when developing and deploying AI systems in HC.

Lack of regulation as a challenge is outlined in a number of reviewed articles: [5, 6, 9, 12, 13, 15, 22], and [25].

4   Solutions

To overcome the challenges of adopting AI in HC discussed in previous section, reviewed articles suggests several solutions to apply. The contribution of the reviewed articles to each of the solutions are described in following subsections.

4.1 Value Based Healthcare

The value-based HC approach serves to increase HC outcomes for patients in a more efficient way compared with the current volume-based approach. Currently, the HC system rewards volume over outcomes or performance, even though the performance of HC is of major importance. Value can be defined as patient health outcomes generated per unit of currency spent. Delivering high value to patients measured by health outcomes is the main purpose of HC and it is believed that value is the only goal that can bring together the interests of all participants in the HC environment and prevent reduced HC services [4].

Value based HC as a solution to overcome challenges in AI adoption in HC is proposed in [17].

4.2 Change Management

Change management is the process of planning, implementing, and monitoring changes to an organization in order to meet specific goals and objectives. It involves identifying the need for change, assessing the impact of the change, developing a plan to implement the change, and then overseeing the execution of the plan. The goal of change management is to minimize disruptions and negative impacts while maximizing the benefits of the change [14].

Change management as a solution to overcome challenges in AI adoption in HC is proposed in [5, 22], and [27].

4.3 Explainable AI

Explainable AI (XAI) refers to AI systems that are able to explain their decision-making processes, reasoning, and actions to users in a way that is understandable. XAI is important because it allows for greater transparency and accountability in AI systems and helps to build trust and confidence in their use [8].

In [23] four principles to XAI are proposed: transparency (users can understand how they work and how they make decisions); interpretability (users can understand the reasoning behind their decisions); accountability (users can understand the consequences of their actions and hold them responsible for any negative impacts); and trustworthiness (users can have confidence in their decisions and actions).

XAI as a solution to overcome challenges in AI adoption in HC is proposed in [1, 3, 11], and [25].

4.4 Teaching AI Fundamentals and Applications

Benefits of teaching AI fundamentals and applications to HC professionals:

- Professionals who understand AI can contribute to the development of new AI applications that can improve patient outcomes, increase efficiency, and reduce costs.
- Understanding AI can help HC professional to keep pace with technological advancements and to use them to improve patient care.
- By understanding AI, HC professionals can work more effectively with data scientists and other AI experts to develop and implement AI solutions.

Teaching AI fundamentals and applications as a solution to overcome challenges in AI adoption in HC is proposed in [2, 5, 7, 13, 16, 17, 22], and [25].

4.5 Data Availability

The challenge of data availability can be overcome by secondary use of health data enabling researchers to discover new knowledge and breakthroughs in medical science. Secondary usage of health data refers to the use of existing health data for purposes other than the original intent of the data collection, such as research and development of new products and services. This approach allows HC providers to leverage existing data to train AI models and to gain new insights into HC.

Data availability as a solution to overcome challenges in AI adoption in HC is proposed in [2, 12, 15, 20], and [21].

4.6 Federated Learning

Federated learning is a method of training machine learning models on decentralized data, where the data is kept on individual devices or local servers, rather than on a centralized server. This allows HC providers to collect and share data without compromising patient privacy or having to transfer large amounts of data to a centralized location. This approach can help to overcome the lack of quality data and labeled data that is often encountered in HC [18].

Federated learning as a solution to overcome challenges in AI adoption in HC is proposed in [20].

4.7 Regulation

Proper regulation is essential for the safe and ethical development, testing, and use of AI in HC for several reasons: patient safety, ethical considerations, transparency and accountability, data privacy and security, and innovation [4, 10].

Proper regulation development as a solution to overcome challenges in AI adoption in HC is proposed in [1, 2, 5, 6, 9, 12, 13, 15, 22], and [25].

5 Conclusions

After a review of the selected articles (N = 19), an analysis of the challenges for the adoption of AI in HC was conducted.

Through this analysis, several key challenges were identified: black-box decision making, data availability, data privacy, perception and acceptance of AI, and lack of regulation. Black-box decision making refers to the inability to understand the reasoning behind the decisions made by AI systems. Data availability and data privacy are closely related, as the availability of high-quality data is crucial for the successful implementation of AI in HC, but it also raises concerns about the privacy and security of sensitive patient information. The perception and acceptance of AI by HC providers and patients is also a significant challenge, as the understanding and trust of AI is crucial for its successful adoption. The lack of regulation is also a major challenge, as it can be difficult to ensure that AI systems are properly tested and validated for safety and effectiveness in HC. Innovation also can be negatively impacted by creating uncertainty what is and is not allowed when developing and deploying AI systems in HC.

To address these challenges, a number of solutions were proposed in the reviewed articles. Value-based HC as a shift in focus from the quantity of care provided to the quality of care provided, which can help to ensure that AI is used to improve patient outcomes. Change management as the implementation of AI in HC requires significant changes in the way HC is delivered. Explainable AI, teaching AI fundamentals and applications, data availability, federated learning, and regulation are all key solutions that can help to address the challenges of black-box decision making, data availability, data privacy, perception and acceptance of AI, and lack of regulation. By implementing these solutions, the successful adoption of AI in HC can be achieved.

References

1. Amann, J., Blasimme, A., Vayena, E., et al.: Explainability for artificial intelligence in healthcare: a multidisciplinary perspective. BMC Med. Inform. Decis. Mak. **20**, 310 (2020). https://doi.org/10.1186/s12911-020-01332-6
2. Babel, A., Taneja, R., Mondello Malvestiti, F., Monaco, A., Donde, S.: Artificial intelligence solutions to increase medication adherence in patients with non-communicable diseases. Front. Digit. Health **3** (2021). https://doi.org/10.3389/fdgth.2021.669869
3. Barredo Arrieta, A., et al.: Explainable Artificial Intelligence (XAI): concepts, taxonomies, opportunities and challenges toward responsible AI. Int. J. Inf. Fusion **58**, 82–115 (2020). https://doi.org/10.1016/j.inffus.2019.12.012
4. Bohr, A., Memarzadeh, K. (eds.): Artificial Intelligence in Healthcare. Academic Press (2020)

5. Choudhury, A., Asan, O.: Impact of accountability, training, and human factors on the use of artificial intelligence in healthcare: exploring the perceptions of healthcare practitioners in the US. Hum. Factors Healthc. **2**(100021), 100021 (2022). https://doi.org/10.1016/j.hfh.2022.100021

6. Dwivedi, Y.K., et al.: Artificial Intelligence (AI): Multidisciplinary perspectives on emerging challenges, opportunities, and agenda for research, practice and policy. Int. J. Inf. Manag. **57**(101994), 101994 (2021). https://doi.org/10.1016/j.ijinfomgt.2019.08.002

7. Esmaeilzadeh, P.: Use of AI-based tools for healthcare purposes: a survey study from consumers' perspectives. BMC Med. Inform. Decis. Mak. **20**, 170 (2020). https://doi.org/10.1186/s12911-020-01191-1

8. Explainable Artificial Intelligence (XAI), DARPA Homepage. https://www.darpa.mil/program/explainable-artificial-intelligence. Accessed 20 Jan 2023

9. Farahani, B., Firouzi, F., Luecking, M.: The convergence of IoT and distributed ledger technologies (DLT): opportunities, challenges, and solutions. J. Netw. Comput. Appl. **177** (2021). https://doi.org/10.1016/j.jnca.2020.102936

10. Girasa, R.: Artificial Intelligence as a Disruptive Technology: Economic Transformation and Government Regulation. Springer, Cham (2020). https://doi.org/10.1007/978-3-030-35975-1

11. Giuste, F., et al.: Explainable artificial intelligence methods in combating pandemics: a systematic review. IEEE Rev. Biomed. Eng. 1–17 (2022). https://doi.org/10.1109/RBME.2022.3185953

12. Hlávka, J.P.: Security, privacy, and information-sharing aspects of healthcare artificial intelligence. In: Artificial Intelligence in Healthcare, pp. 235–270 (2020). https://doi.org/10.1016/B978-0-12-818438-7.00010-1. www.scopus.com

13. Ibeneme, S., et al.: Data revolution, health status transformation and the role of artificial intelligence for health and pandemic preparedness in the African context. BMC Proc. **15** (2021). https://doi.org/10.1186/s12919-021-00228-1

14. Kotter, J.P.: Leading Change, with a New Preface by the Author. Harvard Business Review Press (2012)

15. Laï, M.C., Brian, M., Mamzer, M.F.: Perceptions of artificial intelligence in healthcare: findings from a qualitative survey study among actors in France. J. Transl. Med. **18**, 14 (2020). https://doi.org/10.1186/s12967-019-02204-y

16. Li, J.-O., et al.: Digital technology, tele-medicine and artificial intelligence in ophthalmology: a global perspective. Progr. Retin. Eye Res. **82** (2021). https://doi.org/10.1016/j.preteyeres.2020.100900

17. Lytras, D.M., Lytra, H., Lytras, M.D.: Healthcare in the times of artificial intelligence: setting a value-based context. In: Artificial Intelligence and Big Data Analytics for Smart Healthcare, pp. 1–9 (2021). https://doi.org/10.1016/B978-0-12-822060-3.00011-5. www.scopus.com

18. Nguyen, T.V., et al.: A novel decentralized federated learning approach to train on globally distributed, poor quality, and protected private medical data. Sci. Rep. **12**(1), 8888 (2022). https://doi.org/10.1038/s41598-022-12833-x

19. Page, M.J., et al.: The PRISMA 2020 statement: an updated guideline for reporting systematic reviews. BMJ (Clin. Res. Ed.) n71 (2021). https://doi.org/10.1136/bmj.n71

20. Patel, V.A., et al.: Adoption of federated learning for healthcare informatics: emerging applications and future directions. IEEE Access **10**, 90792–90826 (2022). https://doi.org/10.1109/ACCESS.2022.3201876

21. Pereira, T., et al.: Sharing biomedical data: strengthening AI development in healthcare. Healthcare (Switzerland) **9**(7) (2021). https://doi.org/10.3390/healthcare9070827

22. Petersson, L., Larsson, I., Nygren, J.M., et al.: Challenges to implementing artificial intelligence in healthcare: a qualitative interview study with healthcare leaders in Sweden. BMC Health Serv. Res. **22**, 850 (2022). https://doi.org/10.1186/s12913-022-08215-8

23. Phillips, P.J., et al.: Four principles of explainable artificial intelligence. National Institute of Standards and Technology (2021)
24. Rudin, C., Radin, J.: Why are we using black box models in AI when we don't need to? A lesson from an explainable AI competition. Harv. Data Sci. Rev. **1**(2) (2019). https://doi.org/10.1162/99608f92.5a8a3a3d
25. Sibbald, M., Zwaan, L., Yilmaz, Y., Lal, S.: Incorporating artificial intelligence in medical diagnosis: a case for an invisible and (un)disruptive approach. J. Eval. Clin. Pract. (2022). https://doi.org/10.1111/jep.13730
26. Sunarti, S., Fadzlul Rahman, F., Naufal, M., Risky, M., Febriyanto, K., Masnina, R.: Artificial intelligence in healthcare: opportunities and risk for future. Gac. Sanit. **35**(Suppl 1), S67–S70 (2021). https://doi.org/10.1016/j.gaceta.2020.12.019
27. Yang, Z., et al.: Advancing primary care with artificial intelligence and machine learning. Healthc. (Amsterdam, Netherlands) **10**(1), 100594 (2022). https://doi.org/10.1016/j.hjdsi.2021.100594

An Explainable Deep Network Framework with Case-Based Reasoning Strategies for Survival Analysis in Oncology

Isabelle Bichindaritz[(⊠)] and Guanghui Liu

Intelligent BioSystems Lab, Biomedical Informatics, Department of Computer Science, State University of New York at Oswego, New York, USA
ibichind@oswego.edu

Abstract. Survival analysis models the time-to-event information while handling data censorship. Such technique yields extensive applications in carcinoma treatment and prediction. Deep neural networks (DNNs) are appealing for survival analysis because of their non-linear nature. However, DNNs are often described as "black box" models because they are hard or practically impossible to explain. In this study, we propose an explainable deep network framework for survival prediction in cancer. We utilize strategies from nearest neighbor retrieval in case-based reasoning (CBR) to provide useful insights into the inner workings of the deep network. First, we use an autoencoder network to reconstruct the features of a training input. We create a prototype layer, which can store the weight vector following the encoded input and receive the output from the encoder. In this deep survival model network, the total loss function consists of four terms: the negative log partial likelihood function of the Cox model, the autoencoder loss, and two interpretability prototype distance terms. We use an adaptive weights approach to combine the four loss terms. The network that the prototype layer learns during training naturally comes with an explanation for each prediction. We also introduce Shapley Additive Explanation (SHAP) to explain each feature importance for the model predictions. The results of this study demonstrate on two cancer methylation data sets that the developed approach is effective.

Keywords: Survival Analysis · Deep Network · Case-based Reasoning

1 Introduction

Cancer is the most common disease on the planet. One goal of cancer studies consists in gaining the ability to predict the disease severity through survival prediction. Survival prediction affords to split cases between risk groups for personalized cancer management, allowing to avoid either overtreatment or undertreatment. For instance, cases classified into the high-risk group may benefit from closer follow-up and more aggressive therapies [18]. Among genomic data, DNA methylation levels [17] can be very useful to analyze tumors to identify potential survival risk in a personalized manner.

© The Author(s), under exclusive license to Springer Nature Singapore Pte Ltd. 2023
Y.-W. Chen et al. (Eds.): KES InMed 2023, SIST 357, pp. 63–73, 2023.
https://doi.org/10.1007/978-981-99-3311-2_7

Deep Learning techniques, such as Deep Neural Networks (DNNs), can be used in survival analysis to learn the hazard function and create deep models [1]. Although nonlinearity endows the neural network with high model representation capabilities, it requires sophisticated parameter tuning techniques. If the input and output are explicit, the processing that occurs in-between is obscure, so that a black-box effect is obtained. The large number of parameters and the typical non-linearity of the activation functions are the main reasons why model transparency is practically impossible.

However, interpretable approaches are required in medicine because users are ultimately responsible for their clinical decisions and therefore need to make informed decisions [13]. In this study, we create a DNN survival prediction architecture capable of explaining its own reasoning process for each prediction, with explanations that are faithful to what the network is actually computing. We create a prototype layer to store the weight vector following the encoded input, and to receive the output from encoder layers. Our purpose for using encoder layers is to reduce the dimensionality of the original input features. The prototype layer, inspired by case-based reasoning, utilizes the strategy of the nearest neighbor retrieval in case-based reasoning (CBR) to provide a useful insight into the inner workings of the deep network. Finally, for further model explanation and interpretability, SHapley Additive exPlanation (SHAP) [12] method is applied to reflect the relationship between important features and the model prediction.

2   Research Background

DNA methylation has recently become more prevalent in genetic research in oncology. This paper determines DNA methylation signatures for cancer prognostic survival analysis. Cancer cases can be either censored cases or non-censored cases [3]. For censored cases, the death events were not observed during the follow-up period, and thus their genuine survival times are longer than the recorded data, while for non-censored cases their recorded survival times are the exact time from initial diagnosis to death.

Several survival analysis approaches have been proposed. LASSO method [12, 15] applies the lasso feature selection method for selecting the parts associated with cancer prediction. Random Survival Forests (RSF) [7] calculates a random forest with the log-rank test as the splitting standard. Though much progress has been made, the prediction performance of the previously proposed approaches can be improved.

Deep learning models overcome many of the restrictions of Cox-based models like the proportionality assumption. DeepSurv [9] was developed with a cutting-edge deep neural network based on the Cox proportional hazards method [10]. However, DeepSurv lacks interpretability, which this paper proposes to address.

3   Related Work

3.1   Case-Based Reasoning

Case-based reasoning (CBR) is a method of reasoning based on analogy. Its fundamental idea is to reuse similar previous experiences in order to solve new problems. CBR systems have in common the following processes: retrieve, reuse, revise, and retain. The most used case retrieval strategy is the k-nearest neighbor strategy (kNN). CBR decisions are made by similarity between a new case and solved retrieved cases, which can serve as explanations for a system recommendations. With high dimensional genetic data however, there are thousands of features for a small subset of samples (specifically tens of thousands for the standard chipset used in DNA methylation), and these samples are often imbalanced between cases and controls. Little work has been done so far in genetic survival analysis with case-based reasoning, We can cite Karmen et al., who calculate similarity based on survival functions [8]. Bartlett et al. (2021) consider clinical covariates when retrieving genetic cases for case-based survival prediction [2].

3.2 Features Importance Explanation

Explainable artificial intelligence (XAI) methods have become a growing field, by which machine learning (ML) black boxes are transformed into grey boxes. It gives insight into the reasons behind the outcomes of the ML models. In this study, the used XAI method is SHAP, which can explain features importance for a given model prediction. Essentially, the SHAP method reverse-engineers the output of a predictive machine learning algorithm. The SHAP algorithm observes specific features, then traverses the entire subset, calculates any changes in the output by removing the observed features, and determines the feature contributions in binary form. As for the final heat map that highlights each feature contribution, the simplified input is converted with a binarization function into the original input space. Several recent studies introduced SHAP values for cancer classification, such as [14] in Lung Cancer prediction.

3.3 Synergies Between Deep Learning and CBR

A number of approaches have been proposed to combine case-based reasoning and deep learning. Several systems use deep learning for sub-tasks within a CBR architecture. Eisenstadt et al. classify design cases from labels to select most relevant cases during retrieval [5]. Li et al. construct a prototype layer by adding an autoencoder to deep convolutional networks [11]. Their application processed image data, for which convolutional neural networks are particularly adapted. By contrast, our approach fits clinical and multi-omics data, using Long Short-Term Memory (LSTM) [6], and performs survival prediction tasks. Our approach can also tackle classical classification and regression tasks since LSTM can be adjusted for that purpose as well, even though they excel particularly on sequence data, such as time series and other forms of sequence.

4 Methods

In survival analysis, the goal is to predict the time duration until a certain event occurs, such as death in this study. We propose an interpretable deep network framework for cancer survival prediction using case-based reasoning. Our model architecture features two stages: an autoencoder (an encoder and a decoder) and the custom deep survival model. We use the linear activation function in all autoencoder layers, and a bidirectional Long Short-Term Memory (biLSTM) [6] as the last output layer (see Fig. 1). The autoencoder is used to reduce the dimensionality of the input; then the encoded input is used to produce a deep Cox model through the prototype layer, which receives the output from the encoder. Because the prototype layer output vectors live in the same space as the encoded inputs, we can feed these vectors into the decoder and trace the learned custom network throughout the training process. Inspired by case-based reasoning, we minimize the distance between the output and input of the prototype layer during the model iteration training. The output of the prototype layer can then be used to interpret the input data features and show how the network reaches its predictions.

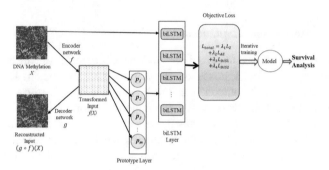

Fig. 1. Deep survival model architecture.

In this deep survival model, the total loss function consists of four terms: the negative log partial likelihood function of the Cox model, the autoencoder loss, and two required distances. These distances ensure that every feature vector in the original input looks like at least one of the prototype layer feature vectors and that every prototype layer feature vector looks like at least one of the feature vectors in the original input. We use an adaptive weights approach to combine the four loss terms. The network that the prototype layer learns naturally provides an explanation for each prediction. The negative log partial likelihood function of the Cox hazard model is defined as follows [16]:

$$L_Z(\theta) = - \sum_{i=1}^{n} \delta_i \left(\theta^T x_i - \log \sum_{j \in R(t_i)} \exp(\theta^T x_j) \right) \tag{1}$$

where $x = (x_1, x_2, \cdots, x_n)$ corresponds to the covariate variable of dimensionality n, δ_i is a binary value indicating whether the event happened or not, and $R(t_i)$ denotes the set of all individuals at risk at time t_i, which represents the set of cases that are still at risk before time t_i. $\theta^T x_i$ is called the risk (or survival) function, in which θ can be estimated by minimizing its corresponding negative log partial likelihood function; n denotes the number of patients.

The autoencoder loss L_{AE} uses the squared L2 distance between the original and reconstructed input for penalizing the autoencoder's reconstruction error:

$$L_{AE} = \frac{1}{n} \sum_{i=1}^{n} \|(g \circ f)(x_i) - x_i\|_2^2 \tag{2}$$

where $(g \circ f)(x_i)$ is the decoder network reconstructed input.

The two required distances loss, which are two interpretability regularization terms, are formulated as follows:

$$L_{DIS1} = \frac{1}{m} \sum_{j=1}^{m} \min_{i \in [1,n]} \left\| p_j - f(x_i) \right\|_2^2 \tag{3}$$

$$L_{DIS2} = \frac{1}{n} \sum_{i=1}^{n} \min_{j \in [1,m]} \left\| f(x_i) - p_j \right\|_2^2 \tag{4}$$

where $f(x_i)$ is the encoded input vector, and p_i is the vector learned from the prototype layer. The prototype layer p computes the squared L_2 distance between the encoded input $f(x_i)$ and each of the prototype layer vectors. Minimization of L_{DIS1} will make each prototype vector as close as possible to at least one training case. The minimization of L_{DIS2} will make each encoded training example as close as possible to some prototype vector. This implements the nearest neighbor strategy method from case-based reasoning in the deep network. We use the two terms L_{DIS1} and L_{DIS2} in our cost function for interpretability. Intuitively, L_{DIS1} approximates each prototype to a potential training example, making the decoded prototype realistic, while L_{DIS2} forces each training example to find a close prototype in the latent space, thus encouraging the prototypes to spread out over the entire latent space and to be distinct from each other.

The objective loss function combines the above 4 loss terms and reads as:

$$L_{total} = \lambda_1 L_Z + \lambda_2 L_{AE} + \lambda_3 L_{DIS1} + \lambda_4 L_{DIS2} \tag{5}$$

where $\lambda_i (i = 1, 2, 3, 4)$ is the regularization weight for the regularization terms. We use these weights as trainable parameters in the deep network for adaptive optimization [3].

This network architecture, unlike traditional case-based learning methods, automatically learns useful features. For methylation data, instance-based methods such as *kNN* tend to perform poorly from raw input space or hand-crafted feature space. Instead, we feed the sequence vectors into the decoder and learn variables during the process, which can explain how the network reaches its predictions.

To understand the importance of specific features for the model predictions, we decided to use SHAP values, since they present several characteristics advantageous to our study. Firstly and most importantly, SHAP values are model agnostic, which was crucial to our comparison of different models. Moreover, SHAP values present properties of local accuracy, missingness, and consistency, which are not found simultaneously in other methods. We chose a random test data partition to compute the SHAP values and to obtain a visualization of the overall feature importance for the models. Then, we generated SHAP dependency plots for each model and compared how the features contributed to the corresponding model output. Lastly, we analyzed the most important interaction effects across features and their insights.

5 Results and Discussions

5.1 Benchmark Datasets

In this section, we assess the performance of the proposed method on two DNA methylation datasets through ten-fold cross validation. We selected Glioma cohort (GBMLGG) cancer and Pan-kidney cohort (KIPAN) cancer, two datasets from Firehose [4]. The

GBMLGG dataset includes 20116 gene-level features for DNA methylation data. The KIPAN datasets contain 20533 DNA methylation features. We also use two clinical variables: survival status ('Deceased' or 'Living') and survival time, representing the number of days between diagnosis and date of death or last follow-up. This study removes cases with survival days that were not recorded or negative. For these reasons, this study extracts 650 samples for GBMLGG and 654 samples for KIPAN having both DNA methylation data and clinical data after merging and filtering. To address the high-dimensionality, we use a multivariate Cox regression preprocess to extract biomarkers. We calculate the log rank of each gene feature and select the genes whose p-value is less than 0.01. By using this methods, we extract 586 methylation features from GBMLGG data and 749 methylation features from KIPAN data. Table 1 shows the genetic and clinical characteristics for the selected cases.

Table 1. Gene and clinical characteristics in two cancers.

Characteristics	GBMLGG	KIPAN
Patient number	650	654
Gene number		
DNA Methylation	20116	20533
Survival status		
Living	434	500
Deceased	216	154
Follow up (days)	1–481	3–5925

We use the Concordance index (C-index) [14] to assess the performance of the survival models. C-index is the probability that the predicted survival time of a random pair of individuals is in the same order as their actual survival time.

5.2 Convergence Analysis and Interpretability

To investigate the convergence of the proposed method, we calculated the corresponding loss curves of Eq. 5 and determined that the four loss terms (L_Z, L_{AE}, L_{DIS1}, and L_{DIS2}) and the total loss value (L_{total}) converge to some stable values after a few iterations. Therefore, our proposed optimization algorithm is reliable and convergent.

Let us investigate the autoencoder loss and the two interpretability prototype distance terms for a test case. We randomly select one test case No. 62 from the GBMLGG dataset and one test case No. 319 from the KIPAN dataset respectively for the experiments. Figure 2 shows the curves of three distance terms (L_{AE}, L_{DIS1}, and L_{DIS2}) during the prediction iterations for one test case of each of the two datasets. In Fig. 3 (a), the values (L_{AE}, L_{DIS1}, and L_{DIS2}) are changed to (0.01671, 2.82664, and 0.02032) when 1000 epochs are completed. As also can be seen from Fig. 2 (b), the three values will converge to 0.005529, 2.0152, and 0.07098.

From Fig. 2, we can see that the curve of L_{AE} (purple) and the curve of L_{DIS2} (pink) both converge to almost the same value after 1000 epochs. The results of the two different datasets are consistent. The autoencoder loss L_{AE} is the distance between the original and reconstructed input. We use the autoencoder to create a latent low-dimensional space. The smaller the distance between the decoder and the original input, the more the encoder output can represent the original input. The interpretability prototype distance L_{DIS2} means the minimum distance between the encoder output and prototype output. Since the output of the prototype layer is generated during the iterative optimization of the model, it represents the characteristics of the training set. Minimizing the distance between the encoder output and prototype output corresponds to finding the nearest neighbor to a test case in the training set. If the minimum prototype distance is found, it means that one prototype case can represent the encoder output of this test case. When the two distances (L_{AE} and L_{DIS2}) tend to be the same, the prototype features will explain the original input data. For each training sample, the linear expression of each feature is calculated and used to construct one prototypical case. Each prototype case would then represent typical DNA methylation patterns present in different samples. The Euclidean distance between each encoder from the case base and its respective prototype is used to determine how similar the prototype is to its sample.

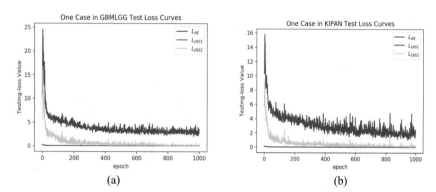

Fig. 2. Three distance curves on two test cases. (a) the curves of distance terms on one test case in GBMLGG dataset; (b) the curves of distance terms on one test case in KIPAN dataset.

Obviously, by searching for the minimum distance L_{DIS2}, for GBMLGG, we can find the most similar case No. 356 in the training set to the test case No. 62. This means that we can use the characteristics of the known cases in the case base to explain the unsolved cases. Similarly, for KIPAN, we can find the most similar case No. 266 in the training set to match the test case No. 319.

Figure 2 also shows that the values of L_{DIS1} and L_{DIS2}, are different, even though their equations (Eq. 3 and Eq. 4) look similar. Actually, L_{DIS1} helps make the prototypes meaningful, and L_{DIS2} keeps the explanations faithful by forcing the network to use nearby prototypes.

We compared our explainable model with its non-explainable counterpart, by removing the autoencoder layers and the prototype layer. We replaced the prototype output

Table 2. C-index performance comparison between two models (with standard deviations)

Models	GBMLGG	KIPAN
Prototype	0.7132 (0.0166)	0.7246 (0.0149)
Without prototype	0.7157 (0.0234)	0.7313 (0.0188)

vectors with original input vectors (without prototype) as the input for the last output layer directly. Table 2 shows the C-index performance comparison between these two models on GBMLGG and KIPAN datasets. Table 2 shows that the C-index of the prototype model is only 0.25% and 0.67% lower on GBMLGG and KIPAN datasets respectively. Hence, we do not sacrifice much C-index when including the interpretability elements into the network.

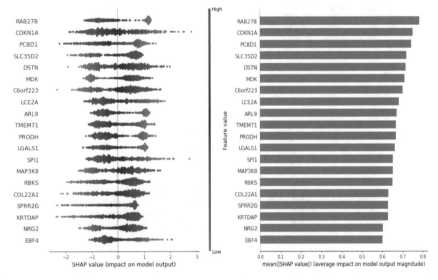

Fig. 3. Summary plots for SHAP values on GBMLGG dataset.

5.3 Gene Importance Analysis

For model interpretation and to identify the most important genes, we apply SHAP values method to perform the experiments. First, we use the SHAP values method to obtain the importance ranking of features and draw importance ranking plots. Figure 3 shows as an example the summary plots of the model SHAP values on GBMLGG. The left subplot illustrates the twenty most important features for the survival model on this dataset and the SHAP value importance is represented by a color from high to low. Each point on the summary plot is a SHAP value for a feature and an instance. For each feature, a point corresponds to a single case. The location of the point along the x-axis (that is, the actual SHAP value) represents the effect of that feature on the model output for that particular case. Mathematically, this corresponds to the relative risk of death between patients (i.e., patients with higher SHAP values have a higher risk of death relative to patients with lower SHAP values). Features are arranged along the y-axis according to their importance, which is given by the average of their absolute SHAP values. In the plot, the higher the position of the feature, the more important it is to the model. The right subplot presents the SHAP values ranking of the most important twenty genes related to the model.

Next, we compare in Table 3 the performance of our model on the 20 most important features identified by SHAP and compare it with the model performance on all features. We see that performance on the 20 selected features is slightly lower than on all features. However, the identified signatures reveal that these methylation profiles can be associated with distinct cancer types and could serve as biomarkers.

Table 3. C-index performance comparison with top 20 features (with standard deviations)

Features	GBMLGG	KIPAN
20	0.7065 (0.0173)	0.7182 (0.0177)
All	0.7132 (0.0166)	0.7246 (0.0149)

5.4 Comparison with Different Survival Prediction Methods

To explore the effectiveness of the proposed method, we compare it with three existing machine learning survival prediction approaches: LASSO, RSF, and DeepSurv. For the sake of fairness, this part of the study runs the same input feature set in all cross-validation tests. Table 4 shows that, compared with LASSO, RSF, and DeepSurv, the C-index of the proposed method improves the survival analysis in all cases.

Table 4. C-index performance comparison with state-of-the-art algorithms

Methods	GBMLGG	KIPAN
LASSO	0.6035 (0.0141)	0.6146 (0.0246)
RSF	0.5836 (0.0238)	0.6133 (0.0233)
DeepSurv	0.6547 (0.0216)	0.6858 (0.0173)
Proposed Method	**0.7132 (0.0166)**	**0.7246 (0.0149)**

6 Conclusions

In this study, we developed an explainable deep network framework for survival analysis of cancer patients. This deep survival prediction architecture can explain its own reasoning process and provide explanations for each prediction. The C-index performance of the model improves on three state-of-the-art methods (i.e., LASSO, RSF, and DeepSurv) while explainability is added. For further model interpretation, we apply the SHAP method to identify the biomarkers associated with the cancer survival model.

References

1. Amiri, Z., Mohammad, K., Mahmoudi, M., Zeraati, H., Fotouhi, A.: Assessment of gastric cancer survival: using an artificial hierarchical neural network. Pak. J. Biol. Sci. **11**, 1076–1084 (2008)
2. Bichindaritz, I., Bartlett, C., Liu, G.: Predicting with confidence: a case-based reasoning framework for predicting survival in breast cancer. In: The International FLAIRS Conference Proceedings, vol. 34, 18 April 2021 (2021)
3. Bichindaritz, I., Liu, G., Bartlett, C.: Survival prediction of breast cancer patient from gene methylation data with deep LSTM network and ordinal cox model. In: The Thirty-Third International Flairs Conference (2020)
4. Bichindaritz, I., Liu, G., Bartlett, C.: Integrative survival analysis of breast cancer with gene expression and DNA methylation data. Bioinformatics **37**, 2601–2608 (2021)
5. Farzindar, A.A., Kashi, A.: Multi-task survival analysis of liver transplantation using deep learning. In: The Thirty-Second International Flairs Conference (2019)
6. Eisenstadt, V., Langenhan, C., Althoff, K.-D., Dengel, A.: Improved and visually enhanced case-based retrieval of room configurations for assistance in architectural design education. In: Watson, I., Weber, R. (eds.) ICCBR 2020. LNCS (LNAI), vol. 12311, pp. 213–228. Springer, Cham (2020). https://doi.org/10.1007/978-3-030-58342-2_14
7. Hochreiter, S., Schmidhuber, J.: Long short-term memory. Neural Comput. **9**, 1735–1780 (1997)
8. Ishwaran, H., Kogalur, U.B., Blackstone, E.H., Lauer, M.S.: Random survival forests. Ann. Appl. Stat. **2**, 841–860 (2008)
9. Karmen, C., Gietzelt, M., Knaup-Gregori, P., Ganzinger, M.: Methods for a similarity measure for clinical attributes based on survival data analysis. BMC Med. Inform. Decis. Mak. **19**, 1–14 (2019)
10. Katzman, J.L., Shaham, U., Cloninger, A., Bates, J., Jiang, T., Kluger, Y.: Deep survival: a deep cox proportional hazards network. stat 1050, 2 (2016)
11. Katzman, J.L., Shaham, U., Cloninger, A., Bates, J., Jiang, T., Kluger, Y.: DeepSurv: personalized treatment recommender system using a Cox proportional hazards deep neural network. BMC Med. Res. Methodol. **18**, 24 (2018)
12. Li, O., Liu, H., Chen, C., Rudin, C.: Deep learning for case-based reasoning through prototypes: a neural network that explains its predictions. In: Thirty-Second AAAI Conference on Artificial Intelligence (2018)
13. Lin, D.Y., Wei, L.-J., Ying, Z.: Checking the Cox model with cumulative sums of martingale-based residuals. Biometrika **80**, 557–572 (1993)
14. Lundberg, S.M., Lee, S.-I.: A unified approach to interpreting model predictions. Adv. Neural Inf. Process. Syst. **30** (2017)
15. Mayr, A., Schmid, M.: Boosting the concordance index for survival data. Ulmer Informatik-Berichte **26** (2014)

16. Ramos, B., Pereira, T., Moranguinho, J., Morgado, J., Costa, J.L., Oliveira, H.P.: An interpretable approach for lung cancer prediction and subtype classification using gene expression. In: 2021 43rd Annual International Conference of the IEEE Engineering in Medicine & Biology Society (EMBC), pp. 1707–1710. IEEE (2021)
17. Shao, W., Cheng, J., Sun, L., Han, Z., Feng, Q., Zhang, D., Huang, K.: Ordinal multi-modal feature selection for survival analysis of early-stage renal cancer. In: Frangi, A.F., Schnabel, J.A., Davatzikos, C., Alberola-López, C., Fichtinger, G. (eds.) MICCAI 2018. LNCS, vol. 11071, pp. 648–656. Springer, Cham (2018). https://doi.org/10.1007/978-3-030-00934-2_72
18. Sy, J.P., Taylor, J.M.G.: Estimation in a Cox proportional hazards cure model. Biometrics **56**(1), 227–236 (2020)
19. Suzuki, H., Maruyama, R., Yamamoto, E., Kai, M.: DNA methylation and microRNA dysregulation in cancer. Mol. Oncol. **6**, 567–578 (2012)
20. Yu, K.-H., et al.: Predicting non-small cell lung cancer prognosis by fully automated microscopic pathology image features. Nat. Commun. **7**, 12474 (2016)

Projects, Systems, and Applications of Smart Medicine/Healthcare

Healthcare Under Society 5.0: A Systematic Literature Review of Applications and Case Studies

Jean Paul Sebastian Piest[1]([✉]) [iD], Yoshimasa Masuda[2,3] [iD], and Osamu Nakamura[2]

[1] University of Twente, Drienerlolaan 5, 7522 NB Enschede, The Netherlands
j.p.s.piest@utwente.nl
[2] Keio University, 2 Chome-15-45 Mita, Minato City, Tokyo 108-8345, Japan
[3] Carnegie Mellon University, 5000 Forbes Ave, Pittsburgh, PA 15213, USA

Abstract. Current challenges in healthcare urge the need for more productive and efficient healthcare. Healthcare technologies are expected to address these challenges as part of the Society 5.0 (S5.0) vision. Earlier research revealed a variety of digital architectures under S5.0. However, most research is based on single case studies and no cross-case analysis has been conducted in healthcare. Therefore, this paper aims to identify and analyze health-related applications that are developed and evaluated in case studies under S5.0. More specific, this paper focuses on alignment between the research and development work of the Open Healthcare Platform 2023 (OHP2023) consortium and the S5.0 reference architecture using the Adaptive Integrated Digital Architecture Framework (AIDAF). The PRISMA2020 guidelines were used to conduct a Systematic Literature Review (SLR) regarding healthcare applications and evaluations in case studies under S5.0. The initial search included 94 documents of which 23 documents were selected for this SLR. The SLR extracted 18 applications and six case studies. Based on the SLR, the use of the AIDAF by the OHP2030 consortium is visualized and described for the development of applications under S5.0 and alignment with the S5.0 reference architecture. The main limitation of the SLR is the limited depth of the cross-case analysis. In spite of this limitation, this study contributes to creating a common ground for the OHP2030 consortium, interested healthcare scholars, and professionals, to develop applications under S5.0 and align with the S5.0 reference architecture. Future research may contribute to developing a case study protocol for in-depth and cross-case analysis.

Keywords: AIDAF · Healthcare · OHP2030 · Society 5.0 · Reference Architecture · PRISMA2020 · Systematic Literature Review

1 Introduction

The healthcare sector (in Japan) faces many challenges, including an aging population, increased life expectation, labor shortages, and a continuous pressure on social health costs [1, 2]. Thus, one of the main challenges is to deliver healthcare to more people with less workforce and minimal resources. Healthcare technology is expected to contribute

© The Author(s), under exclusive license to Springer Nature Singapore Pte Ltd. 2023
Y.-W. Chen et al. (Eds.): KES InMed 2023, SIST 357, pp. 77–87, 2023.
https://doi.org/10.1007/978-981-99-3311-2_8

to addressing these challenges and solving related problems. The envisioned use of healthcare technologies has been positioned, amongst other initiatives, in the Society 5.0 (hereafter S5.0) vision of a "human-centered supersmart society" [3] and specific propositions for citizens and professionals in healthcare [4]. Although some solutions are already available for use, realizing the S5.0 vision is a long-term effort. Given the urgency of the current problems in healthcare, it is important to develop solutions for both the short- and mid-long term to overcome the identified main challenges and ensure the availability and quality of healthcare.

Earlier work regarding digital architectures under S5.0 illustrated a variety of digital architectures in different domains and, more specifically, shows how the Adaptive Integrated Digital Architecture Framework (AIDAF), amongst alternative approaches, is used in healthcare [5, 6]. Currently, the AIDAF is applied to establish the architecture vision and strategy for the Open Healthcare Platform 2030 (hereafter OHP2030) [7]. The OHP2030 consortium develops healthcare solutions under the umbrella of Industry 4.0 and evaluates the effectiveness and societal implications via case study research under S5.0 [8]. This research paper seeks alignment with current research and development of the OHP2030 consortium.

As emphasized in earlier and related research [5, 9], the S5.0 Reference Architecture (hereafter S5.0RA) is not yet publicly available. More specifically, principles for designing, constructing, and evaluating digital architectures under S5.0 are lacking. Moreover, related work mainly contains single case studies [1, 2, 5–8] and a systematic cross-case analysis in healthcare is lacking. In order to support short-term development of solutions, earlier work introduced the idea of developing domain-driven approaches using established enterprise architecture frameworks (e.g., AIDAF in healthcare) [5]. Isolated development might however result in substantial changes. To mitigate this risk, the OHP2030 consortium can bundle user needs and engage with the government regarding the development and implementation of the S5.0RA.

This paper aims to identify and analyze health-related applications and case studies under S5.0. More specific, this paper seeks alignment between research and development work of the OHP20230 consortium and the S5.0RA using the AIDAF. Accordingly, the following guiding Research Questions (RQs) have been defined:

- **RQ1:** Which applications have been developed and evaluated in case studies in healthcare under S5.0?
- **RQ2:** How can the AIDAF framework incorporate the S5.0 vision and S5.0RA in the OHP2030 vision and IT strategy to develop solutions for healthcare?

In order to answer RQ1, a Systematic Literature Review (hereafter SLR) was conducted using the PRISMA2020 guidelines and 27-item checklist [10] to identify and analyze applications and case studies in healthcare under S5.0. Next, to answer RQ2, the proposed use of the AIDAF has been described to align research and development in the OHP2030 consortium with the S5.0 vision and the S5.0RA.

This paper is structured as follows. Section 2 summarizes relevant related and earlier work. Section 3 explains the research design and methodology. Section 4 discusses the main results of the SLR and proposed use of the AIDAF for the OHP2030 consortium. Section 5 concludes this paper and positions future research.

2   Related Work

This section summarizes related and earlier work. Section 2.1 reviews healthcare use cases under S5.0 and summarizes earlier work regarding digital architectures. Section 2.2 highlights the current use of the AIDAF in healthcare.

2.1   Healthcare Use Cases Under S5.0

In the fifth science and technology basic plan of Japan, the Society 5.0 vision was introduced along with use cases in different sectors or application domains [1–4]. For healthcare and caregiving, four use cases were positioned under S5.0 [4]. In a conceptual overview, current problems in healthcare and caregiving are addressed and solutions were positioned based on healthcare technologies, including data sharing, big data analytics, artificial intelligence, mobile apps, wearables, and robots. More recent work provided an extensive overview of several healthcare technologies, trends, and issues [2]. The values and envisioned benefits for individuals are briefly emphasized in use cases, including comfortable living, health promotion, optimal treatment, and reduction of burden. Taken together, these use cases are expected to contribute to reduce social costs and address labor-shortage problems in healthcare facilities and on caregiving sites. The habitat innovation framework provides an evaluation framework for S5.0, including metrics and Key Performance Indicators (KPIs). Additionally, S5.0 may contribute to realizing the Sustainable Development Goals (SDGs) [1].

Earlier work revealed a variety of 37 digital architectures that are (being) developed under S5.0, including eight digital architectures in healthcare [5]. Examples include large development initiatives, such as the SMARTAGE platform [11], digital health platforms [6] and ecosystems such as OHP2030 [7], and specific applications, such as an AI-Based Heart Monitoring System [12] or Intelligent Health Service [13]. Furthermore, special attention has been given to cybersecurity and privacy preserving techniques, for example by means of secure data sharing in a delay-tolerant public blockchain network with integrated healthcare systems [14] and, more specifically, cipher policy-attribute-based encryption for smart healthcare systems [15]. In addition, this earlier work revealed that design thinking is utilized in two case studies for human-centered design, innovation, and co-creation with stakeholders [5, 9, 12].

Next, the use of the AIDAF in healthcare will be discussed.

2.2   AIDAF in Healthcare

AIDAF is a strategic enterprise architecture framework that focuses on digital agility and -transformation utilizing digital IT, cloud, and mobile technologies in global companies. The AIDAF has been implemented, amongst other sectors (e.g. energy, government), in healthcare within global enterprises. Here, the use of the AIDAF is evaluated in several single case studies in different countries under S5.0 [6–9].

Currently, the AIDAF is used by the OHP2030 consortium to develop a cross-functional community for digital healthcare [6, 7]. The OHP2030 vision encompasses a variety of use cases and applications, including digital platforms for vaccination management [9], regulated digital pharmacy [16], drug development [17], and several use cases involving the Internet of (Medical) Robotics Things (e.g., robotic nursing, surgery, diagnosis, rehabilitation), and related digital innovation platforms [18, 19].

Now that related and earlier work has been summarized, the methodology of the current study will be explained in the next section.

3   Methodology

This section clarifies the research design and methodology. Section 3.1 highlights the SLR methodology. Section 3.2 documents the use of the PRISA2020 guidelines.

3.1   Overview

The literature review process is guided using the PRISMA2020 guidelines [10] and the software of Covidence (https://www.covidence.org/). First, the topic and scope have been identified. Next, the search was conducted and literature was screened. Lastly, the full-text review took place based on in- and exclusion criteria. Figure 1 provides an overview of the use of the PRISMA2020 guidelines for this study. Next, the application of the PRISMA2020 guidelines will be explained in more detail.

3.2   Application of the PRISMA2020 Guidelines

Following the PRISMA 2020 guidelines and its 27-item checklist, this study was identified as a SLR. The rationale of the SLR was described in the introduction, including the objective and research questions. Next, in- and exclusion criteria were specified and the data extraction protocol was defined. For screening, the title-abstract-keywords should contain the main topics S5.0 and/or health(care) and indicate the presence of an application and/or case study. For inclusion, the full text should provide an original contribution. Next, the SLR was pre-registered [20].

After pre-registration, the search, analysis, and data extraction started. The date of extraction and queries have been specified, as shown in Fig. 1. No restrictions were set. Next, the initial search results were exported (in .ris format) and imported in Covidence for subsequent screening, full-text review, and data extraction. Then, the results of the analysis and synthesis of the selected papers were described and tabulated in Sect. 4.1 in the form of a cross-case analysis of healthcare applications, use cases, and case studies under S5.0. Both the certainty of provided evidence and risks of biases in individual studies and synthesis have been assessed and briefly discussed.

The SLR was conducted independently by the first author without the use of automation tools. The second author assessed the results and the third author assessed the methodology. Both the second and third author conducted an overall review of the research. Additionally, this paper was subject to peer-review by multiple anonymous reviewers. This research was conducted independently and received no funding or financial support. The authors declare no conflict of interest.

Based on the methodology, the next section presents the main results.

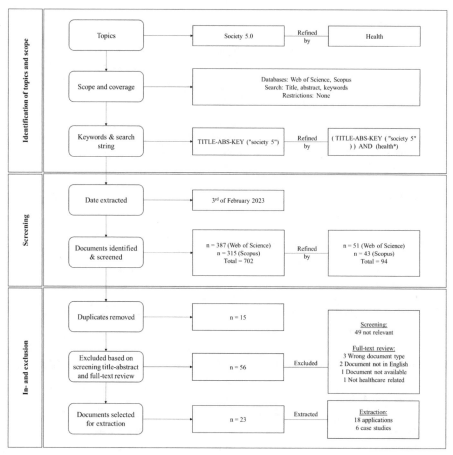

Fig. 1. Overview of the SLR regarding healthcare applications and case studies under S5.0 (adapted from: [10]).

4   Results

This section contains the main results. Section 4.1 presents the identified applications and case studies to answer RQ1. Section 4.2 visualizes and describes the proposed use of the AIDAF for the OHP2030 consortium to answer RQ2.

4.1   Applications and Case Studies in Healthcare

Following the methodology from the previous section, the SLR identified 18 applications and six case studies, as listed in Table 1. The identified 18 applications have been linked to use cases for Comfortable Living (CL), Health Promotion (HP), Optimal Treatment (OT), and Reduction of Burden (RoB), as introduced in Sect. 2.1.

The presented applications show how S5.0 use cases can (partly) be realized and also illustrates how use cases can be connected and combined. The AIDAF has been used in

Table 1. Identified Applications and Case Studies in Healthcare under S5.0.

ID	Name (Source)	Use Case	Status (Year Reported)	Case Study (Country)	Evidence Certainty
1	In-home elderly monitoring system and robots [1]	CL; RoB;	Requirements (2020)	No	N/A
2	Internet of (Medical) Robotics Things and digital platform [18, 19]	CL; OT; RoB;	Conceptualized (2020) and architected (2021)	Planned cases (USA, Japan)	N/A
3	IoT sensor for magnetocardiography applications [25]	HL; OT; RoB;	Developed and tested (2020)	No	N/A
4	i-health care monitoring system [13]	CL; OT; RoB;	Conceptualized (2021)	No	N/A
5	AI-based hearth monitoring system [12]	CL; RoB;	Developed and tested (2021)	No	N/A
6	Physical activity monitoring platform [8]	HL	Developed and validated (2021)	Single case (USA)	Neutral
7	SMARTAGE platform [11]	CL; HL; OT; RoB;	Developed and evaluated (2021)	Single case (Italy)	High
8	Smart pillow [22]	CL; HL; OT; RoB;	Designed and tested (2021)	No	N/A
9	Digital platform for regulated digital pharmacy [16]	OT; RoB;	Developed and evaluated (2021)	Single case (Japan)	Neutral
10	Digital drug development platform [17]	OT; RoB;	Developed and evaluated (2021)	Single case (Japan)	Neutral
11	Blockchain based medical records [2]	OT; RoB;	Designed (2022)	No	N/A
12	Blockchain for COVID-19 patient tracking [2]	HL; RoB;	Designed (2022)	No	N/A
13	Delay-tolerant public blockchain network [14]	OT; RoB;	Developed and tested (2022)	No	N/A

(*continued*)

Table 1. (*continued*)

ID	Name (Source)	Use Case	Status (Year Reported)	Case Study (Country)	Evidence Certainty
14	HCI-AI Digital Healthcare Platform [23]	CL; RoB;	Architected (2022)	Planned case (USA)	N/A
15	Mobile clinic decision support system [26]	CL; HL; OT; RoB;	Developed and tested (2022)	Single case (Italy)	High
16	Multi-sensor device for stress estimation [21]	HL	Developed and tested (2022)	No	N/A
17	Online escape room for digital mindset [24]	CL; OT;	Designed (2022)	No	N/A
18	Vaccination management system [9]	OT; RoB;	Evaluated and redesigned (2022)	Single case (Japan)	Neutral

multiple digital platforms and case studies, mostly related to the OHP2030 consortium [8, 9, 16–19, 23]. The SMARTAGE project and related platform provided a detailed description of a case study and a convincing evaluation with multiple stakeholders [11]. The mobile clinic decision support system also provided a detailed description and detailed evidence based on a pilot study evaluation [26].

The number of related case studies (6) is limited and were all based on single case studies. Whereas some case studies provided in-depth descriptions and convincing empirical evidence, others provided a general description, lacked a structured evaluation, and/or did not present (convincing) empirical evidence. Due to the lack of a case study protocol and practical constraints, an in-depth cross-case analysis has not been conducted yet. This is considered as an area for future research and development.

4.2 Applying AIDAF for the OHP2030 Consortium Under S5.0

This section presents the proposed use of the AIDAF for the OHP2030 consortium to establish a healthcare platform ecosystem under S5.0, as shown in Fig. 2.

The top layer aims to bring together the OHP2030 consortium, a cross-functional healthcare community with different stakeholders, and the S5.0RA that is being developed by the government. The OHP2030 consortium conducts research regarding healthcare use cases and develops prototypes and applications in close collaboration with involved stakeholders and the government. Initially, the OHP2030 consortium defined the IT strategy and architecture, supporting guidelines for cloud, services, and security, and provides the infrastructure for the OHP2030 platform. Following the AIDAF, each stakeholder may differentiate and/or complement the adaptive EA cycle with EA processes, deliverables, and principles. Using the AIDAF, the OHP2030 consortium can engage with the government regarding the development and implementation of the S5.0RA. More specifically, the OHP2030 consortium can contribute to evaluating the

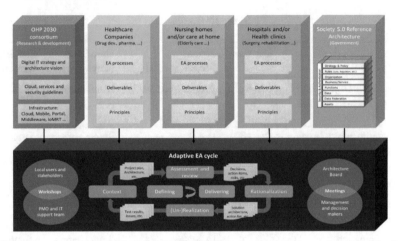

Fig. 2. Proposed use of the AIDAF for the OHP2030 consortium and cross-functional healthcare community under S5.0 (image adapted based on: [6]).

S5.0RA with real-life use cases and applications of involved stakeholders. This way, stakeholders can prepare to adopt the S5.0RA and minimize the risk of substantial architecture and/or system changes to comply with the S5.0RA.

The layer with the adaptive EA cycle facilitates a continuous process of project initiation, review and assessment of project proposals by the architecture board. The architecture board then involves top management for decision making. Following, the delivery starts using agile development practices (or similar). The process of defining projects is facilitated in the form of workshops with local users, stakeholders, the Project Management Office (PMO), and IT support based on the AIDAF design thinking approach and STrategic Risk Mitigation Model (STRMM). Here, the intelligence amplification design canvas and design workshop from earlier work can be integrated [27, 28]. Workshops can be clustered (e.g., by use case) and form the basis for project proposals/plans, architecture specifications, and related deliverables. The PMO is responsible for proposing new projects. The architecture board reviews project proposals using the AIDAF assessment model. The decision making is facilitated in the form of meetings with the architecture board, top management, and involved decision makers based on the Social Collaboration Model (SCM). Following decision making, the introduction of new information systems and (de)commissioning of existing systems is guided by a solution architecture and action list for the PMO and IT support. The Global Digital Transformation Communication (GDTC) model is utilized throughout the adaptive EA cycle to share documents, deliverables, action lists, test results, and issues with involved stakeholders in support of the SCM.

Now that the results have been presented, the study will be concluded.

5 Conclusion

This research identified and analyzed 18 applications and six related case studies in healthcare under S5.0 based on a SLR using the PRISMA2020 guidelines. These applications illustrate how S5.0 use cases (e.g., CL, HL, OT, RoB) can be realized and combined to address current challenges in healthcare. Additionally, the proposed use of the AIDAF for the OHP2030 consortium is visualized and described to develop S5.0 applications on the short-term and align with the S5.0RA on the mid-long term. The main limitation of the SLR is the scope and two selected databases. The analysis has a limited depth due to practical constraints and the lack of a case study protocol for in-depth and cross-case analysis. Despite these limitations, this research paper contributes to creating a common ground for the development of applications in healthcare under S5.0 and alignment with the S5.0RA. The OHP2030 consortium can leverage the results of this study to refine its IT strategy, architecture vision, and roadmap under the S5.0 vision and prepare the implementation of the S5.0RA. Similarly, healthcare professionals and policy makers can utilize this study for the ideation of use cases, the development of applications under S5.0, and alignment with the S5.0RA. Current work focuses on incorporating the intelligence design canvas and workshop as part of the AIDAF for design thinking approach, both for prototyping and enterprise software development, and related models (e.g., STRMM, SCM and GDTC) under S5.0. Future research may contribute to the development of a case study protocol for the in-depth and cross-case analysis of different case studies.

References

1. Deguchi, A., et al.: Society 5.0 A People-Centric Super-Smart Society. Hitachi-UTokyo Laboratory (H-UTokyo Lab.), Japan. Springer, Singapore (2020). https://doi.org/10.1007/978-981-15-2989-4
2. Kansal, V., Ranjan, R., Sinha, S., Tiwari, R., Wickramasinghe, N. (eds.): Healthcare and Knowledge Management for Society 5.0: Trends, Issues, and Innovations, 1st edn. CRC Press (2021). https://doi.org/10.1201/9781003168638
3. Cabinet Office: Society 5.0 (2023). https://www8.cao.go.jp/cstp/english/society5_0/index.html. Accessed 03 Feb 2023
4. Cabinet Office: Examples of Creating New Value in the Fields of Healthcare and Caregiving (Society 5.0) (2023). https://www8.cao.go.jp/cstp/english/society5_0/medical_e.html. Accessed 03 Feb 2023
5. Piest, J.P.S., Masuda, Y., Iacob, M.E.: Digital architectures under society 5.0: an enterprise architecture perspective. In: Sales, T.P., Proper, H.A., Guizzardi, G., Montali, M., Maggi, F.M., Fonseca, C.M. (eds.) EDOC 2022 Workshops. LNBIP, vol. 466, pp. 5–24. Springer, Cham (2023). https://doi.org/10.1007/978-3-031-26886-1_1
6. Masuda, Y., Viswanathan, M.: Enterprise Architecture for Global Companies in a Digital IT Era: Adaptive Integrated Digital Architecture Framework (AIDAF). Springer, Singapore (2019). https://doi.org/10.1007/978-981-13-1083-6
7. Masuda, Y., Zimmermann, A., Sandkuhl, K., Schmidt, R., Nakamura, O., Toma, T.: Applying AIDAF for enabling industry 4.0 in open healthcare platform 2030. In: Zimmermann, A., Howlett, R.J., Jain, L.C., Schmidt, R. (eds.) KES-HCIS 2021. SIST, vol. 244, pp. 211–221. Springer, Singapore (2021). https://doi.org/10.1007/978-981-16-3264-8_20

8. Masuda, Y., Zimmermann, A., Shepard, D.S., Schmidt, R., Shirasaka, S.: An adaptive enterprise architecture design for a digital healthcare platform: toward digitized society – industry 4.0, society 5.0. In: 2021 IEEE 25th International EDOCW, 2021, pp. 138–146 (2021). https://doi.org/10.1109/EDOCW52865.2021.00043

9. Fukami, Y., Masuda, Y.: Society 5.0 as digital strategy for scalability: Tamba's COVID-19 vaccination management system and its expansion. In: Chen, Y.W., Tanaka, S., Howlett, R.J., Jain, L.C. (eds.) Innovation in Medicine and Healthcare. SIST, vol. 308, pp. 27–37. Springer, Singapore (2022). https://doi.org/10.1007/978-981-19-3440-7_3

10. Page, M.J., et al.: The PRISMA 2020 statement: an updated guideline for reporting systematic reviews. BMJ **372**, n71 (2021). https://doi.org/10.1136/bmj.n71

11. Bartoloni, S., et al.: Towards designing society 5.0 solutions: the new Quintuple Helix-Design Thinking approach to technology. Technovation **113**, 102413 (2022). https://doi.org/10.1016/j.technovation.2021.102413

12. Dampage, U., Balasuriya, C., Thilakarathna, S., Rathnayaka, D., Kalubowila, L.: AI-based heart monitoring system. In: 2021 IEEE 4th International Conference on Computing, Power and Communication Technologies (GUCON), pp. 1–6 (2021). https://doi.org/10.1109/GUCON50781.2021.9573888

13. Al Mamun, S., Kaiser, M.S., Mahmud, M.: An artificial intelligence based approach towards inclusive healthcare provisioning in society 5.0: a perspective on brain disorder. In: Mahmud, M., Kaiser, M.S., Vassanelli, S., Dai, Q., Zhong, N. (eds.) BI 2021. LNCS (LNAI), vol. 12960, pp. 157–169. Springer, Cham (2021). https://doi.org/10.1007/978-3-030-86993-9_15

14. Ghosh, T., Roy, A., Misra, S.: B2H: enabling delay-tolerant blockchain network in healthcare for Society 5.0. Comput. Netw. **210**, 108860 (2022). https://doi.org/10.1016/j.comnet.2022.108860

15. Ghosh, T., Roy, A., Misra, S., Raghuwanshi, N.S.: CASE: a context-aware security scheme for preserving data privacy in IoT-enabled society 5.0. IEEE IoT J. **9**(4), 2497–2504 (2022). https://doi.org/10.1109/JIOT.2021.3101115

16. Zhong, J., Mao, Z., Li, H., Masuda, Y., Toma, T.: Regulated digital pharmacy based on electronic health record to improve prescription services. In: Chen, Y.-W., Tanaka, S., Howlett, R.J., Jain, L.C. (eds.) Innovation in Medicine and Healthcare. SIST, vol. 242, pp. 155–170. Springer, Singapore (2021). https://doi.org/10.1007/978-981-16-3013-2_13

17. Masuda, Y., Zimmermann, A., Viswanathan, M., Bass, M., Nakamura, O., Yamamoto, S.: Adaptive enterprise architecture for the digital healthcare industry: a digital platform for drug development. Information (2021). https://doi.org/10.3390/info12020067

18. Masuda, Y., Shepard, D.S., Nakamura, O., Toma, T.: Vision paper for enabling internet of medical robotics things in open healthcare platform 2030. In: Chen, Y.-W., Tanaka, S., Howlett, R.J., Jain, L.C. (eds.) Innovation in Medicine and Healthcare. SIST, vol. 192, pp. 3–14. Springer, Singapore (2020). https://doi.org/10.1007/978-981-15-5852-8_1

19. Masuda, Y., Zimmermann, A., Shirasaka, S., Nakamura, O.: Internet of robotic things with digital platforms: digitization of robotics enterprise. In: Zimmermann, A., Howlett, R.J., Jain, L.C. (eds.) Human Centred Intelligent Systems. SIST, vol. 189, pp. 381–391. Springer, Singapore (2021). https://doi.org/10.1007/978-981-15-5784-2_31

20. Piest, J.P.S.: Review of Society 5.0 use cases, applications, and case studies in healthcare (2023). https://doi.org/10.17605/OSF.IO/HW7J4

21. Imura, I., et al.: A method for estimating physician stress using wearable sensor devices. Sens. Mater. **34**(8), 2955–2971 (2022). https://doi.org/10.18494/SAM3908

22. Li, S., Chiu, C.: Improved smart pillow for remote health care system. J. Sens. Actuator Netw. **10**(1), 9 (2021). https://doi.org/10.3390/jsan10010009

23. Masuda, Y., Ishii, R., Shepard, D., Jain, R., Nakamura, O., Toma, T.: Vision paper for enabling HCI-AI digital healthcare platform using AIDAF in open healthcare platform 2030. In: Chen, Y.W., Tanaka, S., Howlett, R.J., Jain, L.C. (eds.) Innovation in Medicine and Healthcare. SIST, vol. 308, pp. 301–311. Springer, Singapore (2022). https://doi.org/10.1007/978-981-19-3440-7_27

24. Salvetti, F., Galli, C., Bertagni, B., Gardner, R., Minehart, R.: A digital mindset for the society 5.0: experience an online escape room. In: Guralnick, D., Auer, M.E., Poce, A. (eds.) TLIC 2021. LNNS, vol. 349, pp. 290–303. Springer, Cham (2022). https://doi.org/10.1007/978-3-030-90677-1_28

25. Mohsen, A., Al-Mahdawi, M., Fouda, M.M., Oogane, M., Ando, Y., Fadlullah, Z.M.: AI aided noise processing of spintronic based IoT sensor for magnetocardiography application. In: 2020 IEEE ICC, Dublin, Ireland, pp. 1–6 (2020).https://doi.org/10.1109/ICC40277.2020.9148617

26. Ciasullo, M.V., Orciuoli, F., Douglas, A., Palumbo, R.: Putting Health 4.0 at the service of Society 5.0: exploratory insights from a pilot study. Socio-Econ. Plan. Sci. **80**, 101163 (2022). https://doi.org/10.1016/j.seps.2021.101163

27. Piest, J.P.S., Iacob, M.E., Wouterse, M.J.T.: Designing intelligence amplification: a design canvas for practitioners. AFHE Open Access **68**, 68–76 (2022). https://doi.org/10.54941/ahfe1002714

28. Piest, J.P.S., Iacob, M.E., Wouterse, M.J.T.: Designing intelligence amplification: organizing a design canvas workshop. AFHE Open Access **68**, 247–251 (2022). https://doi.org/10.54941/ahfe1002739

Strategic Risk Management for Low-Code Development Platforms with Enterprise Architecture Approach: Case of Global Pharmaceutical Enterprise

Tetsuro Miyake[1]([✉]), Yoshimasa Masuda[2,3], Akiko Oguchi[4], and Atsushi Ishida[4]

[1] Bayer Yakuhin, Ltd., Osaka, Japan
tetsuro.miyake@bayer.com
[2] The Graduate School of Media and Governance, Keio University, Kanagawa, Japan
[3] The School of Computer Science, Carnegie Mellon University, Pittsburgh, PA, USA
[4] Bayer Holding Ltd., Osaka, Japan

Abstract. Global Pharmaceutical Enterprises (GPEs) have increasingly adopted and promoted Low-Code Development Platforms (LCDPs) to aim for higher agility and resilience to the rapidly changing market demands. While LCDPs facilitate rapid application development by democratising application development platforms to non-professional developers ("citizen developers"), these organisations are challenged to establish strategic conformance with Low-Code applications regarding interoperability, scalability, security, and vendor lock-in. Since these LCDP challenges relate to the organisation's enterprise strategy, the organisations should implement mitigations at the strategic level where Enterprise Architecture frameworks play an important role. This paper investigates how the LCDP challenges can be managed with the "Adaptive Integrated Digital Architecture Framework (AIDAF) with Design Thinking Approach." A case project in a GPE verified that the AIDAF with Design Thinking Approach successfully supported managing a Low-Code application project and achieved strategic conformance with the developed Low-Code application. In addition, challenges and future issues for this research area are presented.

1 Introduction

Digital transformation is critical for business organisations to remain competitive in the market. Business organisations have adopted various emerging technologies to thrive in a competitive market. However, they still suffer from solid market pressure to be more agile and resilient to rapidly changing market demands [1]. Nevertheless, it is not realistic for business organisations to hire as many IT developers as they need because there is a need for more skilled IT developers in the market, which also drives the bottom line up and negatively impacts the margin of the business. As a solution to this business challenge, business organisations are inclined to adopt Low-Code Development Platforms (LCDPs) that provide business employees (non-professional developers, so-called "citizen developers") with easy access to application development platforms without extensive and costly training [2].

Y.-W. Chen et al. (Eds.): KES InMed 2023, SIST 357, pp. 88–100, 2023.
https://doi.org/10.1007/978-981-99-3311-2_9

Forrester Research coined the term "Low Code" in 2014, and LCDPs are commonly recognised as cloud-based platforms that enable rapid custom application development by citizen developers with a reduced amount of programming and intuitive usability (e.g., drag-and-drop) [3]. LCDPs are characterised by their benefits: simplicity, reusability, interoperability, lower cost, and faster release time [4]. In addition, Low-Code development benefit from Agile Software Development (ASD) and the Design Thinking (DT) approach. ASD is a software development approach that emphasises an incremental approach, prototyping, and end-user collaboration for quicker release of products. DT is an iterative approach to capturing end-user needs and identifying problems for the rapid realisation of end-user needs and possible solutions. The DT consists of non-sequential phases of "empathise," "define," "ideate," "prototype," and "test." Hence, applying ASD and the DT approach in combination will yield synergies for Low-Code development projects in building user-centric applications in short cycles [5].

On the other hand, recent research revealed that LCDP's advantages, such as speed and cost-effectiveness, often lead to trade-offs regarding interoperability, scalability, security, and vendor lock-in [6–9]. These challenges are subject to enterprise digital strategies, so mitigations must be best implemented strategically. A recent Enterprise Architecture (EA) study proposed "the adaptive integrated digital architecture framework (AIDAF) for Design Thinking Approach" [10]. This model could address the LCDP challenges because it is designed to be harmonised with digital projects that follow the ASD and the DT approach. However, this model has yet to be evaluated against Low-Code application development projects in the pharmaceutical industry, where some authors of this research belong. Since the adoption of LCDPs has been increasingly accelerated in the pharmaceutical industry, like in other industries, evaluating the model in a Low-Code application development project in a pharmaceutical company is worthwhile. Hence, this paper presents a case project of a Low-Code application development in a global pharmaceutical enterprise (GPE), to which some of the authors belong, and verifies how the AIDAF with Design Thinking Approach can address the LCDP challenges. The case project developed an application for regulatory compliance training using an LCDP. The research questions employed in this paper are:

RQ1: How can the Low-Code regulatory compliance training application be built with the AIDAF with Design Thinking Approach in a GPE?

RQ2: How can the Low-Code regulatory compliance training application be managed and improved in alignment with enterprise digital strategy with LCDPs using the AIDAF with Design Thinking Approach in a GPE?

The paper is structured as follows: the next chapter details the background of this study, followed by an explanation of research methodology and a case of a Low-Code application development project. Discussion of the results and outcomes of the case project is presented. Finally, challenges, future studies, and the limitations of the case project are presented, followed by a conclusion.

2   Literature Review

2.1   Related Work – Low-Code Development Platforms (LCDPs)

Since the term "Low-Code" was coined in 2014, many LCDP vendors have been in the market, such as OutSystems, Mendix, salesforce, and Microsoft [3]. The Low-Code industry is expected to constitute about two-thirds of the application development activities by 2024 [2]. LCDPs are referred to as cloud-based platforms that facilitate rapid custom application development by citizen developers with reduced hand-coding and intuitive usability (e.g., drag-and-drop) [3]. The main difference with conventional software development platforms is that LCDPs offer pre-designed software modules that replace most manual-coding efforts [9].

According to a recent systematic literature review study [3], the benefits of LCDPs are characterised by low requirements regarding technical skills, short development time, low cost, and high efficiency. This explains that LCDPs contribute to high productivity in application development. On the other hand, challenges are described as interoperability issues, scalability, and vendor lock-in [3, 6–9]. Interoperability issues are caused by the fact that most LCDPs are proprietary and not interoperable across different LCDPs. This hampers the reuse of the developed Low-Code applications. In addition, LCDPs are not scalable because LCDPs is not intended for large-scale applications [6]. Furthermore, vendor lock-in is also a significant concern for LCDPs because LCDPs are based on proprietary development languages, practices, and Platform as a Service (PaaS) delivery models [11].

2.2   Microsoft Power Platform and Power Apps

Microsoft Power Apps is one of the industry-leading LCDPs [32]. Power Apps is provided as part of Microsoft Power Platform included in Microsoft 365. Power Apps provides a collection of ready-to-use templates that enables users to build applications with relatively little effort by drag-and-drop [12, 34]. As Power Apps is highly user-friendly, there is no need for lengthy training. In addition, Power Apps provides an extensive collection of connectors that allow Microsoft applications (e.g., Excel, Teams, Forms, SharePoint) [33] and third-party systems to be integrated with the workflow [9]. Power Apps' environments are containers that enable administrators to control applications, flows, connections, and other functionalities, in line with permissions for users in the organisation to use the resources. [9].

2.3   Agile Software Development (ASD) Framework

Conventionally, software development processes have been defined with linear process models, such as the waterfall model, characterised by low customer involvement [13]. This often leads to the end-user dissatisfaction with the resulting final product. Agile methods aim to address this point, particularly by working iteratively and incrementally with frequent communication with the end-users to present interim results [14]. Today, ASD evolves within several frameworks and has advanced the basic understanding of ASD. The most important is Scrum of Scrums [15], Large Scale Scrum (LeSS) [16],

Scaled Agile Framework [17], and Disciplined Agile (DAD) [18], migrated to the latest version of this framework called "Disciplined Agile 2.0." From the frameworks' maturity viewpoint, the Scaled Agile Framework has the most significant contributions and integrates an EA role [19]. To cope with high complexity, Large Scale Scrum and Disciplined Agile define less beforehand and give more flexibility for individual solutions [20].

2.4 Design Thinking (DT) Approach

The DT [21–23] is an approach for problem-solving with a user-centric creativity and innovation-oriented mindset [10]. The philosophy of the DT [21] includes essential vital attributes: (1) people-centred, (2) highly creative, (3) hands-on, and (4) iterative processes. More specifically, the DT approach aims to capture what end-users expect, which is technically feasible for businesses, and turn it into both end-user benefit and business value [21]. While the defined initial processes of the DT approach appear in some variations, there cover key phases in common: Empathise, Define, Ideate, Prototype, and Test [21–23]. The empathise phase engages in understanding cultures, attitudes, barriers, behaviours, and emotions. The definition phase incorporates the findings and approaches through systematic identification of user types, a particular combination of needs, and formulation of insights and principles. Developing ideas requires methods for igniting creativity, such as brainstorming, mind-mapping, group synergy, presentation of new ideas, and different idea generation and evaluation. The prototype phase is experimentation to turn ideas into a tangible working prototype of the future concept or system. This process includes a rough illustration of an idea, visualisation, look and feel of solutions, and mainly building working models and artefacts (e.g., minimal viable product (MVP)). The testing phase gathers feedback on the prototype. Complementary lessons learned sessions are conducted to learn more about users, change perspective, refine the prototype, and enable first concrete experiences.

2.5 AIDAF Framework and Strategic Risk Management

EA has become an essential framework for modelling the relationship between enterprise and individual systems. In ISO/IEC/ IEEE42010:2011, an architecture framework is defined as "conventions, principles, and practices for the description of architecture established within a specific domain of application and community of stakeholders" [24]. EA is a vital component of corporate IT planning and offers benefits to companies, like coordination between business and IT [25]. Past research has discussed the integration of EA with service-oriented architecture (SOA) [35]. OASIS, a public standards group [26], has released an SOA reference model. Then, a critical EA research proposed an "Adaptive Integrated Digital Architecture framework (AIDAF)," which facilitates a strategic alignment between digital projects and IT strategy [27]. The AIDAF consists of four phases in the adaptive EA cycle. The adaptive EA cycle should work well with any EA framework, such as TOGAF and a simple EA framework on an operational domain unit [27, 28]. Besides, the AIDAF framework is treated as a digital EA (DEA) framework.

Moreover, the authors of the AIDAF proposed the "STrategic Risk Mitigation Model (STRMM model)" as the risk management framework in the Architecture Board (AB) and verified it with a case project [29]. The STRMM model defines processes and viewpoints that enable digital IT projects to be aligned with IT strategies (e.g., security/privacy policy) and effectively manage risks in the digital IT project. In particular, the STRMM model assists the project team in managing risks by systematic risk assessment referring to IT Strategy by raising risks and proposing mitigations. A recent study also examined whether the AIDAF and STRMM model can effectively manage a Proof of Concept (PoC) project and verified the applicability and validity with a case project [30].

2.6   AIDAF with Design Thinking Approach

In response to the increasing adoption of the DT approach in digital projects, the AIDAF was extended to harmonise with the DT approach and ASD methodologies and turned into a variant model, the "AIDAF Framework for Design Thinking Approach with Strategic Risk Mitigation (STRMM)" [10] consisting of the four steps: [1A]–[4A].

[1A] In the Prototype Development phase, the project team uses the DT approach to identify a potential issue from the viewpoint of users' preferences (e.g., cultural, behavioural, motivational preference, value, and philosophy of project stakeholders). Next, the DT approach captures the functional and non-functional needs. Then, prototypes (i.e., MVP) are developed with ASD methodology. Finally, the prototype is assessed and modified with architecture guidelines such as user interfaces, data privacy, and data security. (The architecture reviews can be held, if necessary.)

[2A] In the Context phase, the project team uses the DT approach to identify unconsidered needs from the viewpoint of production use. Then, the identified needs are used to define necessary enhancements to the prototypes.

[3A] In the Assessment/Architecture Review phase, the Architecture Board (AB) reviews the digital IT project's proposal with enhancements of prototypes to identify risks of deployment in consideration of production environments and Rationalisation (e.g., checking enterprise system portfolio) there.

[4A] In the Realisation phase, the risk management process can be started based on the review's results and necessary policies (e.g., data privacy/data security). In digital IT projects, project teams can mitigate the risks identified by the AB.

3   Research Methodology

A case project was designed to evaluate how effectively the AIDAF with Design Thinking Approach supports Low-Code application developments in a GPE in terms of strategic conformance. Firstly, the authors identified three factors in choosing a case project:

A) The project should aim to develop a business application with Power Apps, the standard LCDP in the GPE.

B) The project should allow the authors to obtain sufficient information about how the project goes through the DT processes. Since the DT activities deal with cultural, behavioural, and motivational aspects of the end-user needs, the authors should know the cultural and business context behind the project to evaluate the DT activities in the project better. In this regard, the authors determined to choose a case project in an organisational unit to which one or some of the authors belong.

C) The project allows the authors to quantitatively evaluate the contribution of the AIDAF with Design Thinking Approach to Low-Code application development. This means that the application to be replaced by the Low-Code application should have the results of end-user satisfaction surveys performed in the past regarding the application's usability so that the authors can compare the end-user satisfaction between the two applications.

Next, the authors chose a case project meeting the above factors. The design of the project was as below:

- The Regulatory Compliance (RC) unit, a function of about 50 employees in a regional affiliate of the GPE to which an author belongs, develops a Power Apps custom application to provide sales representatives with regulatory compliance training.
- The Power Apps custom application is developed to switch from an existing Software as a Service (SaaS) - based training platform.
- The results of the end-user satisfaction surveys performed in the past for the usability of the SaaS-based application are available and accessible.

Then, during and after the project, the authors collected information by interviewing the project team and reviewing project documents. In particular, one of the authors, working in the GPE, conducted all phases of structuring and implementing the Regional Architecture Board (RAB) and was a member of the RAB to mainly support the coordination between the project team with the RAB. More details of the case project and the RAB are presented in the next chapter.

4   Case: Low-Code Application Development with Power Apps

The case project followed the processes of the "AIDAF for Design Thinking Approach," as illustrated in Fig. 1.

The RC unit was responsible for providing sales representatives with training programs in country-specific regulations of sales promotion activities. Conventionally, the RC unit prepared quizzes and provided them as an independent training program on a SaaS training platform. The training programs were provided twice a year, in the first half (1H) and the second half (2H), and the answering period was for one month. After closing the answering period, the RC unit conducted an end-user satisfaction survey for each training program. The SaaS platform was popular across industries and well-accepted by the trainees of the GPE. However, there was a financial burden because subscription fees were charged per trainee for each training program. To address the financial challenge, the RC unit decided to develop a custom training platform with Microsoft Power Apps, the standard LCDP in the GPE. One of the employees in the RC unit built the application

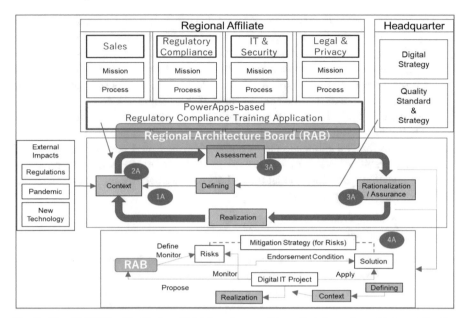

Fig. 1. The "AIDAF with Design Thinking Approach" applied for a Low-Code application development project in a regional affiliate in a GPE.

as a citizen developer. She had some experience in end-user computing (e.g., macro) but did not have experience working as a professional IT developer in her career.

The model in Fig. 1 consists of three parts. The upper part shows that the regional affiliate of the GPE follows the enterprise digital strategy defined by the headquarter. The middle part is an adaptive EA cycle where the project goes through the project phases (i.e., Context, Assessment, Rationalisation, and Realisation) with the DT steps [1A]–[3A] as defined in Chapter 2.6. In addition, the RAB reviews the project documentation and identifies risks in [3A]. The RAB comprises domain experts in IT, Security, Privacy, and Computer System Validation (CSV), providing expert consultation to project teams.

The lower part is the risk management process in [4A] as defined in Chapter 2.6, where the project team copes with each risk mitigation strategy for risks raised by RAB.

5   Discussion

The case project followed [1A]–[4A] as below.

In the step of [1A], before starting development, the project team used the DT approach, reviewed past end-user satisfaction survey results to capture the trainees' real needs or pain points, and identified two critical factors in designing User Interface (UI). One was the trainees' behavioural preferences. Sales representatives are busy with visiting customers and generally prefer brief but concise training material when they have time rather than comprehensive training. Here, the project team recognised that a new training application should adopt quiz-style training rather than long narrative lecture-style training so trainees can save and exit anytime needed. The other key factor was the trainee's natural resistance to 'dry' training contents. Trainees understand regulatory compliance's importance but cannot avoid natural resistance to dry training contents. Then, the project team realised that a new training application should give trainees a sense of fun and motivation, for example, by using cartoon-like illustrations or interactive features such as real-time scoring and ranking. With these empathetic insights, the project team developed an MVP with Power Apps. Moreover, during the development, the project team checked data privacy aspects. For example, the General Data Protection Regulation (GDPR) principles and the regional privacy regulations were considered to make data privacy internationally and locally compliant. Moreover, the project team confirmed that the global headquarter thoroughly assessed Microsoft Power Platform regarding privacy and security and was officially approved as the standard LCDP of the GPE. In addition, the project team referred to seven principles [31] to enhance UI and designed the UI to attract users' attention and simplify error messages.

In the step of [2A], the project team used the DT approach to enhance the prototype in light of scaling to production use. The project team had large-scale exploratory testing that allowed about 150 sales representatives to play with the prototype based on their way of use in the past. This heuristic testing revealed many enhancement points (e.g., legibility when accessed from a smartphone, response speed, and a technical bug of double entry). These unconsidered needs were turned into necessary enhancements to the prototype.

In the step of [3A], the RAB assessed the project proposal submitted by the project team and identified risks in case of deployment to the production environment. The assessment was conducted in the four elements as described in Table 1.

Table 1. Summary of Risk Management of Case Project performed in STRMM Model

Elements of Evaluation Criteria	Review points in each element	Risks [Category]	Solutions [Category]
Enterprise Level Conformance	• Standard LCDP (PowerApps) • Cloud-first (Power Platform) • API-first (Connector)	Vendor Lock-In [Application Architecture]	Process documentation and role assignment [Employee]
Functional Aspect	• Data Flow • Application Design • Interfaces (Connector) • Login (Single Sign On)	No risk identified (due to the adoption of the DT approach)	Not Applicable

(continued)

Table 1. (*continued*)

Elements of Evaluation Criteria	Review points in each element	Risks [Category]	Solutions [Category]
Operational Aspect	• Security (ISO27001) • Privacy (GDPR) • SLA (availability, RTO, platform update) • Scalability (enterprise, ecosystem)	No control in case of system down [Compliance and Validation]	Process documentation for system down [Employee]
Viability Aspect	Applicable Regulations − GxP (Validation, Data Integrity) − Regional regulations − Business Process Criticality	No risk identified (due to non-regulated business process)	Not Applicable

Note: [] denotes the categories defined in Fig. 4 of [28].

Firstly, from the perspective of Enterprise Level Conformance, the RAB assessed whether the technology used for the proposed application complied with the enterprise architectural guidelines. In the case of the project, Power Platform (including Power Apps) was the standard LCDP in the GPE and was a cloud-based service and supported the use of APIs via "connector." Therefore, the technology was compliant with the enterprise architectural guidelines. However, the RAB raised a risk of vendor lock-in, which falls into the "Application Architecture" risk category. While applications developed with Power Apps were interoperable via connectors, the application itself could not be transferred to other LCDPs. Hence, for long-term enterprise architectural conformance, the RAB suggested that the project team establish a process to document specifications as a mitigation measure to enable easier migration to other platforms in the future. This solution falls into the solution category of "Employee."

Secondly, from the viewpoint of Functional Aspect, RAB's assessment was focused on the key functionalities such as Interface and login because the end-user needs and business logic were already reflected in the application design by the DT approach. The application had an interface with other Microsoft 365 applications, as illustrated in Fig. 2, and adopted a single sign-on (SSO) with standard corporate credentials. Since both the Interface and login conformed to the enterprise architectural guidelines, no risk was raised.

Thirdly, from the perspective of Operational Aspect, the RAB confirmed that Microsoft was certified to ISO27001, compliant with GDPR as stated in their privacy statement, and SLA (including availability, maintenance window, and platform update) was available. In addition, the RAB confirmed that the application was intended to be used only at a regional affiliate in the GPE and not to be extended to the level of enterprise-wide or ecosystem. In this regard, the RAB judged that the limited scalability

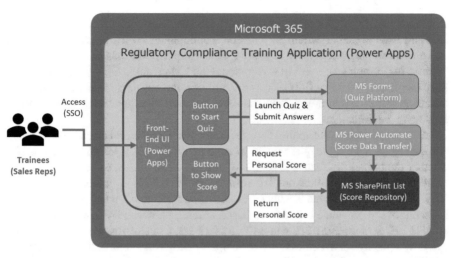

Fig. 2. Application Design of a regulatory compliance training application with Power Apps

of Power Apps was not an issue for the application. However, the RAB raised a potential risk of operational stability, which falls into the "Compliance and Validation" risk category. Microsoft 365 was a cloud-based service, so the operation team had no control over technical problems and automatic platform updates. This could cause a planned periodic regulatory compliance training to be cancelled or postponed. Hence, for stable operations, the RAB suggested that the project team establishes an operational procedure in case the application is compromised due to a platform issue or unintended platform update. This solution falls into the solution category of "Employee."

Lastly, from the perspective of Viability Aspect, the RAB checked whether the application would be regulated by any applicable regulations such as industry-specific regulations (e.g., GxP, Data Integrity). Then, the RAB confirmed that there was no applicable regulation for the application because the regulatory compliance training supported by the application was not a regulatory requirement by itself. Therefore, there was no particular risk identified in this regard. Furthermore, the RAB also made a portfolio assessment as part of the Rationalisation phase and confirmed that the developed application would not replace the existing SaaS training platform because many other business functions will continue to use the Platform. In addition, the training platform is an external cloud service to which each business function directly subscribes. This means no internal stakeholder will be affected by the newly developed application in the case project. Therefore, the RAB determined that there was no critical stakeholder for the project team to communicate with regarding the newly developed application.

In the step of [4A], the project team worked together to implement mitigations for the risks raised in [3A]. For the first risk (vendor lock-in), the project team defined a process to document technical specifications and the business logic embedded in the application design. The assigned responsible member retrospectively prepared the documents. For the second risk (stable operations), the project team performed a risk assessment to determine the level of stable operations in their business context and concluded that they should have a defined process on who decides cancellation or postponement by what criteria and also how and to whom the decision is communicated. Then, process documentation was completed concisely. However, the backup solution was judged unnecessary because the compliance training was optional, and Microsoft's SLA (e.g., availability, Recovery Time Objective (RTO)) was tolerable for the business criticality. Then, with the above-implemented mitigations, the RAB endorsed releasing the application to the production environment.

After the release of the application, the project team conducted an end-user satisfaction survey with the same questions as in the past, which was a yes/no question asking whether the trainee was satisfied with the tool and wanted the next session to be provided with the same application. The result shows that 89% of the respondents (N = 308) were satisfied with the developed Power Apps application, which was higher than the score of the previously used SaaS-based training platform; 84% in 2020 2H, 88% in 2021 1H, 86% in 2021 2H, and 88% in 2022 1H. Considering the new application was developed by a non-professional developer in only four months, it can be seen as a significant success of the Low-Code application development supported by the AIDAF with Design Thinking Approach.

As demonstrated above, RQ1 is verified as the Low-Code application was successfully built by following the steps of [1A]–[4A] in the AIDAF with Design Thinking, especially in terms of capturing end-users' behavioural and motivational preferences, security, and privacy. RQ2 is also verified as strategic risks were successfully raised against the enterprise architectural guidelines and addressed.

6   Challenges, Future Issues

Further study is needed to investigate more Low-Code development projects at different scales (e.g., enterprise-wide, ecosystem) and complexity (e.g., complex business process with large datasets). In addition, the potential challenges in the operational phase still need to be examined (e.g., risks in automatic platform updates and turnover of the citizen developers).

7   Limitations

The primary limitation of this study is the scope of only one case project in a single GPE. In addition, since the business logic is less complex in the case project, the number and variety of risks and solutions are limited.

8   Conclusion

This paper investigated how the LCDP challenges can be managed with the "Adaptive Integrated Digital Architecture Framework (AIDAF) for Design Thinking Approach." Based on the results and progress of the case project for a regulatory compliance training application developed with an LCDP (Power Apps), this research shows that the regulatory compliance training application developed with an LCDP can be built with the

DT approach supported by the AIDAF in a GPE, especially in terms of capturing end-users' behavioural and motivational preferences, security, and privacy, to answer RQ1. Moreover, we demonstrated by this research that the training application developed with an LCDP could be managed and enhanced in alignment with the digital strategy with LCDPs using the AIDAF in a GPE, which can lead to the answer for RQ2.

References

1. Mangalaraj, G., Nerur, S., Dwivedi, R.: Digital transformation for agility and resilience: an exploratory study. J. Comput. Inf. Syst. 1–13 (2021)
2. Vincent, P., Iijima, K., Driver, M., Wong, J., Natis, Y.: Magic quadrant for enterprise low-code application platforms. Gartner Report (2019)
3. Pinho, D., Aguiar, A., Amaral, V.: What about the usability in low-code platforms? A systematic literature review. J. Comput. Lang. 101185 (2022)
4. Sahay, A., Indamutsa, A., Di Ruscio, D., Pierantonio, A.: Supporting the understanding and comparison of low-code development platforms. In: 2020 46th Euromicro Conference on Software Engineering and Advanced Applications (SEAA), pp. 171–178. IEEE, August 2020
5. Pereira, J.C., de FSM Russo, R.: Design thinking integrated in agile software development: a systematic literature review. Proc. Comput. Sci. **138**, 775–782 (2018)
6. Sanchis, R., García-Perales, Ó., Fraile, F., Poler, R.: Low-code as enabler of digital transformation in manufacturing industry. Appl. Sci. **10**(1), 12 (2019)
7. Luo, Y., Liang, P., Wang, C., Shahin, M., Zhan, J.: Characteristics and challenges of low-code development: the practitioners' perspective. In: Proceedings of the 15th ACM/IEEE International Symposium on Empirical Software Engineering and Measurement (ESEM), pp. 1–11, October 2021
8. Bock, A.C., Frank, U.: Low-code platform. Bus. Inf. Syst. Eng. **63**, 733–740 (2021)
9. Heuer, M., Kurtz, C., Böhmann, T.: Towards a governance of low-code development platforms using the example of Microsoft power platform in a multinational company (2022)
10. Masuda, Y., Zimmermann, A., Shepard, D.S., Schmidt, R., Shirasaka, S.: An adaptive enterprise architecture design for a digital healthcare platform: toward digitised society–Industry 4.0, Society 5.0. In: 2021 IEEE 25th International Enterprise Distributed Object Computing Workshop (EDOCW), pp. 138–146. IEEE, October 2021
11. Kaess, S.: Low Code Development Platform Adoption: A Research Model (2022)
12. Khorram, F., Mottu, J.M., Sunyé, G.: Challenges & opportunities in low-code testing. In: Proceedings of the 23rd ACM/IEEE International Conference on Model Driven Engineering Languages and Systems: Companion Proceedings, pp. 1–10, October 2020
13. Alshamrani, A., Bahattab, A.: A comparison between three SDLC models waterfall model, spiral model, and incremental/Iterative model. Int. J. Comput. Sci. Issues (IJCSI) **12**(1), 106 (2015)
14. Beck, K., et al.: Agile Manifesto (2001). https://www.agilealliance.org/wp-content/uploads/2019/09/agilemanifesto-download-2019.pdf
15. Qurashi, S.A., Qureshi, M.: Scrum of scrums solution for large size teams using scrum methodology. arXiv preprint arXiv:1408.6142 (2014)
16. Larman, C., Vodde, B.: Large-Scale Scrum: More with LeSS. Addison-Wesley Professional (2016)
17. Leffingwell, D.: SAFe 4.5 Reference Guide: Scaled Agile Framework for Lean Enterprises. Addison-Wesley Professional (2018)
18. Ambler, S.W., Lines, M.: Disciplined agile Delivery: A Practitioner's Guide to Agile Software Delivery in the Enterprise. IBM Press (2012)

19. Masuda, Y., Viswanathan, M.: Enterprise Architecture for Global Companies in a Digital IT Era: Adaptive Integrated Digital Architecture Framework (AIDAF). Springer, Singapore (2019). https://doi.org/10.1007/978-981-13-1083-6
20. Ebert, C., Paasivaara, M.: Scaling agile. IEEE Softw. **34**(6), 98–103 (2017)
21. Brown, T.: Design thinking. Harv. Bus. Rev. **86**(6), 84 (2008)
22. Dorst, K.: The core of 'design thinking' and its application. Des. Stud. **32**(6), 521–532 (2011)
23. Gruber, M., de Leon, N., George, G., Thompson, P.: Managing by design. Acad. Manag. J. **58**(1), 1–7 (2015)
24. Garnier, J.-L., Bérubé, J., Hilliard, R.: Architecture Guidance Study Report 140430, ISO/IEC JTC 1/SC 7 Software and Systems Engineering (2014)
25. Tamm, T., Seddon, P. B., Shanks, G., Reynolds, P.: How does enterprise architecture add value to organisations? (2011)
26. MacKenzie, C.M., Laskey, K., McCabe, F., Brown, P.F., Metz, R.: Reference Model for SOA 1.0. (Technical Report), Advancing Open Standards for the Information Society (2006)
27. Masuda, Y., Shirasaka, S., Yamamoto, S., Hardjono, T.: Int. J. Enterp. Inf. Syst. IGI Global **13**, 1–22 (2017)
28. Masuda, Y., Shirasaka, S., Yamamoto, S., Hardjono, T.: Architecture board practices in adaptive enterprise architecture with digital platform: a case of global healthcare enterprise. Int. J. Enterp. Inf. Syst. IGI Global **14**, 1 (2018)
29. Masuda, Y., Shirasaka, S., Yamamoto, S., Hardjono, T.: Risk Management for digital transformation and big data in architecture board: a case study on global enterprise. Inf. Eng. Express **4**(1), 33–51 (2018)
30. Miyake, T., Masuda, Y., Deguchi, K., Iwasaki, M., Obanayama, K., Miura, K.: Strategic risk management model for agile software development: case of global pharmaceutical enterprise. In: Innovation in Medicine and Healthcare: Proceedings of 10th KES-InMed 2022. SIST, vol. 308, pp. 261–273. Springer, Singapore (2022). https://doi.org/10.1007/978-981-19-3440-7_24
31. Wewerka, J., Micus, C., Reichert, M.: Seven guidelines for designing the user interface in robotic process automation. In: 2021 IEEE 25th International Enterprise Distributed Object Computing Workshop (EDOCW), Gold Coast, Australia, pp. 157–165 (2021)
32. Cunningham, R.: Gartner magic quadrant names Microsoft Power Apps a leader for low code application platforms. Microsoft (2020). https://powerapps.microsoft.com/en-us/blog/gartner-magic-quadrant-names-microsoft-power-apps-a-leader-for-low-code-application-platforms/
33. Wang, S., Wang, H.: A teaching module of no-code business app development. J. Inf. Syst. Educ. **32**(1), 1 (2021)
34. Lebens, M., Finnegan, R.: Using a low code development environment to teach the agile methodology. In: Gregory, P., Lassenius, C., Wang, X., Kruchten, P. (eds.) XP 2021. LNBIP, vol. 419, pp. 191–199. Springer, Cham (2021). https://doi.org/10.1007/978-3-030-78098-2_12
35. Chen, H.-M., Kazman, R., Perry, O.: From software architecture analysis to service engineering: an empirical study of methodology development for enterprise SOA implementation. IEEE Trans. Serv. Comput. **3**, 145–160 (2014)

Optimized Deployment Planning for Elderly Welfare Facilities Based on Network Theory – A Case Study of Ibaraki Prefecture's Day Care Welfare Facilities for the Elderly

Xiangchu Chen and Sumika Arima[✉]

University of Tsukuba, Tsukuba, Ibaraki, Japan
{s2120483,arima.sumika.fp}@u.tsukuba.ac.jp

Abstract. In this study, based on a survey of previous studies, we once again applied a production engineering perspective and network theory to the problem of overall optimization of day-care welfare facilities for the elderly, considering the demand of elderly customers, local labor force, and aspects of service quality, considering the impact of the facilities on each other. Specifically, the study also aims to reduce regional disparities by solving problems that consider supply, demand, geography, and various other aspects. Now, the purpose of this study is to find the bottleneck facility (Unsatisfactory demand and underutilized facilities) among existing welfare facilities, solve the problem considering the weekly supply-demand balance in the region, and obtain the desired effect (regional equilibration) with minimal facility changes through three measures: facility cooperation, facility integration, or new facility construction. The distribution of facilities and customers is dynamically partitioned into networks according to the algorithm, which finds connections between facilities in the same area to locate bottleneck facilities. Then, improvement measures are applied to the bottleneck facilities, considering the number of optimized facilities and facility losses, on the assumption that fairness and efficiency are ensured, to derive a solution that achieves regional equilibrium with a minimum of facility modification.

Keywords: network theory · bottleneck facilities · region-wide balance

1 Introduction

1.1 Research Background

In terms of the image of welfare 30 years from now, an extremely pessimistic outlook prevails, with only 19% of respondents believing that welfare will be improved. [7] it is necessary to balance service capacities within different areas to improve Japan's welfare standards in the face of extreme labor shortages.

In the location-allocation model, there are p-median and p-center problems, in the classical p-center problem, the objective is set to locate p facilities so that the maximum cost of all vertices is minimized [1]. This study does not involve finding a location, but rather locating the facilities that need improvement in each area to equilibrate the region, so that the maximum facility loss in the area with the worst situation is minimized.

© The Author(s), under exclusive license to Springer Nature Singapore Pte Ltd. 2023
Y.-W. Chen et al. (Eds.): KES InMed 2023, SIST 357, pp. 101–117, 2023.
https://doi.org/10.1007/978-981-99-3311-2_10

1.2 Research Objective

The research objective of this paper is to derive an optimal "area-based" plan for the use of day-care elderly care facilities, considering the impact of facilities on each other. Here, "region" is a geographical administrative division such as Bando City, and within this "region" several "zones" are divided based on the demand point-facility network. For this purpose, based on network analysis using demand and the geography of elderly care facilities and their service supply capacity as inputs, we search for bottleneck facilities in "zones," which represent nearby areas within a region, and after leveling the supply-demand balance in space-time, The target conditions are derived from the following three strategies: 1, facility cooperation, 2, facility consolidation, or 3, facility establishment. In this study, as a numerical experiment, we present proposals based on the three strategies and their effects on fairness, efficiency, and improvement of risk response capability, using Ibaraki Prefecture as a concrete case study.

In general, additional costs are required for new construction or modification of facilities. The more facilities changed, the higher the change fee. Therefore, as a strategy, the recommended order is 1, 2, and 3, in that order.

2 Problem Setup

Elderly welfare facilities should generally be optimized by evaluating fairness and efficiency, and based on this, considering the location of new facilities, facility consolidation and adjustment of facility size. Kondo et al. (2002) [5] Analyzed day-care welfare facilities in Tokushima Prefecture by calculating the fairness and efficiency of the facilities, considering travel time, and waiting time, and proposed improvements through three adjustment methods: new facility location, consolidation, and facility size. In this study each facility exists independently and if a facility closes, the customers of the closed facility are equally distributed to the other facilities, which is not the case in real situations. Kawakami et al. (2012) presented a method for determining the assignment of elderly persons requiring support or care to each existing facility to optimize the total distance for elderly persons to travel from their residences to the facility they use and back [2]. However, the model has a maximum deviation from predictions of facility utilization of 425%, with sparsely populated areas and regions having very low predictive accuracy for remote facilities. Based on this study, we not only consider the distance, but also add the size of the facility and the number of users per person to determine the allocation of elderly persons requiring support and care to each existing facility.

3 Research Methodology

3.1 Parameters

Parameters have three parts. Sets, Input parameters and Judgment parameters. The Set has two parts: the set of existing facilities and the set of demand points. The Input parameters are the parameters related to the elderly welfare facilities and demand points, of which there are eight. Judgment parameters are parameters that determine the status of demand points and facilities when configuring the network.

Sets	Definitions
(1) C : (2) U :	(1) Aggregation of existing facilities $C = \{c_1, c_2, c_3, \ldots c_j \ldots c_n\}$ (2) Set of demand points $U = \{w_1, w_2, w_3 \ldots w_i \ldots w_m\}$

Input parameters	Definitions
(1) $d(i, c_j)$: (2) d_{max}: (3) $f(i)$: (4) $Q(c_j)$: (5) w_i: (6) $p(i, c_j)$: (7) N_j: (8) s_j:	(1) Travel distance from demand point i to facility c_j (2) Distance limitation of service (maximum usage distance) (3) Frequency of use per week of the facility at the demand point (4) Capacity of facility c_j (5) Demand at node i in the area centered on the demand point (6) Probability that a customer at demand point i can go to facility j (7) Number of staff at facility c_j (8) Number of users per employee in charge at facility c_j

Judgment parameters	Definitions
(1) x_i (2) z_j	(1) $x_i = \begin{cases} 0 & \text{Demand for demand point i not satisfied} \\ 1 & \text{Satisfied all the demands of demand point i} \end{cases}$ (2) $z_j = \begin{cases} 1 & \text{Facility j reached full capacity} \\ 0 & \text{Facility j not reached full capacity} \end{cases}$

3.2 Facility Importance Model

Facility Importance Model

The importance of a facility is affected by two variables: the distance from the demand point and the capacity of the facility (Table 1). The longer the distance from the demand point, the lower the importance, and the larger the capacity of the facility, the higher the importance.

Table 1. Determinants of Customers' Facility Choice (adapted from [3])

Projects	n = 217	%	Projects	n = 217	%
1, Proximity to home	72	33.2	5, Friend's invitation	8	3.7
2, Services and facilities	44	20.3	6, Physician Referral	1	0.5
3, Inexpensive usage fees	6	2.8	7, Introduction of government offices	4	1.8
4, Caregiver Referrals	64	29.5	8, others	13	6

Based on the above findings, this study defines the importance of a facility as follows. The importance of the facility $\pi(c_j)$ is expressed by the following equation.

$$\pi(c_j) = \exp(-d(i, c_j)^{\tau}/Q(c_j)) \tag{3-1}$$

τ: Adjustment Parameters

$d(i, c_j)$: Distance from demand point

$Q(c_j)$: Facility Capacity (Personnel) Limitations

The influence items for distance are 1 and for facility size are 3–8. Since the impact on customers is 33.2% and 43.8%, or about 0.7579, we decided to determine τ at 0.76.

The Probability that a Customer will Choose a Facility

When a client chooses a facility, it is not due to a single factor, but to a combination of factors that influence the client's choice.

Table 2. Determinants of customers' facility choice (adapted from [3]).

Projects	n = 133	%	Projects	n = 133	%
1,	18	13.5	2	7	5.3
1,2	17	12.8	4	36	27.1
1,2,4	9	6.8	6	1	0.8
1,4	10	7.5	7	4	3
1,5	3	2.3	9	5	3.8
1,6	0	0	others	23	17.3

According to the MFLP model, membership within a facility cluster is more probable the closer its center is [4] Membership within the same facility cluster is more likely for customers to want to go the higher its degree of importance and the higher its service quality.

$$p(i, c_j) = \frac{\prod_{j \neq k}((1 - \pi(c_j)) * s_j^\varepsilon)}{\sum_{l=1}^{K} \prod_{m \neq l}((1 - \pi(c_m)) * s_m^\varepsilon)} k \in 1 : K \qquad (3\text{-}2)$$

c_j : Elderly welfare facilities

$\pi(c_j)$: Facility Importance

s_j: Number of users per employee in charge

K: Number of all districts in the same area

Table 1 and Table 2 show that (2) is a function of service quality, and the probability of selecting a facility including the factor (2) is 24.9%, and the probability of selecting a facility excluding the factor (2) is 40.7%, or about 0.612, so ε in Eq. (3-2) is set at 0.61.

3.3 Network Creation Methods

Facility Network Configuration

Figure 1 shows the facility network organization procedure used in this study. The basic threshold values used in this study are based on the previous studies (See Fig. 1).

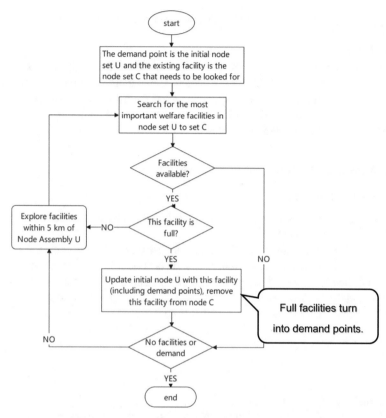

Fig. 1. Facility network organization procedure

Demand Points-Facilities Network

This network includes a population center point (demand point) from which facilities are searched for until there are no facilities or demand, based on whether facilities are available or not, and whether facilities are full or not. Finally, the network is divided into zones based on the relationship between existing facilities and demand points.

Supply and Demand State of the Facilities

X_i is a parameter that determines the state of the demand point. z_j is a parameter that determines the state of the elderly care facility. The demand point-facility network configuration algorithm stops when $\prod_{i=0}^{m} x_i = 1$ and $\prod_{i=0}^{n} z_j = 1$ are satisfied.

How to Connect Convenient Facilities from the Points of Demand

First, find the nearest neighbor day care facility C from node U and connect the facility with the highest importance to the demand point. The importance of the facility is calculated using Eq. (3-1).

$$max \ \pi_j = \max \exp(-d(i, c_j)^\tau / Q(c_j))$$

d_{max}: Distance limit (maximum usage distance) for the service is set at 5 km.

Connection to the Following Facilities
If the demand exceeds the capacity of the first facility connected, the next facility is looked for and the closest facility is connected. When there is no facility or demand to calculate, the algorithm terminates. Interconnected facilities are considered a group of facilities in the same zone. All facilities (even if stand-alone) belong to one of the zones and are automatically divided into zones.

3.4 Elderly Care Facility Optimization Model

3.4.1 Facility Loss Model

(1) Calculate the number of customers that can be served by the staff of one facility per week, i.e., the service rate μ_j.
(2) Calculate the total number of clients arriving per week, i.e., the expected arrival rate λ_j. This is the arrival rate assuming that each customer is set in terms of the number of times he/she uses the facility in a unit of time and that he/she arrives according to a Poisson distribution within a period. Note that in the problem setting of this study, all facilities are assumed to be vacant at time 0.

Arrival Rates:

$$W_i = w_i f(i) \qquad \lambda_j = \sum p(i, c_j) W_i \tag{3-3}$$

i: demand point identifier. $i \in I(i)$
$p(i, c_j)$: Probability that a customer at demand point i can go to facility j
w_i: Weekly demand at demand point

Service Utilization Rate
The service utilization E_j (traffic intensity in the queue) for facility j can be calculated.

$$\rho = \lambda_j / \mu_j \quad E_j = \lambda_j / N_j \mu_j \tag{3-4}$$

N_j: Number of staff at facility j

Customer Waiting Time Calculation
Calculate the average wait time for one facility based on the customer arrival rate, the facility's service rate and the number of staff [5].

$$\text{Waiting Time, } WQ_j = \frac{\rho^{N_j}}{\mu (N_j - 1)!(N_j - \rho)^2} / (\sum_{P_j=0}^{N_j-1} \frac{\rho^{P_j}}{N_j!} + \frac{\rho^{N_j}}{(N_j - 1)!(N_j - \rho)}) \tag{3-5}$$

N_j: Number of staff at facility j
P_j : Number of people in queue at facility j

ρ: Service intensity per staff member

Demand Unsatisfaction Loss
When customer waiting time exceeds the customer's tolerance, the service quality is turned down because the demand cannot be satisfied. (Demand Unsatisfaction Rate = (Arrival Rate - Facility Service Rate)), calculated as an indicator of demand unsatisfaction, and the sum of the two is further summed up.

When the customer arrival rate is greater than the service rate:

$$If \ E > 1 \quad \partial_i = \lambda_j - N_j \mu_j \tag{3-6}$$

Underutilization Loss
If the customer wait time is sufficiently less than the standard wait time, i.e., the workforce is waiting for a long time, then the workforce is underutilized, further exacerbating the labor shortage. Here, when the customer waiting time is less than the standard waiting time, the facility is judged as underutilized. The minimum arrival rate is calculated as an indicator of underutilization using (standard arrival rate - average arrival rate), and the sum of the two is further summed up. δ is set at 0.02. The minimum arrival rate is the arrival rate when the customer waiting time is the standard waiting time.

$$If \ 0 < WQ_i < \delta \quad \theta_j = \lambda_j - \overline{\lambda_j} \tag{3-7}$$

Facility Loss Function
(see Table 3).

Table 3. Facility status judgment.

Terms	Facility Status
$E > 1$	demand-unsatisfied loss
$0 < WQ_i < \delta$	under-utilization loss
$E < 1 \ and \ WQ_i > \delta$	normal facility

K: All are sets of areas.

$$K = \{1, 2, 3, \ldots\ldots\} \ k \in K$$

Minimize the facility loss accumulation in each area and optimize the facility loss accumulation in the kth network. Specifically, the optimization is based on $loss_j$ expressed in the following equation.

$$loss_j = \begin{cases} \pi_j(\lambda_j - N_j \mu_j) & if \ \lambda_j \geq N_j \mu_j \\ \pi_j(\overline{\lambda_j} - \lambda_j) & if \ \lambda_j < N_j \mu_j \end{cases} \tag{3-8}$$

Loss of facilities throughout the same district

$$F(k)_{loss} = \min \sum_{i \in A} \pi_i(\lambda_i - N_j\mu_j) + \min \sum_{j \in B} \pi_j(\overline{\lambda_j} - \lambda_j) = \min(\sum_{i \in A} \pi_i \partial_i + \sum_{j \in B} \pi_j \theta_j)$$
(3-9)

Set A: The set of demand-unsatisfied bottleneck facilities in the k area-facility network area.

Set B: k areas - the set of bottleneck facilities with insufficient utilization in the facility network area.

3.4.2 Search for Facilities in Need of Improvement by Regret Value

Regret Value
Different zones have different facility loss accumulations, and if the facility loss accumulation in one zone is greater than that in another zone, the degree of improvement needed will also be greater. Among all areas, determine the area with the largest loss difference. Here, it is represented by the regret value REGR in the equation below.

$$REGR = \max(F(X)_{loss} - F(Y)_{loss})$$
(3-10)

$$X \in K \quad Y \in K \quad X \neq Y$$

$$s.t. \quad REGR \geq 0$$

Objective Function
To balance the facility losses in all areas, the worst areas need to be improved, i.e., the areas where the regret value in Eq. (3-10) is large.

$$min \; REGR$$

Improve only the worst facilities at a time until the utility reaches 0, achieving the highest effect with the least facility changes. *Change* is the number of facilities that need to be improved.

$$min \; Change$$

Facility Improvement by Regret Value
Step 1: Initialization

$$Change = 0$$

Step 2: Change = Change + 1 Step 3: For a given *Change*, improve the facility with the largest facility loss and solve the following model.

$$min \; REGR$$

Step 4: constraint

$$REGR \geq 0 \quad REGR \leq \gamma$$

is satisfied. If it is satisfied, go to step 5; otherwise, return to step 2. Where γ is the equilibrium criterion.

Step 5:

$$\min \quad Change = \varepsilon \tag{3-11}$$

Outputs the Eq. (3-11) solution and stops.

3.4.3 Cluster of Facilities in Need of Improvement

A facility is clustered if the distance between two facilities in need of improvement falls within a certain range. Facilities in the same cluster are clusters that can cooperate with each other.

K center point facilities are set

$$1 \leq K < n(n \text{ is the number of facilities that need improvement}) \quad K \in N \quad K = \{1, 2, \ldots, n\}$$

Step 1: Initialization (1) All combinations of center point facilities are computed and recorded in the same array. (2) In the distance matrix, all distances are set sufficiently large $M = 0$.

Step 2: Randomly select a combination from the list of combinations, calculate the total cost, and replace it with a distance that meets the distance criteria in the distance matrix. These two partner facilities are then classified into the same cluster.

$$dis_{ij} < d_{max} \quad Cost = \sum_{i \in C} \sum_{j \in c_i} dis_{ij} \tag{3-12}$$

Step 3: Eq. (3-12) If the total cost is less than the existing cost, replace the existing cost; if the total cost is greater than the existing cost, assume $M = M + 1$ and return to Step 2.

However, if $M > L$ for the end condition of the specified number of times L, proceed to 4.

Step 4: Output the best result obtained because of clustering the facility and stop execution.

3.4.4 Improvement Program

Facility Cooperation (Facility Scale Change)

When an under-utilized facility is adjacent to an undemanding facility, each facility may select a portion of its workforce as a co-member to be utilized at the facility in need. The facilities cooperate with each other and transfer staff from the underutilized facility to be used at the underutilized facility. Cooperation game theory is used to find the optimal

Table 4. Facility Classification and Solutions

Facility Status		Solutions
Not a bottleneck facility next door	demand-unsatisfied facilities	New Facility Locations
	underutilized facilities	Facility closures and consolidation
Bottleneck facility next door	Unsatisfactory demand and underutilized facilities	Facility Cooperation and consolidation
	Unsatisfactory and Unsatisfactory Demand Facilities	New Facility Locations
	Underutilized and underutilized facilities	Facility consolidation

state of cooperation. After cooperation staffing is balanced according to facility needs. (Distance between is within 3 km)

$$\frac{\sum_{i \in C} \lambda_i}{\sum_{i \in C} \mu_i} = \frac{\lambda_i}{\mu'_i} \quad C = \{1, 2, \ldots\}$$

Procurement Personnel:

$$\partial_i = \frac{\mu_i - \mu'_i}{\sigma} \quad \text{Min} \, \aleph = \sum_{i \in c} \partial_i \tag{3-13}$$

where λ_i is the arrival rate of customers at one facility, μ_i is the service rate, μ_i' is the service rate after procuring personnel, and Eq. (3-13). $\aleph$ is the total number of people to procure. Based on the service rate, the number of people required to be procured is calculated, expressed as ∂_i. The higher the efficiency of personnel procurement, the lower the cost, and the smaller the total number of people to be procured, the better.

Facility Consolidation (Facility Closure)
If adjacent facilities are also bottleneck facilities, create a situation where multiple bottleneck facilities can complement each other. Calculate the utility after integration and apply the optimal integration method. This is based on the strategy of increasing the service rate that can be handled at the same inventory level by consolidating the inventories of multiple locations into a single inventory in production management. For example, the aim is to significantly reduce the inventory level by consolidating multiple inventory levels from a situation where each location is responding to variations in demand. (Unutilized rate is more than 50%).
    Before consolidation

$$loss_o = \sum_{i \in O} \pi_i loss_i \quad O = \{1, 2, \ldots\}$$

After consolidation

$$N = \sum_{j=1}^{j \in H_i} N_j \qquad \mu_{combine} = \sigma N \qquad \lambda_{combine} = \sum_{combine} p_j w_i$$

$$loss_o' = \begin{cases} \pi_i(\lambda_{combine} - \mu_{combine}) if \ \lambda_{combine} > \mu_{combine} \\ \pi_i(\overline{\lambda_{combine}} - \lambda_{combine}) if \ \lambda_{combine} < \overline{\lambda_{combine}} \\ 0 \end{cases}$$

Utility calculation, optimization:

$$\max v_o = loss_o - loss_o' \qquad (3\text{-}14)$$

where $\mu_{combine}$ is the service capacity after facility integration and $\lambda_{combine}$ is the customer arrival rate after facility integration. The best integration method is selected by calculating the facility loss after integration and the improvement effect formula (3-14).

Facility Establishment
If, after implementing the above two improvement measures, demand is still significantly higher than services in the same area and demand is unsatisfactory, a new facility will need to be located. By locating a new facility, the customers in the area will have more freedom in choosing a facility. In this section, the optimal location of a new location is derived based on demand data. (Shortage is at least 10 people).

Required capacity.

$$\beth = w_i - \sum_{j \in k} c_j \qquad p_{best} = \frac{\beth}{w_i}$$

Optimal position

$$p_{best} = \frac{\prod_{j \neq k}((1 - \pi(c_{best}, i)) * s_j^\varepsilon)}{\sum_{l=1}^k \prod_{m \neq l}((1 - \pi(c_{best}, i)) * s_m^\varepsilon)} \rightarrow d(i, c_{best}) \qquad (3\text{-}15)$$

$\beth$ is the portion of this area lacking facility capacity, and $\beth$ can be used to calculate the probability of getting customers to the new facility based on $\beth$. Finally, the optimal distance is calculated based on Eq. (3-15).

4 Numerical Experiments

4.1 Analysis and Improvement Simulation Using Actual Data

Figure 2 shows the population estimates for Bando City. This data is used to establish the population distribution of demand [9] (See Fig. 2).

Elderly Population Situation
Adapted from [6] the use of welfare facilities for the elderly. These are referenced as

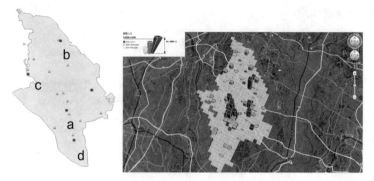

Fig. 2. Population projection (Bando City) [8]

the utilization rate of day-care facility services for the elderly relative to the elderly population.

According to the elderly population of Bando City, as well as the ratio of elderly who use day-care and day-rehabilitation services and the ratio of those who need nursing care, to estimate the population in need of nursing care.

Demand Point Situation
Table 5 shows the estimated results of the degree of demand considering the density and ratio of the population starting from the demand point in Bando City, the population distribution.

Table 5. Population projection of need points

Demand point number	a	b	c	d	e
Level of need	307	97	85	19	164

Population density (per square kilometer): 417.7 (as of July 1, 2022) [8].
Area: 123.03 square kilometers (as of April 1, 20).

Bando City Demand Points - Facility Network Configuration
Figure 3 shows the results of the analysis of the Demand Point-Facility Network Organization, using data from Bando City. In the same figure, the zones are shown as ovals. Blue dots are population center points of demand points, red dots are unsatisfactory demand elderly care facilities, black dots are underutilized facilities, and green dots are facilities in normal operation. The probability Eq. (3-2) that a customer wants to go to a facility is displayed on the line, constituting a network from the demand point to the facility. (See Fig. 3).

Figure 4 shows an example of facility loss and classification of facilities. The red columns are facility losses for unsatisfied demand facilities, and the black columns are facility losses for underutilized facilities. And the results of the analysis of Eqs. (3-11) and (3-12) (See Fig. 4).

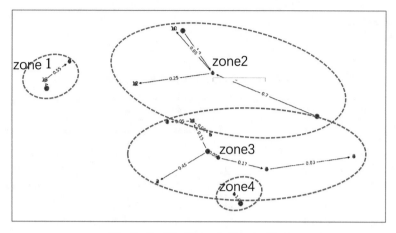

Fig. 3. Facility Network (Bando City)

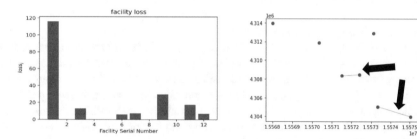

Fig. 4. Facility Loss and Cluster of facilities in need of improvement (Bando City)

Searching for facilities in need of improvement by regret value and clustering facilities in need of improvement. From among the facilities that need improvement, those that should be retained and those that should be eliminated are selected, the optimal staffing and network configuration are redefined. Based on these results, the optimal strategy is determined. (See Fig. 4).

Factual Comparison
(See Table 6).

Table 6. Bando City Actual Situation

Facility No.	1	2	3	4	5	6	7	8	9	10	11	12	13
Actual number of people	186	128	51	24	18	24	11	10	28	14	28	52	36
Simulation	211	138	52	20	18	27	15	9	46	8	46	41	38

Improvement Program
(See Table 7).

Table 7. Facility Improvement Program

Facility cluster	zone number	Improvement method	Criteria
Facility 1, 9	2	New Facility Locations	The shortage is at least 10
Facility [7, 11] [3, 6]	3	Facility Cooperation	Distance is within 3 km
Facility 12	2	Facility Expansion	The shortage is only 5 persons

Based on the proposed solutions in Table 4, we summarized how to improve facilities in need of improvement in each area.

Evaluation of Improvement Effectiveness

Figure 5 shows the results of building 14(120 capacity) and 15(10 capacity) near facilities 1 and 9 according to the improvement plan, adjusting the number of employees by cooperating with facilities 3 and 6, and adjusting the size and number of employees of facilities 12 and 11. In the figure, the blue dots indicate the population center points of the demand points, and the green dots indicate the elderly care facilities. As a result of the network from the demand point to the facility, the numbers on the arrows indicate the probability that a customer wants to go to.

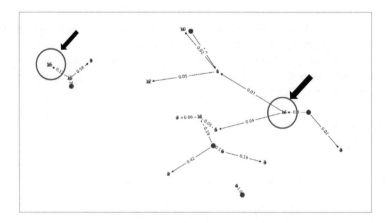

Fig. 5. Predicted Effects of Improvements

5   Comparison and Discussion of Previous Studies

Hu Feiyu, & Kawakami Mitsuhiko [2] developed a model that handles the admission capacity and available area of day care facilities in a facility utilization model and includes the concepts of maximum distance and weekly frequency of use to determine the facilities to be used to achieve the minimum total distance. Model 1 is the model of Hu Feiyu, & Mitsuhiko Kawakami [2], Model 2 is my model. Error rates for facilities are the difference between the simulated and actual number of people divided by the actual number of people for separate facilities (Table 8).

Table 8. Simulation results of the comparative model

Facility No.	1	2	3	4	5	6	7	8	9	10	11	12	13
actual	189	128	51	24	18	24	11	10	28	14	28	52	36
Simulation	159	46	21	3	12	6	30	49	24	7	24	114	6
Model 1	0.16	0.64	0.6	0.86	0.33	0.75	1.73	3.9	0.14	0.5	0.14	1.19	0.8
Model 2	0.12	0.78	0.2	0.17	0	0.13	0.36	0.1	0.64	0.42	0.64	0.21	0.06

Result Analysis

Comparing the two models, the model2 performs better for each facility and is smaller with respect to the mean error; only for facilities 2 and 11 the error rate is higher than in model 1.

6   Conclusions and Issues

6.1   Conclusion

There are three research strengths of this study. The first is that the original model was modified to determine customer choice not only by distance, but also by the importance of the facility. Large-scale facilities tend to be built far from the population due to land costs and size. By taking this factor into account, the model has the advantage that simulation results do not deviate significantly from those of facilities in less populated areas.

Second, facilities are automatically classified according to demand points, and the impact between facilities is also considered. The model considers the impact of changes in size, quality of service, etc. on other facilities when new facilities are built or when facilities are consolidated.

The third was to minimize the costs required to achieve the objectives while optimizing the placement-allocation of facilities. Previous studies have not considered how to reduce change costs while achieving objectives when improving facility allocation-allocation. The present study then further improves the feasibility of the model based on previous studies.

There are two weaknesses of this study: first, the distribution of elderly customers in an aging society does not actually exist on a point-by-point basis. The distribution of the elderly population varies from region to region, with some areas being very concentrated and others scattered. Since the distribution does not exactly match the distribution of the entire population, there are some situations where generalizations cannot be made.

Second, if the amount of data is very large, the model results will be unstable. Calculations using all the data for Ibaraki Prefecture will result in unstable calculation times, and continuous improvement of the algorithm is necessary.

6.2 Future Issues

There are three main challenges for the future. First, it is recommended that facilities and clients be classified according to the level of care needed, considering factors such as local population, facility location and capacity, labor force as well as local economy, topography, etc.; when networking demand and facilities, add the interaction of clients and facilities and arrange staffing and hours; provide each client and facility with specific reference information, etc. are recommended. Second, it is not sufficient to consider only the current situation based on existing data. What is more important in considering improvement measures, including new construction, is to predict the future welfare situation, such as decades from now, and to optimize based on the prediction. For this purpose, it is desirable to simulate the automatic evolution of facilities using machine learning and models that predict the future elderly population and mobility status. Third, the impact of policies in different regions should also be considered. This is because different policies lead to different directions of development of community welfare facilities. In a situation where the cost of care is increasing, the economic situation of the elderly should also be considered.

References

1. Bhattacharya, B., Kameda, T., Song, Z.: Minmax regret 1-center algorithms for path/tree/unicycle/cactus networks. Discrete Appl. Math. **195**, 18–30 (2015)
2. Feiyu, H., Mitsuhiko, K.: A study on demand distribution and allocation planning of welfare facilities for the elderly using a mathematical model: a case study of Kanazawa City. City Plan. Rep. **11**(2), 67–72 (2012)
3. Hatakeyama, T.: Location of long-term care insurance day care facilities and decision conditions at the time of facility selection. Hum. Geogr. **57**(3), 332–346 (2005)
4. Iyigun, C., Ben-Israel, A.: The multi-facility location problem: a probabilistic decomposition method. Comput. Optimiz. Appl. (2013). www.optimization-online.org/DB_FILE/2012/08/3555.pdf
5. Kondo, M., Takahashi, K., Himeno, T., Otani, H., Hirose, Y.: A study on evaluation and layout planning of day-care type welfare facilities for the elderly. City Plan. Rev. **37**, 769–774 (2002)
6. Matsumura, Naomichi, Date, & Yoshihiko.: Basic indicators and evaluation of geriatric health and welfare planning in municipalities in Ibaraki Prefecture. Annual Report of the Research Institute for Regional Studies, Ibaraki University, vol. 29, pp. 45–77 (1996)

7. Yokota, T.: Study on the applicability of DEA model to the proper layout planning of welfare facilities for the elderly: a study on the layout planning of regional facilities by DEA model Part 1. J. Archit. Inst. Jpn. **64**(523), 189–194 (1999)
8. WAM NET
9. https://kaigodb.com/ranking/user_per_staff/08/082287/8/

Characterizing Groups of Patients with Depression using Clustering Techniques

Ma. Sheila A. Magboo$^{(\boxtimes)}$ ⓘ and Vincent Peter C. Magboo ⓘ

University of the Philippines Manila, Manila, Philippines
{mamagboo,vcmagboo}@up.edu.ph

Abstract. Depression is a disorder characterized by a variety of symptoms that includes changes in psychomotor function, weight changes, sleep disturbance, difficulty concentrating, suicidal thoughts, fatigue, and extreme feelings of guilt or worthlessness persisting for at least two weeks affecting more than 300 million people worldwide. However, this is believed to be an underestimate as many people are not seeking professional help due to many reasons such as lack of resources, lack of access to mental health professional, and due to social stigma associated with the condition particularly in low-income countries. The aim of the study is to identify patient subgroups with distinct characteristics from a patient group with depression using clustering techniques. The characterization of patients in the subgroup would assist the mental health professional in instituting a more personalized treatment plan for the patient in each subgroup as there is a no "one size fits all" type of treatment for depression. Furthermore, the resulting clusters may be used as a screening tool to identify patients with a more severe type of depression and thus, be given an urgent attention when seeking professional help with a mental health provider. In this study Partitioning Around Medoids and K-modes clustering were used to identify clusters among patients labelled as having depression. Two groups were identified, and cluster characterizations were formed to describe and differentiate the clusters as well as formulate specific treatment regimens appropriate to each cluster. The identified clusters and their characterizations have a potential to be used as a screening tool to prioritize patients who may have a more severe type of depression. The collaboration of machine learning enthusiasts with mental health professionals is a step forward to the deployment and acceptability of machine learning tools in clinical practice.

Keywords: Depression · Clustering · Partitioning around Medoids · K-modes

1 Introduction

Depression, more particularly major depressive disorder, is characterized by a variety of symptoms that includes changes in psychomotor function, weight changes, sleep disturbance, difficulty concentrating, suicidal thoughts, fatigue, and extreme feelings of guilt or worthlessness [1]. These symptoms need to be persistent for at least two weeks according to the American Psychiatric Association's Diagnostic and Statistical Manual

Y.-W. Chen et al. (Eds.): KES InMed 2023, SIST 357, pp. 118–130, 2023.
https://doi.org/10.1007/978-981-99-3311-2_11

of Mental Disorders (DSM-5) [2]. Depression is a very common mental health condition affecting more than 300 million people worldwide [3]. It is believed however that the actual statistic is much higher since many of these people are not seeking professional help due to many reasons such as lack of resources, lack of access to mental health professionals, and due to social stigma associated with the condition particularly in low-income countries [4, 5]. COVID-19 pandemic worries on many issues such as health effects of the virus, loss of employment due to economic slowdown, and prolonged isolation contributed further to the rise of cases of depression. Several published studies on depression use data from high-income countries due to its easy accessibility. However, higher number of people with depression are also noted in low-income countries brought about by poverty, natural disasters (earthquakes, tsunamis), unemployment, famine, armed conflicts, epidemics, cultural and institutional biases especially in women and certain sections or the community [2, 6, 7]. In many of these countries, minimal attention is given to mental health due to limited budget for healthcare. Unfortunately, the global economic burden for mental health problems is projected to rise to 6 trillion USD by 2030 [8]. World Health Organization (WHO) set the ideal ratio of 10 psychiatrists per 100,000 population. Unfortunately, Japan was the only Asian country able to meet this criterion with 13.6 per 100,000 population while all other Asian countries reported very low ratio with Bangladesh and Pakistan having the lowest scores at 0.12 and 0.19 respectively [9]. Adding more psychiatrists or psychologists to alleviate this shortage is difficult to achieve as it is not easy to produce trained psychiatrists or psychologists. It takes years of education and training to produce competent psychiatrists or psychologists. Thus, it is of paramount importance to increase support and investments in mental health from various institutions to improve access to quality care. This includes funding for research and advocacies dealing with understanding and treatment of mental health, promoting mental health awareness, reducing the stigma among people seeking treatment, and providing training to primary care physicians, other non-mental health professionals and perhaps even schoolteachers on how to recognize and manage mental health conditions.

Due to the proliferation of publicly available healthcare datasets mostly from high-income countries, a few studies had been made about the feasibility of applying artificial intelligence methods, more specifically machine learning (ML) in clinical decision support systems, electronic health records, and genetics [10–16]. Many of these studies employed supervised learning to generate disease predictions with superior classification performance. Supervised learning is a machine learning technique that is well suited for problems with an available large, labelled dataset where the aim is to predict an outcome based on known inputs. There are also studies that utilize unsupervised learning more particularly in cases where labelled data is scarce or when the relationship between input and output is unclear, or when the objective is to uncover hidden structures and patterns in the data [17, 18]. Unsupervised learning specifically clustering is used to identify patterns in data that is not obvious leading to the discovery of new information about the disease. Clustering can be used to identify patient subgroups with similar characteristics, useful for the administration of more personalized treatment plans [19].

The objective of the study is to identify patient subgroups with distinct characteristics from a patient group with depression using clustering techniques. The characterization of patients in the subgroup would assist the mental health professional in instituting a more personalized treatment plan for the patient in each subgroup. It is strongly believed that there is a no "one size fits all" type of treatment as patients respond differently to various treatments. Hence, the need to do further analysis using clustering approaches to identify to which subgroup a patient with depression belongs to, given his clinical characteristics.

2　Literature Review

In recent years, supervised machine learning techniques have been applied to depression dataset. Aleem et al. [20] made a review of various ML techniques (classification, deep learning, and ensemble) to detect depression as well as the limitations of these published studies in depression prediction. Shunmugan et al. [21], reported various ML algorithms such as Naïve Bayes (NB), Support Vector Machines (SVM) and random forest (RF) in the classification of major depressive disorders. In [3], several ML models were applied to a publicly available and anonymized depression dataset with logistic regression (LR) as the model with the best performance (91% accuracy, 93% sensitivity, 85% specificity, 93% precision, 93% F1-score and 0.78 Matthews correlation coefficient). Authors also utilized explainable artificial intelligence method using LIME that will help the health professional in understanding the reasoning behind the model's classification of depression. In [22], authors applied several ML models to predict risk of depression in Korean college students. Results showed LR, SVM and RF generated excellent prediction probabilities as well as identified family and individual factors related to depression. In [23], authors applied various ML models to predict major depressive disorders on a publicly available depression dataset. In this study, the top features were identified to determine which attributes have high predictive power. These top features were also believed to be the important precursors of stress contributing directly to development of depression. Qasrawi et al., used ML techniques to predict the risk of depression and anxiety among school children [24]. SVM and RF showed to be the top performing models for depression with accuracy rates of 92.5% and 76.4%, respectively. The results further showed that school violence and bullying, home violence, academic performance, and family income to be the most important factors affecting the depression scales.

Likewise, unsupervised ML methods have also been applied to depression prediction. In the study by Kung et al. [25], Latent Dirichlet Allocation (LDA) was used to identify five subtypes of depression within symptom data. The five subtypes were psychotic, severe, mild, agitated, and anergic-apathetic and these subtypes were characterized by clusters of unique symptoms. In [26], authors used unsupervised deep learning algorithms on minute-level actigraphy data taken from wearable sensors on persons with depression, schizophrenia, and normal controls. Results showed unsupervised clustering of naturalistic data aligns with existing diagnostic constructs. Iqbal et al. [27], studied various unsupervised learning clustering classifiers for implementation in stress monitoring wearable devices. Their results showed that unsupervised machine learning classifiers can also generate good classification performance when compared to the supervised ML models but without the need for time-consuming training phase. Chen et al. utilized ML methods to replicate three symptom clusters of patients with depression [28]. Results showed that antidepressants demonstrate different treatment effects for each symptom profile and thus can help physicians in selecting personalized treatment for patients with depression. Finally, Yang et al. [29], used unsupervised ML method using K-means clustering to construct depression classifications among Chinese middle and high school students. Authors listed the benefits of K-means clustering method as the ability to set a fixed number of meaningful and practically useful clusters, little need for parameter adjustment, and its low computational complexity.

3   Materials and Methods

The study consisted of 3 phases. In Phase 1, all features in the original dataset of patients classified as having depression were used in clustering. In Phase 2, only the top 13 features identified in the previous work in [3] underwent clustering. In Phase 3, a consultation with a mental health professional was done to assist in the characterization of the clusters.

The original dataset was obtained from a publicly available anonymized online machine learning repository. The dataset was consists of 604 records of patients labeled as either "with depression" or "without depression". Only those records that were labelled "with depression" were included in the machine learning pipeline. A check for existence of null values was done. Furthermore, duplicate records were eliminated resulting in the inclusion of only 391 records. Since the objective of the study is to identify potential clusters of patients among those classified as having depression, the target feature was also removed. In Phase 1, the resulting reduced dataset underwent preprocessing (scaling and normalization) and then checked for cluster tendency using Hopkins statistic and Visual Assessment of Cluster Tendency (VAT). After the verification of cluster tendency, the optimal number of clusters was determined using the Bayesian Information Criterion (BIC) as specification of the optimal number of clusters is a requirement in most clustering algorithms. Two popular clustering techniques, the Partitioning Around Medoids (PAM) and K-modes, were used to determine the clusters. In Phase 2, The same approach was repeated but using only the top features identified in the previous work in [3]. In Phase 3, a mental health professional was consulted to assist in the characterization of the resulting clusters. As there is a no "one-size fits all" type of treatment applicable to all patients with depression, identification of clusters among patients with depression would help any mental health professional device a more appropriate, more tailor-fit type of treatment regimen. All computations were done using R version 4.0.2 (2020–06-22). The machine learning pipeline corresponding to this study is shown in Fig. 1.

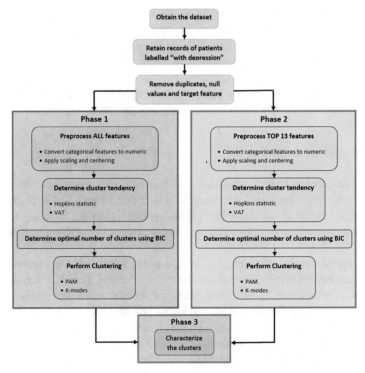

Fig. 1. Machine Learning Pipeline for Characterization of Clusters of Patients with Depression

3.1 Dataset Description

A publicly available anonymized depression dataset retrieved from github was used in the study [30]. The dataset contains 604 records with 455:149 male–female sex ratio, 30 predictor variables and one target variable (depressed or not) based on Burns Depression Checklist. The description of the attributes is in the previous work in [3] As the objective of the study was to identify potential subgroups among patients with depression, patients labelled without depression were removed. Records with null values were also removed resulting to a reduced dataset of only 391 out of the 604 records.

3.2 Phase 1–Clustering using all features provided in the dataset.

After selecting the records that will be included in this study, data preprocessing was performed on the reduced dataset containing 391 records. The categorical features were converted to numeric then normalized and scaled to compute the Hopkins statistic (from hopkins package). This was used to assess for the presence of cluster tendency. Visual Assessment of Cluster Tendency (VAT) test was also performed to visualize the clusters. After confirming the clustering tendency, the optimal number of clusters was determined using Bayesian Information Criterion (BIC). Clustering algorithms using the Partitioning Among Medoids (PAM) and K-modes were used to identify the different clusters among patients with depression.

3.3   Phase 2–Clustering Using Only the Top 13 Features.

In Phase 2, the processes performed in Phase 1 were repeated but this time utilizing only the top 13 features identified in the previous work in [3]. This was to determine if there will be changes in the cluster characterizations identified in Phase 1.

3.4   Phase 3–Cluster Characterization

In Phase 3, the clusters identified in Phases 1 and 2 were presented to a mental health professional for assistance in cluster characterization to determine their clinical significance and severity of depression.

4   Results and Discussion

A total of 391 patients with depression were subjected to clustering techniques. The computed Hopkins statistics were 0.86 and 0.70 in Phase 1 where clustering was obtained using all features and in Phase 2 containing only the top 13 features, respectively. These values indicated that both datasets have good clustering tendency. VAT was also performed to visualize presence of the clusters in both datasets as shown in Fig. 2 a) for the dataset consisting of all features and in Fig. 2b) for the dataset with only top 13 features. The resulting VATs clearly suggested clusterable data as there were visible blocks along the diagonal. The red block represented high similarity (i.e., low dissimilarity) while the violet areas represented low similarity (i.e., high dissimilarity). Additionally, the VAT from the dataset with complete list of features generated better results than that of top 13 features as the red blocks were more clearly delineated. Moreover, Fig. 2a) seemed to suggest presence of two clusters. The BIC of the mclust package was executed to determine the optimal number of clusters which eventually confirmed the presence of two clusters for both datasets as shown in Fig. 3. After confirming 2 optimal clusters, clustering algorithms specifically PAM and K-modes were performed.

In the two datasets with all features and only top 13 features, all features were categorical. As such, these datasets must be label-encoded as integers to use a K-medoids algorithm such as PAM to partition the datasets into k clusters. The resulting clusters for the dataset with all the features are shown in Table 1. Likewise, for the dataset containing the top 13 features are seen in Table 2. PAM performed well on datasets with categorical attributes as seen in this study. However, according to [31] clustering accuracy decreases when PAM is used on datasets with mixed attribute types or with numeric attributes where Manhattan distance is not used. K-modes clustering was also used to determine the clusters for the two datasets containing categorical features. Unlike K-means which utilizes the means to represent the clusters, K-modes uses the modes or the most frequently occurring values to represent the clusters. The K-modes algorithm computes the dissimilarity measure of categorical variables and assigning each point to the cluster whose dissimilarity measure is the smallest. K-modes is an effective technique for categorical datasets while retaining the efficiency of the original k-means clustering algorithm suited for numerical datasets [32, 33]. Tables 3 - 4 show the resulting clusters using K-modes for the dataset consisting of all features and the dataset with only the top 13 features, respectively. The highlighted features in Tables 1 - 4 were believed to be contributory to the severity of depression.

Upon consultation with a mental health professional, PAM applied to the depressed dataset consisting of all features (PAM Cluster 1) was characterized as patients with mild depressive symptoms since the only features prominently seen in

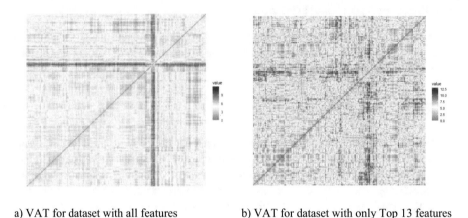

a) VAT for dataset with all features   b) VAT for dataset with only Top 13 features

Fig. 2. Visual Assessment of Cluster Tendency (VAT)

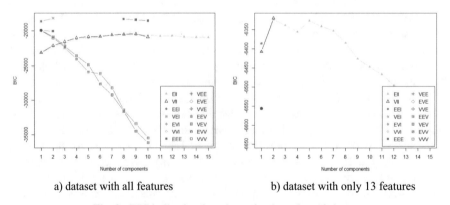

a) dataset with all features   b) dataset with only 13 features

Fig. 3. BIC indicating 2 as the optimal number of clusters.

this group were: have lost a loved one, has some financial difficulty, and is not satisfied with his current position. Psychotherapy sessions and/or starting dose medication as well as other non-pharmacological forms of treatment such as lifestyle–based interventions may be prescribed [34, 35]. Psychotherapy is an effective treatment for depression as it identifies and validates possible reasons for depressive feelings and learn new coping skills. On the other hand, PAM Cluster 2 was characterized as patients with more severe depressive symptoms. In this cluster, patients exhibited more symptoms such as anxiety,

Table 1. PAM clusters for the dataset using all features.

Features	PAM Cluster 1	PAM Cluster 2	Features	PAM Cluster 1	PAM Cluster 2
AGERNG	21-25	21-25	PREMED	No	Yes
GENDER	Male	Male	EATDIS	No	No
EDU	Graduate	HSC	AVGSLP	7 hours	Below 5 hours
PROF	Student	Student	INSOM	No	Yes
MARSTS	Unmarried	Unmarried	TSSN	5-7 hours/day	2-4 hours/day
RESDPL	Town	Village	WRKPRE	Mild	Mild
LIVWTH	W/o Family	With Family	ANXI	No	Yes
ENVSAT	Yes	No	DEPRI	No	Yes
POSSAT	No	No	ABUSED	No	No
FINSTR	Yes	Yes	CHEAT	No	Yes
DEBT	No	Yes	THREAT	No	Yes
PHYEX	Sometimes	Sometimes	SUICIDE	No	Yes
SMOKE	No	No	INFER	No	Yes
DRINK	No	No	CONFLICT	No	Yes
ILLNESS	No	Yes	LOST	Yes	No

insomnia, unhappy with its living environment nor with its current position or academic achievement, felt deprived of something that it deserves and likewise felt cheated. Additionally, this cluster seemed to have finished only up to higher secondary school, and thus expectedly experienced inferiority complex. This group was also in conflict with either friends or family and at some point, and had suicidal thoughts. As such, patients in PAM Cluster 2 would require more psychotherapy sessions, higher dose medications and possibly be subjected to other forms of treatment such as electroconvulsive therapy as compared to PAM Cluster 1 since this group may have suicidal tendencies [34]. Likewise, patients in this cluster lived with his family and had conflict with them, a family therapy approach may be pursued to educate family members about depression [36]. For PAM applied only to the top 13 features, PAM Cluster A was characterized with the following symptoms: presence of anxiety, financial difficulty, feelings of deprivation of something he deserved, and unsatisfactory feelings with his position in society or achievements. Psychotherapy or a combination of psychotherapy and low dose medications and other non-pharmacological interventions such as lifestyle-based interventions may be pursued to address these symptoms [34, 35]. On the other hand, PAM Cluster B was characterized as a more severe form of illness by having more depressive symptoms on top of all the symptoms of PAM Cluster A such as unsatisfied with current environment, felt abused and cheated, presence of inferiority complex, and conflict with family and friends. Presence of more symptoms of negative feelings and perceptions about self and society require a combination of more frequent psychotherapy and medications and other forms of treatment [34].

In K-modes Cluster 1, patients with depression were characterized as having experienced anxiety and financial difficulty, not satisfied with their position in society nor

Table 2. PAM clusters for the dataset using the top 13 features.

Features	PAM Cluster A	PAM Cluster B	Features	PAM Cluster A	PAM Cluster B
ENVSAT	Yes	No	INSOM	No	No
POSSAT	No	No	THREAT	No	No
FINSTR	Yes	Yes	SUICIDE	No	No
ANXI	Yes	Yes	INFER	No	Yes
DEPRI	Yes	Yes	CONFLICT	No	Yes
ABUSED	No	Yes	LOST	No	No
CHEAT	No	Yes			

their achievements, had experienced moderate pressure from work and felt deprived. For this group, counseling and/or medication and other lifestyle–based interventions can be instituted [34, 35]. On the other hand, K-modes Cluster 2 was characterized as more severe with symptoms such as: experienced anxiety and financial difficulty, currently in debt, felt deprived and experienced severe work pressure. For this group, a combination of psychotherapy and antidepressants plus other forms of treatment may be given particularly to address work productivity problems [34]. Several complications may occur due to a loss of work or study opportunity. Generally, the patient can be given counselling to improve on his coping mechanisms especially at work or be advised to have a job change to relieve him of the stress [35]. For K-modes applied only to the top 13 features, K-modes Cluster A was characterized with the following symptoms as: has anxiety, feels deprived, not satisfied with current position in society and experiencing financial difficulty. This was very similar to K-modes Cluster 1 and thus, the same treatment regimen may be administered. Similarly, K-modes Cluster B had all the symptoms in Cluster A plus other symptoms such as presence of insomnia, had lost a loved one recently, felt abused and cheated, had inferiority complex and recently in conflict with family or friends. All of these pertain to a more severe form of the illness and would require more frequent counselling, higher dose medications and other treatment forms [34].

Table 3. K-modes clusters for the dataset using all features.

Features	K-modes Cluster 1	K-modes Cluster 2	Features	K-modes Cluster 1	K-modes Cluster 2
AGERNG	21-25	21-25	PREMED	No	No
GENDER	Male	Male	EATDIS	No	No
EDU	Graduate	Graduate	AVGSLP	6 hours	7 hours
PROF	Student	Student	INSOM	No	No
MARSTS	Unmarried	Unmarried	TSSN	2-4 hours/day	2-4 hours/day
RESDPL	City	Town	WRKPRE	Moderate	Severe
LIVWTH	With Family	With Family	ANXI	Yes	Yes
ENVSAT	Yes	Yes	DEPRI	Yes	Yes
POSSAT	No	Yes	ABUSED	No	No
FINSTR	Yes	Yes	CHEAT	No	No
DEBT	No	Yes	THREAT	No	No
PHYEX	Sometimes	Sometimes	SUICIDE	No	No
SMOKE	No	No	INFER	No	No
DRINK	No	No	CONFLICT	No	No
ILLNESS	No	No	LOST	No	No

Table 4. K-modes clusters for the dataset using the top 13 features.

Features	K-modes Cluster A	K-modes Cluster B	Features	K-modes Cluster A	K-modes Cluster B
POSSAT	No	No	ENVSAT	Yes	No
FINSTR	Yes	Yes	THREAT	No	No
INSOM	No	Yes	SUICIDE	No	No
ANXI	Yes	Yes	INFER	No	Yes
DEPRI	Yes	Yes	CONFLICT	No	Yes
ABUSED	No	Yes	LOST	No	Yes
CHEAT	No	Yes			

5 Conclusions and Recommendations

Clusters among patients with depression using two different clustering techniques, PAM and K-modes were determined. With the guidance of a mental health professional, the characterization of these clusters was determined and in consonance with the clinical assessment of severity of depression. Both PAM and K-modes were able to highlight the differences between the clusters and can thus be useful in the institution of potential treatment approaches appropriate for these patients. Additionally, the generated clusters can be used as potential screening tool to determine extent of the illness which could be utilized to identify patients with a more severe type of depression and thus, be given an urgent attention when seeking professional help. The collaboration of ML enthusiasts with the mental health professionals is a step forward to the deployment and acceptability of ML tools in clinical practice. As the machine learning calculations were obtained using a publicly available depression dataset, it is highly recommended to do more analysis using local depression datasets for an in-depth characterization of patients in local practice.

References

1. Chand, SP., Arif, H.: Depression. [Updated 2022 Jul 18]. In: StatPearls [Internet]. Treasure Island (FL): StatPearls Publishing; 2022 Jan-. Available from: https://www.ncbi.nlm.nih.gov/books/NBK430847/
2. Ridley. M., Rao, G., Schilbach, F., Patel, V.: Poverty, depression, and anxiety: Causal evidence and mechanisms. Science, 370(6522), eaay0214 (2020). https://doi.org/10.1126/science.aay0214
3. Magboo, V.P.C., Magboo, M.S.A.: Important Features Associated with Depression Prediction and Explainable AI. In: Li, H., Ghorbanian Zolbin, M., Krimmer, R., Kärkkäinen, J., Li, C., Suomi, R. (eds) Well-Being in the Information Society: When the Mind Breaks. WIS 2022. Communications in Computer and Information Science, vol 1626 (2022). Springer, Cham. https://doi.org/10.1007/978-3-031-14832-3_2
4. Brouwers, E.P.M.: Social stigma is an underestimated contributing factor to unemployment in people with mental illness or mental health issues: position paper and future directions. BMC Psychol, 8(36) (2020). https://doi.org/10.1186/s40359-020-00399-0
5. Martinez, A.B., Co, M., Lau, J., Brown, J.S.L.: Filipino help-seeking for mental health problems and associated barriers and facilitators: a systematic review. Soc. Psychiatry Psychiatr. Epidemiol. **55**(11), 1397–1413 (2020). https://doi.org/10.1007/s00127-020-01937-2
6. Herrman, H., Patel, V., Kieling, C., et al.: Time for united action on depression: a Lancet-World Psychiatric Association Commission. Lancet (London, England) **399**(10328), 957–1022 (2022). https://doi.org/10.1016/S0140-6736(21)02141-3
7. Rathod, S., Pinninti, N., Irfan, M., et al.: Mental Health Service Provision in Low- and Middle-Income Countries. Health services insights **10**, 1178632917694350 (2017). https://doi.org/10.1177/1178632917694350
8. Proudman, D., Greenberg, P., Nellesen, D.: The Growing Burden of Major Depressive Disorders (MDD): Implications for Researchers and Policy Makers. Pharmacoeconomics **39**(6), 619–625 (2021). https://doi.org/10.1007/s40273-021-01040-7
9. Isaac, M., Ahmed, H.U., Chaturvedi, S.K., et al.: Postgraduate training in psychiatry in Asia. Curr. Opin. Psychiatry **31**(5), 396–402 (2018). https://doi.org/10.1097/YCO.0000000000000444
10. Javaid, M., Haleem, A., Singh, R.P., Suman, R., Rab, S.: Significance of machine learning in healthcare: Features, pillars and applications. International Journal of Intelligent Networks **3**(2022), 58–73 (2022). https://doi.org/10.1016/j.ijin.2022.05.002
11. Magboo, M.S.A., Coronel, A.D.: Data Mining Electronic Health Records to Support Evidence-Based Clinical Decisions. In: Chen, Y.-W., Zimmermann, A., Howlett, R.J., Jain, L.C. (eds.) Innovation in Medicine and Healthcare Systems, and Multimedia. SIST, vol. 145, pp. 223–232. Springer, Singapore (2019). https://doi.org/10.1007/978-981-13-8566-7_22
12. Magboo, V.P.C., Magboo, M.S.A.: Machine Learning Classifiers on Breast Cancer Recurrences. Procedia Computer Science **192**, 2742–2752 (2021). https://doi.org/10.1016/j.procs.2021.09.044

13. Magboo, V.P.C., Magboo, M.S.A.: Classification Models for Autism Spectrum Disorder. In: Kumar, A., Fister Jr., I., Gupta, P.K., Debayle, J., Zhang, Z.J., Usman, M. (eds) Artificial Intelligence and Data Science. ICAIDS 2021. Communications in Computer and Information Science. 2022; 1673. Springer, Cham. https://doi.org/10.1007/978-3-031-21385-4_37

14. MacEachern, S.J., Forkert, N.D.: Machine learning for precision medicine. Genome **64**(4), 416–425 (2021). https://doi.org/10.1139/gen-2020-0131

15. Magboo, M.S.A., Magboo, V.P.C.: Explainable AI for Autism Classification in Children. In: Jezic, G., Chen-Burger, YH.J., Kusek, M., Šperka, R., Howlett, R.J., Jain, L.C. (eds) Agents and Multi-Agent Systems: Technologies and Applications 2022. Smart Innovation, Systems and Technologies. 2022; 306. Springer, Singapore. https://doi.org/10.1007/978-981-19-3359-2_17

16. Magboo, V.P.C., Magboo, M.S.A.: Prediction Models for COVID-19 in Children. In: Chen, YW., Tanaka, S., Howlett, R.J., Jain, L.C. (eds) Innovation in Medicine and Healthcare. Smart Innovation, Systems and Technologies. 2022; 308. Springer, Singapore. https://doi.org/10.1007/978-981-19-3440-7_2

17. Eckhardt, C.M., Madjarova, S.J., Williams, R.J., et al.: Unsupervised machine learning methods and emerging applications in healthcare. Knee surgery, sports traumatology, arthroscopy : official journal of the ESSKA **31**(2), 376–381 (2023). https://doi.org/10.1007/s00167-022-07233-7

18. Wagner, M., Bodenstedt, S., Daum, M., et al.: The importance of machine learning in autonomous actions for surgical decision making. Artificial Intelligence Surgery, 2(2):64–79 (2022).https://doi.org/10.20517/ais.2022.02

19. Lau, K.Y., Ng, K.S., Kwok, K.W., et al.: An Unsupervised Machine Learning Clustering and Prediction of Differential Clinical Phenotypes of COVID-19 Patients Based on Blood Tests-A Hong Kong Population Study. Front. Med. **8**, 764934 (2022). https://doi.org/10.3389/fmed.2021.764934

20. Aleem, S., Huda, N., Amin, R., Khalid, S., Alshamrani, S.S., Alshehri, A.: Machine Learning Algorithms for Depression: Diagnosis, Insights, and Research Directions. Electronics **11**(7), 1111 (2022). https://doi.org/10.3390/electronics11071111

21. Shunmugam, M., Pavaiyarkarasi, R., Seethalakshmi, E., Shabanabegum, S.K., Anusha, P.: A comparative study of classification of machine learning algorithm for depression disorder: A review. AIP Conf. Proc. **2519**, 050036 (2022). https://doi.org/10.1063/5.0110221

22. Minji, G., Suk-Sun, K., Jeong, M.E.: Machine learning models for predicting risk of depression in Korean college students: Identifying family and individual factors. Frontiers in Public Health, 10 (2022). https://www.frontiersin.org/articles/, https://doi.org/10.3389/fpubh.2022.1023010

23. Magboo, V.P.C., Magboo, M.S.A.: Major Depressive Disorder Prediction Using Data Science. Philippine Journal of Health Research Development, 26 (3), 41 – 50, (2022). https://pjhrd.upm.edu.ph/index.php/main/article/view/647

24. Qasrawi, R., Vicuna Polo, S.P., Abu Al-Halawa, D., Hallaq, S., Abdeen, Z.: Assessment and Prediction of Depression and Anxiety Risk Factors in Schoolchildren: Machine Learning Techniques Performance Analysis. JMIR Formative Research **6**(8), e32736 (2022). https://doi.org/10.2196/32736

25. Kung, B., Chiang, M., Perera, G., Pritchard, M., Stewart, R.: Unsupervised Machine Learning to Identify Depressive Subtypes. Healthcare Informatics Research **28**(3), 256–266 (2022). https://doi.org/10.4258/hir.2022.28.3.256

26. Price, G.D., Heinz, M.V., Zhao, D., Nemesure, M., Ruan, F., Jacobson, N.C.: An unsupervised machine learning approach using passive movement data to understand depression and schizophrenia. J. Affect. Disord. **316**, 132–139 (2022). https://doi.org/10.1016/j.jad.2022.08.013

27. Iqbal, T., Elahi, A., Wijns, W., Shahzad, A.: Exploring Unsupervised Machine Learning Classification Methods for Physiological Stress Detection. Frontiers in Medical Technology, 4 (2022). https://www.frontiersin.org/articles/, https://doi.org/10.3389/fmedt.2022.782756

28. Chen, Y., Stewart, J., Ge, J., Cheng, B., Chekroud, A., Hellerstein, D.: Personalized symptom clusters that predict depression treatment outcomes: A replication of machine learning methods. Journal of Affective Disorders Reports **11**, 100470 (2023). https://doi.org/10.1016/j.jadr.2023.100470

29. Yang, Z., Chen, C., Li, H., Yao, L., Zhao, X.: Unsupervised Classifications of Depression Levels Based on Machine Learning Algorithms Perform Well as Compared to Traditional Norm-Based Classifications. Frontiers in Psychiatry, 11, (2020) https://www.frontiersin.org/articles/https://doi.org/10.3389/fpsyt.2020.00045

30. Sabab31/Depression-Repository,   https://github.com/Sabab31/Depression-Repository.git, last

31. Dixon, M.-G., Genov, S., Hnatyshin, V., Thayasivam, U.: Accuracy of Clustering Prediction of PAM and K-Modes Algorithms. In: Arai, K., Kapoor, S., Bhatia, R. (eds.) FICC 2018. AISC, vol. 886, pp. 330–345. Springer, Cham (2019). https://doi.org/10.1007/978-3-030-03402-3_22

32. Saxena, A., Singh, M.: Using Categorical Attributes for Clustering. International Journal of Scientific Engineering and Applied Science (IJSEAS), 2 (2): 324 - 329, (2016). https://ijseas.com/volume2/v2i2/ijseas20160238.pdf

33. Harous, S., Harmoodi, M.A., Biri, H.: A Comparative Study of Clustering Algorithms for Mixed Datasets," 2019 Amity International Conference on Artificial Intelligence (AICAI), Dubai, United Arab Emirates, 484–488 (2019). https://ieeexplore.ieee.org/document/8701347

34. Bains N, Abdijadid S. Major Depressive Disorder. [Updated 2022 Jun 1]. In: StatPearls [Internet]. Treasure Island (FL): StatPearls Publishing; 2022 Jan-. Available from: https://www.ncbi.nlm.nih.gov/books/NBK559078/

35. Marx, W., Manger, S., Blencowe, M., et al.: Clinical guidelines for the use of lifestyle-based mental health care in major depressive disorder: World Federation of Societies for Biological Psychiatry (WFSBP) and Australasian Society of Lifestyle Medicine (ASLM) taskforce. The World Journal of Biological Psychiatry, https://doi.org/10.1080/15622975.2022.2112074

36. Katsuki, F., Watanabe, N., Yamada, A., Hasegawa, T.: Effectiveness of family psychoeducation for major depressive disorder: systematic review and meta-analysis. BJPsych open **8**(5), e148 (2022). https://doi.org/10.1192/bjo.2022.543

Automatic Recognition of Check-Points for NCPR Video Review

Noboru Nihshimoto[1]([✉]), Mitsuhito Ando[1], Haruo Noma[1], and Kogoro Iwanaga[2]

[1] Ritsumeikan University, Shiga, Japan
nnishimoto@mxdlab.net
[2] Kyoto University, Kyoto, Japan

Abstract. The goal of the Neonatal Resuscitation Promotion Project is to promote neonatal cardiopulmonary resuscitation (NCPR), which is an indispensable skill to help doctors and nurses save the life of a newborn whose respiratory circulation is unstable immediately after birth. Workshops are held throughout Japan consisting of lectures, scenario training, and review in support of this goal. In the NCPR workshop, it is recommended to review student activities in the scenario practice by using video. However, the time available for review is limited, which makes it somewhat difficult to play and review the entire video. Our concept is to save review time by automatically detecting essential scenes in scenario practice. In this study, we tackled the detection of essential scenes the instructor wanted to emphasize. First, we developed and experimented with an annotation tool and analyzed the results to identify the essential scenes. Second, we utilized two techniques to detect student behavior, namely, sensor recognition and image recognition, and investigated which was more suitable. In future work, we plan to create a system that automatically generates video teaching materials from automatically extracted scenes.

Keywords: NCPR · Review · Sensor · Object detection

1 Introduction

The Japan Society of Perinatal and Neonatal Medicine aims to ensure that "medical personnel trained in neonatal cardiopulmonary resuscitation (NCPR) are present at all deliveries". In 2007, the Society initiated a project to promote the widespread implementation of NCPR [1], but its success so far has been limited, mostly due to a lack of NCPR instructors and equipment. This study aims to facilitate the widespread usage of NCPR through information technology. The NCPR workshop consists of three key elements: lectures, where the instructor imparts basic knowledge to the students; scenario training, where the instructor teaches the NCPR procedure using a simulated newborn; and review, where the instructor explains the good and bad points of the scenario training to the students [2]. There are various methods to facilitate "awareness" among students in terms of errors and the implications of their actions, one of which is a video review. We previously developed a video review system with a manual bookmark function for highlighting key scenes to facilitate the video review. However, as most instructors were unfamiliar with the manual bookmark function, efficiency was reduced and it could not be utilized to perform other tasks [3].

Our current research aim is to automate the bookmark function through image recognition. As a first step, we want to identify the specific scenes instructors feel should be emphasized. We therefore developed annotation tools and asked instructors to mark the relevant scenes. Our analysis of the annotation data showed that the instructors typically wanted to emphasize scenes including errors in knowledge, good technique, bad technique, delayed decisions, and rapid decisions. These findings represent an important milestone in the automation of the bookmarking function and enabled us to establish recognition categories using previous experiments and NCPR textbooks. We implemented the recognition of NCPR procedures using two techniques, sensor recognition and image recognition, and found that sensor recognition (specifically, GVI) was the superior approach. To further improve the recognition accuracy, we investigated the recognition of multiple and single categories of procedures and the selection of training data by the implementation scenario.

2 NCPR Simulator

Two types of simulator are used in NCPR workshops: an expensive high-function one and an inexpensive low-function one. High-function simulators can reproduce vital signs and low-function ones cannot, but due to budget limitations, general hospitals often use the low-function simulator. As a result, when instructors conduct an NCPR workshop with a low-function simulator, they typically utilize alternative simulation techniques such as reproducing the heart rate by tapping on a desk or imitating a baby's cry by using their own voice (Fig. 1).

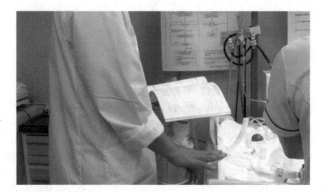

Fig. 1. Reproducing heart rate by tapping on a desk

Previous studies have shown there are two challenges when it comes to using low-function simulators in the classroom setting: the heavy burden on the instructor and the lack of realism. To resolve these, we previously proposed augmenting low-function simulators with simulated medical devices (Fig. 2) [3] consisting of electronic components

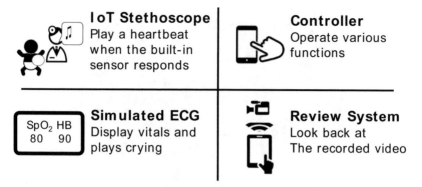

Fig. 2. NCPR simulator (taken from The Development of Simulator Using Neonatal Doll for the Neonatal Cardiopulmonary Resuscitation Training Workshop, TDP vol. 3, no. 4, Noboru Nishimoto; 2022).

and smartphone applications. This approach was able to improve the learning effect while reducing the implementation cost.

The 2020 Guidelines of the NCPR recommend using video reviews to help students view procedures objectively [1]. However, as mentioned earlier, the usage of video reviews is not widespread due to a lack of equipment and the heavy workload imposed on instructors. For example, if instructors cannot recall the exact timing of a scene, they typically have to replay the entire video, resulting in wasted time and potentially a break in the students' concentration. Moreover, students are forced to watch irrelevant scenes, which can reduce the effectiveness of video review even further.

Although we developed a video-review system with a bookmark function to address these issues (Fig. 3) [3], our evaluation with an instructor showed that he could not recall the content of the bookmarked scenes because he was too busy with multitasking. The instructor suggested that "automating the bookmarking function could reduce this burden on the instructors", so our current goal is to automate the bookmarking function by applying recognition technology.

As a first step, we defined a comprehensive list of attention points based on the input of several instructors. We denote these scenes that the instructor wishes to emphasize as "check-points". Our concept is that automatically recognizing and presenting these check-points to the students will reduce the instructor's workload as well as the time it takes to complete the review.

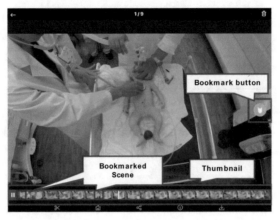

Fig. 3. Video review system (taken from The Development of Simulator Using Neonatal Doll for the Neonatal Cardiopulmonary Resuscitation Training Workshop, TDP vol. 3, no. 4, Noboru Nishimoto; 2022).

3 Check-Points in NCPR Scenario Training

In this section, we explain our analysis of the annotation data and how we identified check-points. As a first step, we developed a check-point collection system (Fig. 4) [4] to determine the types of scenes instructors want to emphasize during video review. In this system, users select a video from a drop-down menu and watch it using the play/pause buttons at the top of the timeline. They then assign three rating tags using buttons at the bottom, specifically, "Requires improvement", "Not so good," and "Excellent". They can also view the list of rating tags and add comments at any time.

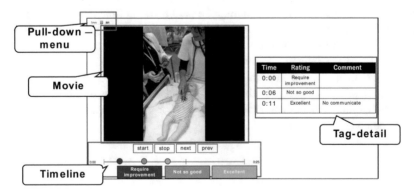

Fig. 4. Check-point collection system (taken from Trial of automatic review point recognition in NCPR workshop, IPSJ Interaction 2020, Kana Tamura; 2020).

We evaluated the system by conducting an experiment in which instructors were asked to specify check-points in videos from an NCPR workshop and comment freely on the scenes. They were particularly encouraged to comment on significant scenes. The experimental conditions included a total of four participants (all of whom were certified NCPR instructors and neonatologists) and 27 NCPR workshop videos. We categorized the free-text comments into the following three categories.

1. Knowledge based on NCPR algorithm
2. Teamwork of students performing the procedure
3. Accuracy of procedures performed by the students

We analyzed the scenes pointed out by the instructors in the comments and videos and identified the categories of scenes that the instructors wanted to emphasize. In total, 386 annotated items of data were obtained: 296 related to the procedure, 37 to communication between students, 12 to the knowledge of NCPR, 18 to time management, and 23 to other items. As the target of this study is automatic recognition, we focused on items related to "procedure" and divided the check-points into two categories:

1. When the procedure was performed and what it was
2 The quality of the procedure

First, we describe which procedure was performed at which time. Note that we focus on auscultation, ventilation, chest compressions, and tracheal intubation procedures, as these are the ones most frequently selected by instructors as check-points in the annotation data (auscultation: 90, artificial respiration: 104, chest compressions: 21, tracheal intubation: 81) and are essential components of the NCPR algorithm (Fig. 5).

Second, we describe the quality of the procedure. In NCPR scenario training, it is essential that students perform the procedure appropriately. For example, if chest compressions are not performed properly, blood cannot be pumped throughout the body and the neonate will die. It is therefore necessary to evaluate the overall quality of the procedure, including pressure, timing, and position of pressure application. The results of our analysis of the annotation data also indicated that many instructors emphasized the accuracy of the procedure. In the next section, we present two techniques for recognizing the procedure types and procedure accuracy: sensor-based recognition and image-based recognition.

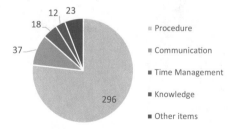

Fig. 5. Essential scenes in NCPR workshop videos pointed out by instructors.

4   Automatic Recognition Techniques

4.1   Technique Based on Image Recognition

Two image recognition techniques for action recognition, specifically, YOLOv5 [5] and Google Video Intelligence (GVI) shot analysis [6], were evaluated to determine which was more suitable for action recognition. We utilized 300 NCPR training videos as training data and set four recognition categories: auscultation, ventilation, chest compressions, and tracheal intubation.

First, we trained with YOLOv5 for 100 epochs and yolo5m weights without implementing any padding process. We chose yolo5m because it is a well-balanced model in terms of accuracy and detection speed, and it also provides high recognition accuracy even with relatively small datasets. We selected procedural scenes from the videos and then assigned bounding boxes to the video frames to create a dataset composed of images. We split the data into a 7:2:1 ratio for training, validation, and testing. The specific data breakdown was 1361 for tracheal intubation, 5526 for ventilation, 10,846 for auscultation, and 5026 for chest compressions. The recognition results of YOLOv5 under these conditions are shown in Fig. 6(a).

Second, we trained with Google Video Intelligence (GVI) for action recognition. No padding process was applied. We selected procedural scenes from the videos and split the training, validation, and test data in a ratio of 7:2:1. The specific data breakdown was 137 for tracheal intubation, 188 for ventilation, 527 for auscultation, and 148 for chest compressions. The recognition results of GVI under these conditions are shown in Fig. 6(b).

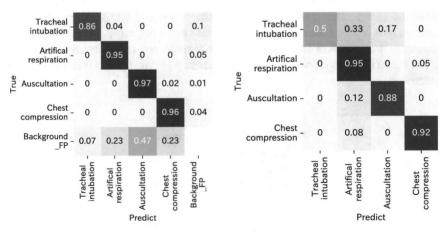

a) Recognition results of YOLOv5   **b)** Recognition results of GVI

Fig. 6. Image recognition results. **a)** Recognition results of YOLOv5 **b)** Recognition results of GVI

We used the created model to perform recognition on video data and then evaluated the accuracy (Table 1). The results showed that YOLOv5 had a low recognition

Table 1: Recognition accuracy for real data.

	Tracheal intubation		Artificial respiration	
	Recall	Precision	Recall	Precision
YOLOv5	0.69	0.56	0.41	1.00
GVI	0.77*	0.77*	0.83*	0.83
	Auscultation		Chest compression	
	Recall	Precision	Recall	Precision
YOLOv5	0.78	0.73	0.77	1.00
GVI	0.68	0.43	0.91*	1.00*

accuracy on video data, possibly due to overfitting. GVI showed a superior recognition rate, presumably because it utilizes temporal convolutional long-short memory (TCLL), which allows comparison between two videos (Fig. 7) [8]. In detail, TCLL implements a nearest-neighbor method for classifying procedures in videos by comparing the frames of one video with the closest matching frame in another video and determining that they belong to the same category if they are cycle-consistent. This approach also allows for the optimization of video uniformity by selecting the frame that minimizes the loss function. As a result, GVI can recognize the initial movements of the procedure. Moreover, since GVI is a web-based API service, it does not require any local computing power. For these reasons, we consider GVI a more suitable choice for the automatic recognition of the video review system than YOLOv5.

However, it is difficult to measure the quality of the procedure (e.g., the timing and pressure of chest compressions) by image recognition. In the next section, we present the sensor recognition technique for measuring the procedure quality.

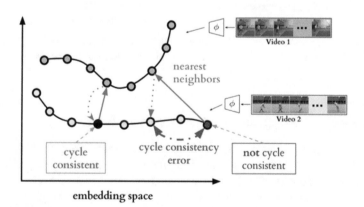

Fig. 7. Temporal convolutional long-short memory (taken from Temporal Cycle-Consistency Learning, IEEE Xplore 2019, Debidatta Dwibedi; 2019).

4.2   Technique Based on Sensor Recognition

The following subsections provide further details on our recognition approach. To start with, sensor-based procedure recognition has the following two key advantages.

1. Sensors can easily measure the quality of the procedure.
2. Sensors can reliably provide accurate measurement results.

We utilized air pressure and pressure sensors to recognize chest compressions and artificial respiration (Fig. 8) [8]. The M5Stack device was used to display pressure values. We also utilized a proximity sensor to recognize auscultation. By placing the sensor on the tube, the system is able to recognize intubation.

This sensor technology enables us to detect the occurrence and timing of procedures by analyzing the electrical signals emitted by the sensors. We can also quantify the quality of the procedure by examining the voltage levels of the sensors. Three specific steps are identified from the sensor data: the initiation of chest compression pressure, the cessation of that pressure, and the timing of the release. These sensors also have higher reliability than image recognition methods.

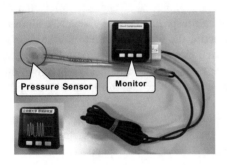
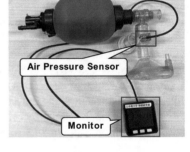

| a) Chest compression recognition system | b) Artificial respiration recognition system |

Fig. 8. Sensor recognition system (taken from Self-Skill Training System for Chest Compressions in Neonatal Resuscitation Workshop, KES International 2020, vol. 192, Noboru Nishimoto; 2020).

4.3   Appropriate Recognition Techniques for Check-Points

Our aim in this study is to automatically identify check-points to aid in the video review. This subsection discusses the appropriate recognition techniques for two types of check-points: which procedure was performed at which time, and the quality of the procedure.

First, we discuss the recognition of the type and timing of the procedure. Both image and sensor recognition are effective here, but sensor recognition has problems related to implementation cost, specifically, the price of sensors, maintenance costs, and complexity of settings. Therefore, image recognition, which is less expensive to implement, is more appropriate. Among the image recognition techniques we examined,

GVI is the most suitable because it is a web API and does not require the power of a local machine.

Second, we discuss the recognition of the quality of the procedure. Here, it is necessary to measure the timing of the procedure, the pressure, and the position of the pressure. Image recognition cannot identify the pressures and positions, whereas sensor recognition can, thus making sensor recognition more appropriate.

Instructors had asked to be able to highlight the behavior of two students individually, but it is difficult to handle multiple students with sensor recognition alone. Doing so might be possible if we used a combination of image recognition and sensor recognition (e.g., image recognition technology that can identify individuals, such as ByteTrack [9], and the sensor recognition utilized in this study). In future work, we will combine these methods to achieve more accurate scene awareness.

	Tracheal intubation	Artifical respiration	Auscultation	Auscultation +Artifical respiration	Chest_comp +Artifical respiration
Tracheal intubation	0.91	0.09	0	0	0
Artifical respiration	0	0.97	0	0.03	0
Auscultation	0	0.06	0.75	0.19	0
Auscultation +Artifical respiration+	0	0.03	0.07	0.83	0.07
Chest_comp +Artifical respiration	0	0	0	0	1

True / Predict

Fig. 9. GVI recognition results. **a)** Artificial respiration and auscultation **b)** Artificial respiration and chest compression.

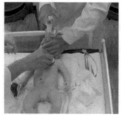 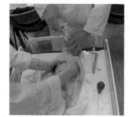

a) Artificial respiration and auscultation

b) Artificial respiration and chest compression

Fig. 10. Composite categories.

5 Accuracy Improvement

Google Video Intelligence (GVI) compares and recognizes items on the entire screen, so separating composite categories from a single category would presumably improve the accuracy. Examples of composite categories include scenarios where two students perform procedures A and B simultaneously, while a single category would refer to instances where one student is performing only one procedure. We therefore re-trained with a more realistic dataset of learning categories and were able to achieve a higher accuracy (Fig. 9).

In general, there are four single categories, and the maximum number of combinations of composite categories is six. However, in this study, we set three single categories and two composite categories for recognition. Therefore, we chose to focus on recognizing three single categories and two composite categories rather than targeting four single categories and six composite categories, for two reasons.

1. The complexity of performing procedures simultaneously at the same site (such as the combination of artificial respiration and intubation on the head or chest compressions and auscultation on the chest).
2. The limited prevalence of certain procedures in NCPR training (such as the combination of artificial respiration and auscultation or artificial respiration and chest compressions (Fig. 10)).

6 Conclusion

In this study, we aimed to automate the bookmark function using image recognition to facilitate training in NCPR workshops. First, we asked an instructor to identify scenes in a video he wanted to emphasize so that we could get an idea of which scenes were important. We then came up with two models for recognizing four types of procedures and experimentally showed that GVI was suitable for performing the recognition. In future work, we plan to detect three additional types of scenes (the status of the knowledge base, the students' teamwork, and the procedure's accuracy), with the ultimate goal of creating a system that can automatically recognize check-points for NCPR video review.

References

1. Neonatal Cardiopulmonary Resuscitation Homepage Accessed 27 JAN 2023. https://www.ncpr.jp/eng/
2. Shigeharu Hosono, Neonatal Resuscitation Instructor Manual based on the Japanese Guidelines for Emergency Resuscitation 2020 (2021)
3. Noboru Nishimoto, The Development of Simulator Using Neonatal Doll for the Neonatal Cardiopulmonary Resuscitation Training Workshop, TDP vol. 3(4) (2022)
4. Kana Tamura Trial of automatic review point recognition in NCPR workshop, IPSJ Interaction 2020 (2020)
5. Redmon, J., Once, Y.O.L.: Unified. Real-Time Object Detection, IEEE CVPR **2016**, 779–788 (2016)
6. Google Inc. Auto ML Intelligence Document. Accessed 27 JAN 2023. https://cloud.google.com/video-intelligence/automl/docs?hl=en

7. Dwibedi, D.: Temporal Cycle-Consistency Learning, In: IEEE Xplore 2019 (2019)
8. Noboru Nishimoto, Self-Skill Training System for Chest Compressions in Neonatal Resuscitation Workshop, KES International 2020, 192, pp. 81–89 (2020)
9. Zhang, Y., et al.: ByteTrack: Multi-Object Tracking by Associating Every Detection Box, ECCV 2020, 1–21 (2020) https://doi.org/10.1007/978-3-031-20047-2_1

Speech Recognition in Healthcare: A Comparison of Different Speech Recognition Input Interactions

Eugenio Corbisiero, Gennaro Costagliola(ID), Mattia De Rosa(✉)(ID),
Vittorio Fuccella(ID), Alfonso Piscitelli(ID), and Parinaz Tabari(ID)

Department of Informatics, University of Salerno, Via Giovanni Paolo II,
84084 Fisciano, SA, Italy
matderosa@unisa.it

Abstract. Speech recognition (SR) in healthcare has the potential to improve clinical documentation and communication among healthcare providers. In this respect, there are different ways of voice interaction. The purpose of this study is to compare four different speech recognition input interactions for healthcare form filling, without implying a specific SR algorithm, and thus to measure which interaction is the best in terms of time spent, error rate, and participant preference.

We conducted a user study involving 15 participants, divided into three groups according to their computer usage expertise. During the experiment, participants filled out forms using four different SR interactions and traditional typing.

The results showed that the interaction in which participants say all the data in a single sentence has the lowest time spent by participants, with an 83% advantage over the traditional keyboard/mouse interaction. Despite this, the System Usability Scale questionnaire revealed that the participants preferred the interaction in which they converse with a vocal assistant. Our results also found that SR interaction reduces the difference in input time between occasional and expert users.

Keywords: Speech recognition · Vocal assistant · User study · Healthcare

1 Introduction

Speech recognition (SR) is a multidisciplinary area that includes physiology, psychology, linguistics, computer science, and signal processing, as well as body language analysis, with the ultimate objective of achieving natural language communication between humans and machines. Speech recognition is slowly but steadily becoming a crucial component of human-machine interaction. This technology allows a machine to convert a voice signal into words or commands by identifying and interpreting it as well as enabling natural voice communication [15]. In the subject of voice recognition, researchers have concentrated on a variety of input interactions. In a typical interaction, users speak verbal orders to a system, and the system subsequently carries out the instructions. This is known as command-and-control. Several systems employ a natural language interface, which allows users to converse more freely with the system and allows the system to interpret the speaker's meaning rather than merely transcribing it [13].

Researchers have recently started using voice recognition technology in the medical industry in a variety of ways. One area of application is using speech recognition to enable patients to provide self-report through phone calls or mobile applications [14]. Another interaction is dictation, where users speak to a system, which transcribes their speech into a written text. Dictation interaction and its use in healthcare is a common application of speech recognition but not the only one, it's widely used in many other fields such as legal, media, and education. This type of interaction is commonly used in the healthcare field, where doctors and nurses need to transcribe patient information into electronic medical records. Another application is using speech recognition to create virtual assistants for patients. For instance, the VRA, a virtual reality assistant, can use a wearable device to communicate with the user and guide them through a series of tasks. If the user deviates from the expected results of these tasks, it may indicate that they are at risk for developing Alzheimer's Disease (AD). [19]. Additionally, researchers are exploring the use of speech recognition to create more sophisticated and accurate diagnostic tests [18].

In general, speech recognition technology can enhance the usability rate of electronic medical documentation. User acceptance, required client cognitive effort, simplicity of use, ergonomic features, and other factors may all be used to quantify usability [10].

The aim of this paper is to evaluate which speech input interaction (regardless of a specific SR algorithm) is the most efficient one for medical form filling in terms of time spent, error rate, and user preference. Five input modes including four SR interaction techniques and traditional keyboard typing were compared. The paper is organized as follows: the related work is highlighted in Sect. 2, the form-filling input methods are described in Sect. 3, the experiment and its results are illustrated in Sects. 4 and 5. Finally, Sect. 6 concludes the paper by discussing the study and providing some comments on future work.

2   Related Work

SR's application in the healthcare domain, especially in clinical documentation, has been increasing lately. There are some reports that hospitals tend to utilize front-end SR platforms. One prevalent idea is to populate free-text fields of EHRs by direct dictation [1]. In this respect, there have been several studies on the application of SR in the medical field in recent years. Some areas of focus include improving the accuracy of speech recognition systems, developing systems that can recognize a wider range of accents and languages, and creating systems that can recognize speech in noisy or adverse environments. Other research has focused on using machine learning techniques to improve the performance of speech recognition systems as well as on developing ways to integrate speech recognition into a variety of applications, such as virtual assistants, language translation software, and automated customer service systems. To illustrate a few, in a study conducted in 2022, Zuchowski and Göller compared data from voice recognition with conventional typing techniques for medical recording using a prospective, non-randomized methodology [21]. The data was gathered by directly observing only the physicians who regularly utilized either this technique or typing for medical note recording, since speech recognition technology may take some time to become acclimated to. Data acquisition by physicians is regarded as an expensive activity with a high risk of burnout [6], and technologies such as SR could be beneficial to them.

The clinicians used "Dragon Naturally Speaking" by Nuance Communications and "Indicda easySpeak" by DFC Systems. Direct observation was also used to keep track of the number of errors per field on the form and the time it took to correct errors. The findings of the mentioned research demonstrated that using speech recognition technology rather than text input for clinical documents had benefits in both time and money. However, the level of staff acceptance of this technology was low [21]. In an interventional study by Peivandi et al., errors in nursing notes taken with two modes of speech recognition and handwriting methods were assessed. Online (Speechtexter) and offline (Nevisa) speech recognition software were reported to be more accurate compared to the paper method. However, the latter was prone to fewer errors [17]. Hodgson and Coiera, in a systematic review [20], analyzed the pros and cons of using speech recognition to compile clinical documentation; they arrived at the results that SR was a promising technology but with some margins of improvement. In another research project, the accuracy of cloud-based speech recognition Korean Application Programming Interfaces (APIs) in the context of medical terminology was evaluated. Naver Clova SR, Google Speech-to-Text, and Amazon Transcribe were used in their study. The recognition accuracy of all transcripts was finally compared to those created by humans as a gold standard (nursing student and physician). Naver Clova SR proved to be the most accurate system [12]. Quality and usability of documentation through two methods of typing and speech recognition were also studied in Blackley et al.'s controlled observational research. In a randomized order, two types of notes (typed and dictated) were entered into the Electronic Health Record (EHR). Afterward, the participants were asked to offer their opinions about each mode. The researchers measured documentation time spent, error count, correction count, word count, vocabulary size, and quality. Compared to dictated documents, typed notes contained more unresolved mistakes per note. In some factors like time savings and efficiency, participants were in favor of SR, although in some aspects they still preferred typing [2]. Error incidence in the SR technique was also analyzed in a study by Goss et al. First, the notes were dictated using the SR system, and then some physicians annotated the dictated notes and analyzed them to extract probable errors [9]. In another article conducted by Hodgson et al., the usability of SR was compared to that of the keyboard and mouse (KBM) technique in EHR documentation. To obtain the participants' views on working with both modes, a system usability scale (SUS) questionnaire was used [10].

There are also some commercial applications related to speech recognition in the field of medicine. 1) Nuance Dragon Medical One: an app for speech recognition that utilizes the built-in speech capabilities to accelerate routine activities like navigating, placing orders, and signing notes [16], 2) DrChrono speech-to-text software: any specialty may benefit from the speech-to-text software, which also learns speaking styles while using it [7].

Although there have been some studies in the field of speech recognition in health, and some of them compared this technology with conventional entry methods, none of them addressed the comparisons between more than two modes of data acquisition.

3   The Form Filling Input Modes

This paper presents and compares different filling modes for medical forms through speech recognition. The decision to do this study was influenced by the relevant literature, in which there is little regarding the comparison of different speech input interactions in the medical field. The four types of interaction we studied were designed after a preliminary analysis of the different speech interactions available both in the literature and software. In this paper, hybrid approaches in which the user may, for example, use voice interaction in conjunction with the use of a mouse, keyboard, or other physical devices are not covered/studied because we considered touching physical devices a possible impediment to the medical practitioner (e.g., for hygiene reasons).

The choice was also influenced by some pilot tests conducted during the development of the experiment's software that implements the different SR input modes (and also to the traditional keyboard mode). This software is a web application that uses the Google Chrome web speech API for the speech recognition part.

In the following, we describe the proposed interaction modes; the experiment and its results are described in Sects. 4 and 5. There they are also compared to the traditional mode, which involves writing on a computer keyboard. The modes have been given the following names: command mode, discursive mode, visual mode, and dialogue mode.

Command Mode. In this mode, the voice assistant stays awake to receive commands from the user. This vocal assistant is able to understand these commands:

- *insert into [field_name] value [field_value]*: with this action, the vocal assistant put [field_value] into the form field called [field_name];
- *clear*: with this command, the vocal assistant clears the entire form;
- *clean [field_name]*: with this command the vocal assistant removes a value from the [field_name] field.

Discursive Mode. The discursive mode allows the user to provide the voice assistant with all field values in a single sentence. For example, it is possible to say "name Paul surname McCartney role Nurse" and the vocal assistant will understand that in the field *name* it has to put the value *Paul*, in the field *surname* the value *McCartney* and in the field *role* the value *Nurse*.

Visual Mode. In the visual mode, the voice assistant highlights (on the screen) the field to be filled in. To start filling in, the user must say "Start filling". The voice assistant then starts by highlighting the first field and, one at a time, the remaining fields. Unlike the previous modes, the user does not have to say the name of the field or a command.

Dialogue Mode. In this mode, the user can fill out the form by having a conversation with the voice assistant. The voice assistant asks the user, for each field on the form, which values to enter, and the participant has to respond with the value of the field.

4   Experiment

We carried out a user study aimed at comparing the time spent and accuracy of the different modes to fill medical forms using the SR described above. To that end, we also include in the comparison the traditional keyboard/mouse technique. In the experiment, we asked participants to use all modes to complete three medical forms, each with a different number of fields.

4.1   Participants

For the experiment, we recruited 15 participants (3 female) either students or workers between 22 and 55 years old ($M = 31.87$, $SD = 11.99$), who agreed to participate for free. Participants were divided into three groups of five people based on their expertise in using computers:

- *Expert.* In this group, there are participants who use computers for at least 8 h a day.
- *Intermediate.* Participants in this group do not use computers frequently (7-20 h per week).
- *Occasional.* Participants in this group rarely use computers, only a few hours per month (0-10 h per month).

Regarding prior use of voice assistants, occasional participants all stated that they had no (or very limited) experience with voice assistants, while intermediate and expert participants predominantly stated that they had some experience with voice assistants, with experts reporting a higher level.

4.2   Apparatus

The experiment was conducted in two different approaches: six participants did the experiment in a laboratory, while nine participated from their homes, due to the COVID-19 pandemic. Participants who took part remotely utilized laptops with a 15-inch screen except for one with a 17-inch screen; participants who participated in the lab used a laptop with the following configuration: an Acer Aspire A315-55G with Windows 11 Professional, an Intel Core i5 2.11 GHz processor, 16 GB of RAM, a 15-inch screen with a 1920×1080 resolution, an external keyboard, and an external mouse.

The link to the experimental web application was sent to each participant, to open it in the Chrome web browser. For the participants that did the experiment in the lab, the laptop's internal microphone was used to allow the vocal assistant to "listen" to the user's voice. Participants that did the experiment remotely shared the computer screen through the Microsoft Teams video calling feature.

4.3   Procedure

Before starting the experiment, participants were instructed on the aims and procedures of the experiment; they were then asked to complete a brief survey asking for their name or nickname, age, gender, whether they were left- or right-handed, the average time they spent using a computer, and the frequency with which they declared to use voice recognition software.

Before beginning the experiment, participants went through a brief (30-minute) training session in which they learned about all the input modes. At the end of the training phase, each participant received the link to start filling out the different forms. Each one had to fill out three forms: the first one had 6 fields (4 free-text fields, 2 select from list fields), the second had 11 fields (9 text, 2 select), and the last one has 14 fields (10 text, 4 select). The start and end time of user input for each form was recorded. Each participant received a sheet, which they printed, containing the data to enter in each form. They could also watch the sheet during the experiment.

At the end of the experiment, for each of the vocal assistant's modes, participants were required to complete a SUS [11] questionnaire. Respondents are required to rate their agreement with ten statements in the SUS on a five-point Likert scale, which alternates between positive and negative. The scores on each SUS questionnaire, which range from 0 to 100, were averaged across all participants. Finally, individuals were required to respond to a questionnaire that inquired about their feedback across each input interaction and their voice assistant comments.

4.4   Design

The experiment was a two-factor design, with one between-subjects factor and one within-subjects factor. The between-subjects factor was the participant expertise, which included three levels (expert, intermediate, occasional), while the within-subjects factor was the input method, which included five levels (traditional, command, discursive, visual, dialogue).

Our dependent variables are the overall task completion time (the sum of the time required to fill in the three forms) and the number of errors (wrong text

Table 1. Counterbalancing scheme used in the user study.

Participants	Input mode order
E1, I1, O1	Traditional, Command, Discursive, Visual, Dialogue
E2, I2, O2	Command, Discursive, Visual, Dialogue, Traditional
E3, I3, O3	Discursive, Visual, Dialogue, Traditional, Command
E4, I4, O4	Visual, Dialogue, Traditional, Command, Discursive
E5, I5, O5	Dialogue, Traditional, Command, Discursive, Visual

entered in a form field). So the total number of tasks was (5 participants ×3 expertise) ×5 input modes = 75 tasks. The total task time was calculated as the sum of the time (not including rests and breaks) spent on the three forms. We counterbalanced the experiment by randomly assigning a different order mode to each participant and arranging the sessions according to the order shown in Table 1.

5   Results

All participants completed the experiment. For each participant, the experiment lasted about half an hour, excluding training. We tested significance using an analysis of repeated variance measures (ANOVA) [8].

5.1   Task Time

Regarding the time spent by participants to complete each task of the experiment, the grand mean was 274.2 s. Participants were fastest with the *discursive* mode (179.9 s), followed by *command* (258.7 s), *dialogue* (262.5 s), *traditional* (329.0 s), and *visual* (340.9 s). Moreover, as expected, expert participants were the fastest (214.7 s), followed by intermediate (248.1 s) and occasional participants (359.8 s). The chart in Fig. 1 shows the average time spent by participants, grouped according to their computer usage expertise.

The ANOVA results showed that there was a significant effect of the participant expertise ($F_{2,12} = 41.124$, $p < .0001$). The main effect of the input method on the overall task completion time was also statistically significant ($F_{4,48} = 63.910$, $p < .0001$). The interaction effect between the two factors was also statistically significant ($F_{8,48} = 10.266$, $p < .0001$).

5.2   Errors

Regarding the number of errors, the chart in Fig. 2 shows the average number of errors for each mode divided by participant expertise. The grand mean was 2.3 errors per task, and, as for task time, participants were more accurate with the *discursive* mode (1.4), followed by *command* (1.5), *dialogue* (2.4), *visual* (2.9), and *traditional* (3.1). Moreover, also in this case, the expert participants did fewer errors (1.5) than the intermediate (2.4) and occasional participants (2.8).

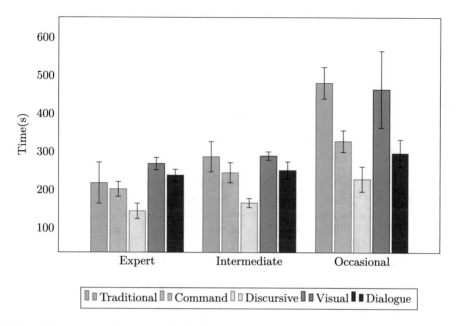

Fig. 1. Average time (in seconds) used in each mode, grouped by participant expertise. Error bars show the standard deviation.

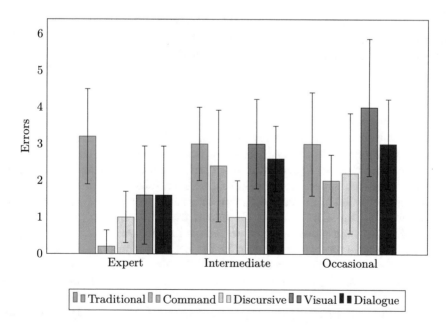

Fig. 2. Average error number for each mode, grouped by participant expertise. Error bars show the standard deviation.

Table 2. SUS results for each mode.

Mode	SUS Score (mean)
Traditional	76.2
Command	63.5
Discursive	75.7
Visual	62.7
Dialogue	82.3

The ANOVA results showed that there was a significant effect of the participant expertise ($F_{2,12} = 5.944$, $p < .05$). The main effect of the input method on the overall task completion time was also statistically significant ($F_{4,48} = 6.445$, $p < .0005$). The interaction effect between the two factors was however not statistically significant ($F_{8,48} = 1.473$, $p > .05$).

5.3   User Satisfaction and Free-form Comments

At the end of the experiments, all involved people filled out a SUS questionnaire in order to measure participant satisfaction for each mode of usage of the vocal assistant. Table 2 shows the mean SUS score for each mode.

The questionnaire revealed that participants preferred Dialogue Mode, despite the fact that Discursive Mode had the lowest time spent and errors. From the open-feedback questionnaire, we recorded some observations about each mode, and some participants reported that the tool could be more helpful with online help containing instructions on how to use it.

5.4   Discussion

The time required by the participants to complete tasks in the traditional mode exemplifies how each class of users usually interacts with computers. According to the data, expert users finished tasks considerably faster than intermediate and occasional participants. When SR interactions were used, a decrease in the time difference between expert and occasional users was observed. This reduction is positively correlated with the decrease in time required by occasional users who benefit from SR input interaction. For expert users, this happens only with the faster SR input interactions such as *discursive* input interaction.

The discursive mode turns out to be the best mode in terms of time spent and errors for all levels of user experience, as it takes less time to fill out forms than the other modes, and also has far fewer errors. The dialogue mode with the voice assistant, on the other hand, is the preferred one, according to participant feedback, as a participant only needs to speak the values requested by an assistant instead of additionally stating the form field name.

Regarding also the speech recognition performed during the experiment, the used API is of a generic type (instead of one trained on medical data) and the experiment was performed in quiet environments without significant external sound interference. We however assume that the use of a different speech recognition algorithm and a more noisy environment will affect the different interaction modes compared in our experiment in a similar way. Nevertheless, this will need to be further investigated.

6   Conclusions and Further Works

Voice assistants have increased the use of SR techniques and can improve data entry for medical records. In this study, different SR input modes were tested by different participants to see which mode is best for them. The results showed that the mode most appreciated by users (the dialogue mode) is different from the less time-consuming and less error-prone one (the discursive one). Another interesting finding is the reduction in the difference in time spent between participants with different degrees of experience to fill out the forms with SR compared to that observed with the traditional method. Future work will mainly involve further experimentation with additional form types and different types of users who already fill medical forms (e.g. physicians), and for example already use speech recognition in medical settings. We also plan to experiment on mobile devices such as smartphones, smartwatches, and tablets, which have smaller screens than the notebooks used in our experiment and offer a touchscreen-based mode of interaction where typically the default text entry is based on various soft keyboards [3–5]. Another area of further work involves improving input interactions that have been found to be faster but less popular among participants in order to improve the user experience and reduce time spent and errors.

Acknowledgment. This work was partially supported by grants from the University of Salerno (grant number: PON03PE_00060_5).

References

1. Blackley, S.V., Huynh, J., Wang, L., Korach, Z., Zhou, L.: Speech recognition for clinical documentation from 1990 to 2018: a systematic review. J. Am. Med. Inform. Assoc. **26**(4), 324–338 (2019)
2. Blackley, S.V., Schubert, V.D., Goss, F.R., Al Assad, W., Garabedian, P.M., Zhou, L.: Physician use of speech recognition versus typing in clinical documentation: a controlled observational study. Int. J. of Med. Informatics **141**, 104178 (2020)
3. Costagliola, G., De Rosa, M., D'Arco, R., De Gregorio, S., Fuccella, V., Lupo, D.: C-QWERTY: a text entry method for circular smartwatches. In: The 25th Int. DMS Conference on Visualization and Visual Languages, pp. 51–57 (2019). https://doi.org/10.18293/DMSVIVA2019-014
4. Costagliola, G., De Rosa, M., Fuccella, V., Martin, B.: BubbleBoard: a zoom-based text entry method on smartwatches. In: Kurosu, M. (eds.) Human-Computer Interaction. Technological Innovation. HCII 2022. Lecture Notes in Computer Science, vol. 13303, pp. 14–27. Springer, Cham (2022). https://doi.org/10.1007/978-3-031-05409-9_2

5. De Rosa, M., et al.: T18: an ambiguous keyboard layout for smartwatches. In: 2020 IEEE International Conference on Human-Machine Systems (ICHMS), pp. 1–4 (2020). https://doi.org/10.1109/ICHMS49158.2020.9209483

6. Dillon, E.C., et al.: Frontline perspectives on physician burnout and strategies to improve well-being: Interviews with physicians and health system leaders. J. Gen. Intern. Med. **35**(1), 261–267 (2020)

7. DrChrono Inc.: Medical speech-to-text. https://www.drchrono.com/features/speech-to-text/. Accessed 12 Dec 2022

8. Girden, E.: ANOVA: Repeated Measures. No. 84 in ANOVA: Repeated Measures, SAGE Publications (1992)

9. Goss, F.R., Zhou, L., Weiner, S.G.: Incidence of speech recognition errors in the emergency department. Int. J. of Medical Informatics **93**, 70–73 (2016)

10. Hodgson, T., Magrabi, F., Coiera, E.: Evaluating the usability of speech recognition to create clinical documentation using a commercial electronic health record. Int. J. Med. Informatics **113**, 38–42 (2018)

11. John, B.: Sus: a "quick and dirty" usability scale. Usability Eval. Ind **189**, 4–7 (1995)

12. Lee, S.H., Park, J., Yang, K., Min, J., Choi, J.: Accuracy of cloud-based speech recognition open application programming interface for medical terms of Korean. J. Korean Med. Sci. **37**, 18 (2022)

13. Liu, C., Xu, P., Sarikaya, R.: Deep contextual language understanding in spoken dialogue systems. In: Sixteenth Annual Conference of the International Speech Communication Association (2015)

14. Maharjan, R., Doherty, K., Rohani, D.A., Bækgaard, P., Bardram, J.E.: Experiences of a speech-enabled conversational agent for the self-report of well-being among people living with affective disorders: an in-the-wild study. ACM Trans. Interact. Intell. Syst. (TiiS) **12**(2), 1–29 (2022)

15. Meng, J., Zhang, J., Zhao, H.: Overview of the speech recognition technology. In: 2012 Fourth International Conference on Computational and Information Sciences, pp. 199–202. IEEE (2012)

16. Nuance Communications, Inc.: Nuance dragon medical one clinical documentation companion. https://www.nuance.com/healthcare/provider-solutions/speech-recognition/dragon-medical-one.html. Accessed 12 Dec 2022

17. Peivandi, S., Ahmadian, L., Farokhzadian, J., Jahani, Y.: Evaluation and comparison of errors on nursing notes created by online and offline speech recognition technology and handwritten: an interventional study. BMC Med. Inform. Decis. Mak. **22**(1), 1–6 (2022)

18. Sadeghian, R., Schaffer, J.D., Zahorian, S.A.: Towards an automatic speech-based diagnostic test for Alzheimer's disease. Front. Comput. Sci. **3**, 624594 (2021)

19. Tariuge, T.: Speech-based virtual assistant for treatment of Alzheimer disease patient using virtual reality environment (VRE). In: Salvendy, G., Wei, J. (eds) Design, Operation and Evaluation of Mobile Communications. HCII 2022. Lecture Notes in Computer Science, vol. 13337, pp. 378–387. Springer, Cham (2022). https://doi.org/10.1007/978-3-031-05014-5_31

20. Tobias Hodgson, E.C.: Risks and benefits of speech recognition for clinical documentation: a systematic review. J. Am. Med. Inform. Assoc. **23**, 169–179 (2016)

21. Zuchowski, M., Göller, A.: Speech recognition for medical documentation: an analysis of time, cost efficiency and acceptance in a clinical setting. British J. Healthcare Manag. **28**(1), 30–36 (2022). https://doi.org/10.12968/bjhc.2021.0074

Medical Image Processing

Improved Diagnostic Accuracy of Rheumatoid Arthritic by Image Generation Using StyleGAN2

Tomio Goto[1,2]([✉]), Reo Kojima[1,2], and Koji Funahashi[1,2]

[1] Dept. of Computer Science, Nagoya Institute of Technology, Gokiso -cho,
Showa-ku, Nagoya 466 -8555, Japan
`t.goto@nitech.ac.jp, r.kojima.485@nitech.jp`
[2] Orthopaedic Surgery, Kariya Toyota General Hospital, 5-15 Sumiyoshi-cho, Kariya,
Aichi 448-8505, Japan
`http://iplab.web.nitech.ac.jp/, http://iplab.web.nitech.ac.jp/`

Abstract. By generating images using StyleGAN2, we aimed to increase the number of test and training images. We also aimed to further improve diagnostic accuracy by generating targeted types of joint images through image manipulation. Experimental results show that image generation with StyleGAN2 is effective and improves the diagnostic accuracy of the system.

Keywords: Rheumatoid Arthritis · Automatic Measurement · Joint Space Distance

1 Introduction

With the recent development of medical technology and information processing technology, there are increasing opportunities to use various medical images such as endoscopic, MRI, and radiographic images in the field of medicine. In actual medical practice, however, physicians identify symptoms and determine the progress of medical conditions by checking these medical images directly with their own eyes, in other words, by subjective evaluation.

As mentioned earlier, there are many opportunities to use medical images. For example, multiple images are used just to assess the progression of a patient's condition. This places a heavy burden on the physician when he or she has to judge all the images of all the patients. In addition to subjective evaluation by the physician's eyes, objective evaluation using a computer is also required. In addition, considering the effects of radiation on patients, X-ray and CT images are often taken in a short period of time, resulting in low-resolution images. Therefore, there is a growing demand for the development of applications for medical image processing using computers.

Early detection and early treatment are important because early detection and appropriate treatment can control symptoms and prevent the progression

© The Author(s), under exclusive license to Springer Nature Singapore Pte Ltd. 2023
Y.-W. Chen et al. (Eds.): KES InMed 2023, SIST 357, pp. 155–163, 2023.
https://doi.org/10.1007/978-981-99-3311-2_14

of joint destruction. Therefore, it is important to detect and treat rheumatoid arthritis at an early stage. In a previous study, we developed an application to measure the distance between joints from X-ray images of patients using the characteristics of symptoms of rheumatoid arthritis, in which cartilage and bones of joints are destroyed, to determine whether patients have rheumatoid arthritis by objective evaluation, thereby contributing to early detection of rheumatoid arthritis [1–5]. However, there are many problems with this application. One problem is that some joint images do not correctly measure the distance between joints. For example, if two edges are detected that are not between joints, the distance is not measured between the upper and lower joints, but between the two edges that are not between joints. Other problems include the fact that rheumatoid arthritis has other characteristics besides the distance between joint fissures, and that the distance measurement cannot be performed on joint images in which only the upper or lower joint edges can be detected.

Therefore, a method for detecting abnormalities in rheumatoid arthritis images was proposed using a convolutional neural network with normal joint images as training images, extracting features and using a one-class SVM [6]. First, normal joint images used as training images are extracted between joints and blurred using a Gaussian filter so that feature extraction using a CNN becomes more advantageous. Then, AlexNet is used to extract the feature values of the image-processed normal joint image, and the feature area of the normal joint image is created by a one-class SVM, and the difference in features from the joint image to be diagnosed is output as an abnormality score. The system is superior in that it can diagnose rheumatoid arthritis by considering inter-articular features other than the inter-articular gap distance, it can perform diagnosis using all joint images, the system is fully automated, and it outputs an objective evaluation in the form of an abnormality score. The diagnostic accuracy of the system was measured using 20 abnormal joint images and 80 normal joint images, and the accuracy was 97%. However, the X-ray images of joints used for training are difficult to obtain, and the number of images that can be used for experiments is small, and the reliability of diagnostic accuracy is low due to the small number of test images. Therefore, we will expand the variations of training and test images by image generation and image manipulation using the GAN method proposed in this paper. In order to further improve diagnostic accuracy, we will also review the selection of the optimal convolutional neural network and the diagnostic system itself.

GANs are a type of AI called Generative Adversarial Networks [7]. The network structure of a GAN consists of a generator and a discriminator, and they compete with each other to improve accuracy. The specific GAN training process consists of preparing a "training dataset", which is a sample of data to be generated, a "generator", which is a neural network model with randomly adjusted weights, and a "discriminator". The appropriate generated data generated by the generator using random noise vectors as input values, and a certain number of training data extracted from the training dataset are input to the discriminator. The discriminator predicts whether the image is data generated from the generator or from the training dataset, and adjusts the weights of the neural network of the discriminator based on the results using error back propagation. Next, a certain number of data are generated by the generator, and they are again classified and predicted by the discriminator. Based on the results, the neural network weights of the generator are adjusted by the error back propagation method so that the discriminator mistakes the predictions for training data. The specific learning process of GAN is a system that improves the accuracy of image generation by repeating these processes a specified number of times as a set. This paper uses a type of GAN, StyleGAN2 [8], for image generation and image manipulation; StyleGAN2 is an improved version of StyleGAN [9]. StyleGAN is capable of generating very high-quality images at high resolution based on PGGAN [10], which progressively increases the resolution of the generated images. Like PGGAN, StyleGAN can not only generate high-resolution images, however, can also use algorithms to control the separation of high-level, global attributes (e.g., facial contours, presence of glasses) to local attributes (e.g., wrinkles, skin texture) in a person image [8]. This paper utilizes this characteristic to perform image manipulation to generate images of various normal and abnormal joint images. Image manipulation is performed by generating images of 20,000 joint images and identifying the dimension with the largest difference between the latent variables of normal and abnormal joint images.

2   StyleGAN2

StyleGAN [9] is a method for generating high-resolution images based on PGGAN [10]. It is characterized by its ability to control the segmentation of human images from high-level, global attributes (e.g., facial contours, glasses) to local attributes (wrinkles, skin texture) using algorithms. The network of StyleGAN2 is shown in Fig. 1, where the latent variable z is transformed nonlinearly into the latent variable W by a fully coupled neural network called the Mapping Network, and then transformed into the latent variable Style. In this paper, image manipulation was performed by changing the value of the latent variable W. Figure 2 shows the specific image manipulation of the joint images used in this paper. First, 20,000 joint images are randomly generated, and the top 100 and bottom 100 abnormality scores output by the diagnostic system are sorted on the 20,000 generated joint images, and the average latent variable W is calculated from both 100 abnormality scores. Next, the difference in the average latent variable between the top 100 and the bottom 100 abnormality scores is calculated, and the dimension of the latent variable W with the largest difference is estimated. Finally, image manipulation of rheumatoid arthritis is achieved by changing the parameters of the estimated dimensions.

3   Evaluation of Image Generation

In image generation of joint images, it is necessary to prove that it is possible to use the generated images instead of the real images, since the human eyes

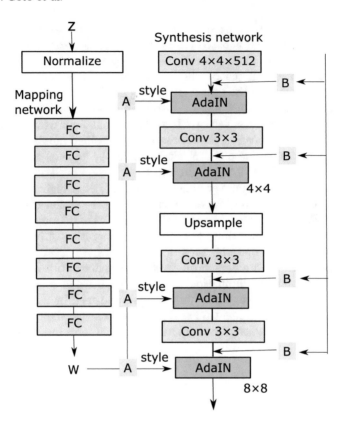

Fig. 1. Network of StyleGAN2.

can only subjectively evaluate the authenticity of the independently generated images. FID (Frechet Inception Distance) [11], a common evaluation index for GAN, was considered insufficient as an evaluation index because the model is not optimal for joint images, a large number of sample images are required, and more than 10,000 images are recommended, while joint images have been cited as a problem due to the small number of sample images. Therefore, it is important to define the criteria for successful image generation. In this paper, we define image generation as successful when the diagnostic system itself proves that the real image is mistaken for the generated image. We then used GoogLeNet [12], which is used in diagnostic systems, to classify the real images and the generated images, and visualized the diagnostic basis using a heat map as shown in Fig. 3. As a result, the generated images were judged to be real images in 85 out of 100 images. This result suggests that GoogLeNet is not able to distinguish between real and generated images.

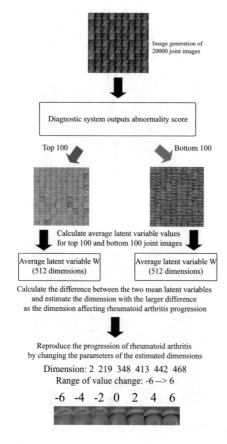

Fig. 2. Block diagram of image manipulation.

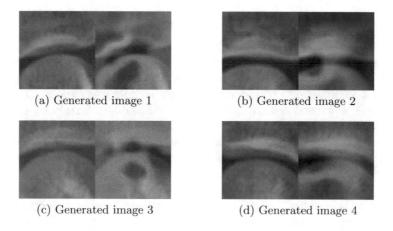

(a) Generated image 1

(b) Generated image 2

(c) Generated image 3

(d) Generated image 4

Fig. 3. Experimental results of heat-map evaluations.

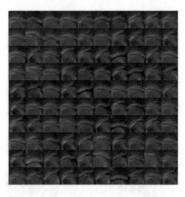

(a) Reproduced image of abnormal joint images

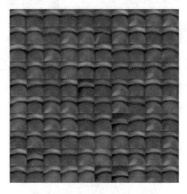

(b) Reproduced image of normal joint images

Fig. 4. Comparison of image generation.

4   Experimental Results

First, an explanation of the generated images used in the training and test images is given. From a total of 28 X-ray images of rheumatoid arthritis patients provided by a doctor, the second joint of the middle finger was clipped, and 50 real joint images were used as experimental images. Although 50 real images are too few for training images, the difficulty of adding real images made it necessary to increase the number of generated images in order to improve diagnostic accuracy. The generated images were manipulated by StyleGAN2 to generate images of abnormal joints with advanced rheumatoid arthritis and normal joints without advanced rheumatoid arthritis. The experimental condition was to generate 100 normal joint images and to confirm whether abnormal joint images could be created by image manipulation of the normal joint images. Figure 4 (a) reproduces an abnormal joint image, and Fig. 4 (b) reproduces a normal joint image. The ability to manipulate the space between joint clefts has enabled the generation

Table 1. Diagnostic results when 100 real images are used for testing.

Conditions	Diagnostic accuracy	Number of Misdiagnosis (Normality)	Number of Misdiagnosis (Abnormality)
50 real images	98%	1	1
50 generated images	98%	2	0
100 generated images	99%	0	1
1000 generated images	98%	2	0

Table 2. Diagnostic results when 1000 generated images are used for testing.

Conditions	Diagnostic accuracy	Number of Misdiagnosis (Normality)	Number of Misdiagnosis (Abnormality)
50 real images	95.8%	3	39
50 generated images	96.9%	17	14
100 generated images	98.0%	2	18
1000 generated images	97.1%	0	29

of a wide variety of normal joint images. As an evaluation experiment of the generated images, GoogLeNet was used to determine the success or failure of using them as a substitute for the real images.

We trained four patterns of images: 50 real images, 50 generated images, 100 generated images, and 1,000 generated images, and extracted the features of normal joint images using GoogLeNet. A diagnostic system that outputs an abnormality score based on the extracted features and a one-class SVM was created, and tests were conducted using two patterns of test images: 100 real images and 1,000 generated images. Table 1 shows the diagnostic results when 100 real images are used for testing, and Table 2 shows the results when 1000 generated images are used for testing. Since there is no difference in diagnostic accuracy from Table 1, it is assumed that the test images are insufficient. Table 2 shows that the test images are sufficient because of the difference in diagnostic accuracy. The highest diagnostic accuracy was obtained when 100 generated images were used as training images, confirming that the more training images are used, the better the result is. Therefore, to further improve the accuracy of diagnosis, a multi-layered diagnostic system as shown in Fig. 5 was used to prevent the combination of images for training from degrading the accuracy of diagnosis. The results are shown in Table 3. Table 3 shows a significant improvement in diagnostic accuracy, from 97.2% to 99.1%. This proves that when all training images are used at the same time, the relationship between the training images has a negative impact on the accuracy of diagnosis.

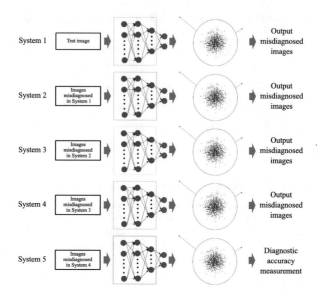

Fig. 5. Multi-layered diagnostic system.

Table 3. Experimental results when 1000 generated images are used for testing.

Conditions	Diagnostic accuracy	Number of Misdiagnosis (Normality to abnormality)	Number of Misdiagnosis (Abnormality to normality)
Previous system	97.2%	0	28
Proposed system	99.1%	0	9

5   Conclusion

In this paper, we reproduced a wide variety of diagnostic environments for rheumatoid arthritis by generating images and improved the accuracy of diagnosis. Comparisons of FID scores and GoogLeNet showed that joint images generated using StyleGAN2 can substitute for real images. Furthermore, by using a multi-layered diagnostic system, a diagnostic accuracy of 99.1% could be achieved. Future prospects include the consideration of a system that mechanically determines the balance between the quality and quantity of images for training and the use of a more optimal CNN than GoogLeNet, with the aim of further improving diagnostic accuracy.

References

1. Shimizu, M., Kariya, H., Goto, T., Hirano, S., Sakurai, M.: Super-resolution for X-ray Images. In: IEEE 4th Global Conference on Consumer Electronics (GCCE), pp.246–47 (2015)

2. Goto, T., Mori, T., Kariya, H., Shimizu, M., Sakurai, M., Funahashi, K.: Super-resolution technology for X-ray images and its application for rheumatoid arthritis medical examinations. Smart Innov. Syst. Technol. **60**, 217–226 (2016)

3. Goto, T., Sano, Y., Funahashi, K.: Improving measurement accuracy for rheumatoid arthritis medical examinations. Smart Innov. Syst. Technol. **71**, 157–164 (2017)

4. Sano, Y., Mori, T., Goto, T., Hirano, S., Funahashi, K.: Super-resolution method and its application to medical image processing. In: IEEE Global Conference on Consumer Electronics (GCCE), pp.771–772 (2017)

5. Goto, T., Sano, Y., Mori, T., Shimizu, M., Funahashi, K.: Joint Image Extraction Algorithm and Super-Resolution Algorithm for Rheumatoid Arthritis Medical Examinations. Smart Innov. Syst. Technol. **98**, 267–276 (2018)

6. Kojima, R., Goto, T.: Abnormality detection in rheumatic images using convolutional neural networks. In: IEEE Global Conference on Consumer Electronics (GCCE), pp.477–478 (2021)

7. Ian, J., et. al.: Generative adversarial networks. IEEE Signal Processing Magazine **35**(1), 53–65 (2018)

8. Karras, T., Samuli Laine, S., Aittala, M., Hellsten, J., Lehtinen, J., Aila, T.: Analyzing and improving the image quality of StyleGAN'. In: IEEE Conference on Computer Vision and Pattern Recognition (CVPR)

9. Karras, T., Laine, S., Aila, T.: A Style-based generator architecture for generative adversarial networks. In: IEEE Conference on Computer Vision and Pattern Recognition (CVPR). pp.4401–4410 (2019)

10. Karras, T., Aila, T., Laine, S., Lehtinen, J.: Progressive growing of GANs for improved quality, stability, and variation. In: International Conference on Learning Representations (ICLR), pp. 1–10 (2018)

11. Heusel, M., Ramsauer, H., Unterthiner, T., Nessler, B., Hochreiter, S.: GANs Trained by a Two Time-Scale Update Rule Converge to a Local Nash Equilibrium. In: Advances in Neural Information Processing Systems. pp.1–12, 2017

12. Szegedy, C., et al.:IEEE Conference on Computer Vision and Pattern Recognition (CVPR). pp.1–9 (2015)

BrainFuse: Self-Supervised Data Fusion Augmentation for Brain MRI's via Frame Interpolation

Robert Herscovici[✉] and Cristian Simionescu

"Alexandru Ioan Cuza" University, Iasi, Romania
hhroberthdaniel@gmail.com, cristian@nexusmedia.ro

Abstract. Deep learning has been successfully applied to medical image analysis tasks, however, the field faces unique challenges related to data scarcity. Medical datasets tend to be considerably smaller than what is accessible in the general computer vision domain. Recent state-of-the-art data augmentation techniques take advantage of combining multiple samples to create new ones. In this paper, we present such a technique and show that it can significantly improve brain age prediction from Magnetic Resonance Imaging (MRI) data. We use self-supervision to learn spatially coherent brain MRI features, and utilize that to fuse together different brain samples.

Keywords: Data Augmentation · Brain MRI · Self-Supervised Learning

1 Introduction

Deep learning has received considerable attention from the research community, which has led to many developments in a wide selection of domains and tasks. Machine learning is being used for offering diagnosis suggestions, identifying regions of interest in images, or augmenting data to remove noise and improve results. Patient privacy, along with the prohibitive costs of medical imaging, makes it difficult to procure large labeled datasets required to train deep neural networks.

An essential tool for alleviating this shortcoming is making use of data augmentation techniques. In this paper, we present such a method that has been tailored specifically for 3D medical images, in this case for the task of brain age prediction. The difference between the real age and the predicted age is an important indicator for detecting accelerated atrophy and brain diseases.

1.1 Self-Supervised Learning

Self-supervised learning is a general framework that, at its core, uses the data itself as the predictive signal to generate qualitative representations. There are two main ways of doing this:

Y.-W. Chen et al. (Eds.): KES InMed 2023, SIST 357, pp. 164–174, 2023.
https://doi.org/10.1007/978-981-99-3311-2_15

- Predictive Self-Supervised Learning (PSSL) - by hiding parts of the input data and asking the model to predict what is missing.
- Constrastive Self-Supervised Learning (CSSL) [1] - popular in the computer vision space, where a single image is augmented with two different data augmentation functions.

1.2 Semi Supervised Learning

Semi-supervised learning is a framework that allows models to use less labeled data, by leveraging unlabeled data. This is done by adding a loss term that is computed on the unlabeled data, with the aim of improving generalization. This loss term is usually in one of 2 categories: entropy minimization [2] which asks the model for confident predictions and Consistency Regularization Semi-Supervised Learning (CRSSL) which, similarly to contrastive learning, asks the model to predict similar outputs for a sample when two different augmentation functions are applied.

1.3 Contribution

Our main contribution lies in the following areas:

1. We propose a training procedure using PSSL on brain MRIs to obtain a model that can generate interpolated two-dimensional slices of the scan; (This will be detailed in the **Training the Frame Interpolation Model** Section)
2. We present an algorithm to fuse two brain scans to create a novel one using this model, by predicting the region of fusion. Using this method we can generate both label-preserving and label-free samples; (This will be detailed in the **Generating new samples** Section)
3. Using the generated data by applying self-supervised and semi-supervised learning we obtain significant improvements on the task of brain age prediction;

2 Related Work

Deep learning has been widely used for modeling brain MRIs. Model architectures range from 2D CNNs (Convolutional Neural Networks) to 3D CNNs and more modern Transformer Architectures. Regardless of the architecture used, data scarcity is a deterrent for the model's performance, making data augmentation policies a very decisive factor. As reported in [3], data augmentation methods for brain MRI are divided in the following main categories: affine transformations such as flip, rotation, translation, and scaling, elastic image transformations such as distortions, pixel-level transformations - such as adding random noise, modifying the pixel intensities, etc. Another data augmentation procedure is generating artificial data [4]. Although our method is not directly generative - such as Generative Adversarial Networks (GAN) or Variational Autoencoders, we do end up generating diverse regions of fusion.

A recent successful method to combine multiple images in order to augment the dataset is CutMix [5]. In short, new samples are created by linearly interpolating two samples. However, as it has been shown in [5], samples are locally ambiguous and unnatural.

In [6], the authors have slightly modified the Mixup procedure by pairing images with the highest amount of foreground information with the images that have the lowest. This paper is similar to BrainFuse in terms of exploiting the particularities of brain MRI images for creating a custom technique of pairing samples. However, since the generated samples are still linearly interpolations, they remain unnatural and locally ambiguous.

Another related augmentation technique is CutMix [5]. It relies on cutting and pasting image patches among training samples. This is similar to Brain-Fuse in terms of copying and pasting parts of the data, except for the following differences:

– BrainFuse makes use of a self-supervised technique to generate smooth, spatially coherent regions between the pasted patches belonging to different samples, thus making the generated samples more natural;
– While CutMix only combines two samples we go as far as mixing up to 40 samples;

The task of Video Frame Interpolation has been successfully tackled with deep neural networks [7]. In short, the frames at position i and $i+2$ are provided as input, and the frame $i+1$ is expected as output. We take inspiration from this by modelling brain MRI's which are also 3-dimensional (excluding the channels dimension), like videos. Our method effectively trains a Frame Interpolation Model on the MRI data. We than use the resulting model to generate new samples.

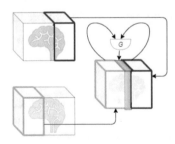 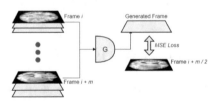

(a) How new brains are being generated. The red brain represents one sample and the green one represents a different sample. A new sample is generated by keeping the first part from the green brain and the last part from the red brain. The region in-between is generated with a model G.

(b) How the model G that generated the transition sequence (the yellow region from the left figure) has been trained. Note that when the model is trained, Frame i and Frame $i+m$ belong to the same brain, and when the model is actually used, Frame i belongs to one brain (green) and Frame $i+m$ belongs to another brain.

Fig. 1. Overview.

3   BrainFuse

In essence, our work focuses on the following 2 aspects:

- Training a frame interpolation model to learn the structural properties of the brain (1);
- Using this trained model to naturally combine multiple brains. (2);

In this section, we will present a summary of how both (1) and (2) are achieved, to give the reader a general idea about the complete mechanism. In the first part we will describe in detail the procedure for (1) and in the second part, we will detail the procedure for (2).

Let $x = (x_1, ...x_n), x \in \mathbb{R}^{\mathbb{D} \times \mathbb{C} \times \mathbb{W} \times \mathbb{D}}, x_i \in \mathbb{R}^{\mathbb{C} \times \mathbb{W} \times \mathbb{D}}$ denote a training sample (a 3D Brain MRI), and x_i denote an image at position i. We want to combine two samples $x_a = (x_{a1}, ...x_{an}), x_b = (x_{b1}, ...x_{bn})$ and their labels (y_a, y_b) to create a new sample $\tilde{x}, \tilde{y}$ in the following way:

$$\tilde{x} = (x_{a_1}, ...x_{a_k}; \alpha_{k+1}.., \alpha_{k+m}; x_{b_{k+m+1}}, ..x_{b_n}) \tag{1}$$

$$\tilde{y} = \frac{k + m/2}{n} * y_a + (1 - \frac{k + m/2}{n}) * y_b \tag{2}$$

$$\alpha_i = G(x_a, x_b, i; \theta) \tag{3}$$

where $\alpha = (\alpha_{k+1}, ..\alpha_{k+m})$ represents a sequence of m generated images that provide a spatially coherent transition between the 2 regions $(x_{a_1}, ...x_{a_k})$ and $(x_{b_{k+m+1}}, ..x_{b_n})$ (Fig 1).

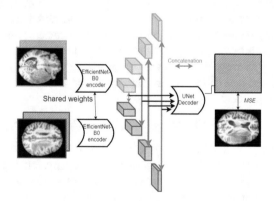

Fig. 2. Frame Interpolation Model Architecture.

This sequence is generated by G, which is a procedure that utilizes a frame interpolation model g parametrized by θ. This model is trained in the following way, given a training sample x, with frames x_i, g is a model such that the following Mean Squared Error (MSE) loss is minimized:

$$L = MSE(g(x_{i-p}, x_{i+p}; \theta), x_i) \tag{4}$$

To minimize this loss, g will have to learn the spatial structure in order to provide smooth transitions between different brain regions. Starting from two different train samples x_a, x_b, each being composed from multiple slides: $(x_{a_1}, ..x_{a_k}) \in x_a$, and $(x_{b_{k+m+1}}, ..x_{b_n}) \in x_b$, we can use the trained model to generate an intermediary frame $\alpha_{k+(m+1)/2} = g(x_{a_k}, x_{b_{k+m+1}}, \theta)$ Note that this is not the actual procedure used, but rather a simplified version to showcase the core mechanism.

3.1   Training the Frame Interpolation Model

In Sect. 3 we have defined g as a model that minimizes the loss in (5). There is a parameter p that describes the distance between the 2 interpolated frames. If we train this model for a small value of p, we obtain a model that can interpolate nearby frames. Since the brain is a "smooth" organ, nearby frames are very similar to each other. However, remember that we ultimately want to use this model to "merge" 2 brain regions belonging to different samples. This means that we need a model that can generate intermediary frames between two dissimilar frames. Therefore, we need a model trained with a high value of p. However, this comes with a few challenges:

1. Since the input frames are no longer close to each other, the model does not have a sense of the local flow of information. For example, let's say that a brain contains a spherical tumor. This tumor will appear as circles in each frame, with smaller circles appearing at the beginning and the end of the tumor and larger circles at the middle of the tumor. If we train the model with a large value of p, and x_i (the first frame) contains a small circle of the tumor, and the x_{i+p} contains a region without the tumor, it is impossible for the model to know if the small circle from the first frame represents the start of a tumor – case in which the intermediary frame should also contain a tumor – or the end of a tumor – case in which the intermediary frame should not contain any tumor. We solve this by providing multiple frames from both the start and the end of the brain. Based on our tests, 2 frames are enough. Therefore g now becomes:

$$L = MSE(g((x_{i-p}, x_{i-\frac{p}{2}}, (x_{i+\frac{p}{2}}, x_{i+p}); \theta), x_i) \tag{5}$$

2. For large values of p, the task naturally becomes very difficult. Training directly on this task leads to models with poor performance. Curriculum learning is a learning technique in which tasks of gradually increasing complexity are presented to a model [8]. This has been shown to increase both the speed and quality of learning. Our approach makes use of Curriculum Learning to gradually increase the value of p –the distance between the interpolated frames. More exactly, we start with $p = 1$ and when we stop getting any improvements, we increase p. For each value of p, we save a checkpoint of that model θ_p. Whenever we want to generate an intermediary frame with a distance of p between the 2 frames we load the corresponding model.

The model architecture that we have used can be seen in Fig 2. Since the output is an image, we have selected the UNet model [9]. The encoder has been

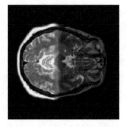 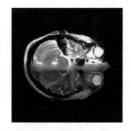 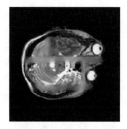

(a) Generated brain by fusing two patients.

(b) Generated brain by fusing eight patients.

(c) Deformed brain obtained from fusing 6 images.

Fig. 3. Example of slices from BrainFuse generated brains.

changed to incorporate two branches – a branch for $(x_{i-p}, x_{i-\frac{p}{2}})$ and a branch for $(x_{i+\frac{p}{2}}, x_{i+p})$. The resulting structure is similar to a Siamese Neural Network [10] using EfficientNet-B0 [11] as the backbone for the encoder.

We have trained different models for each axis of the brain MRI – depth, width, height, each of them for 100 epochs, with a *learning rate* of 1e-3, *batch size* of 16 and *Adam* optimizer [12].

Algorithm 1. Generate Brain

function GENERATE-BRAIN(x_a, x_b, k, m)
    $\alpha \leftarrow [0]_{m \times n \times n}$
    $\tilde{x} \leftarrow (x_{a_1}, .. x_{a_{k-m/2}}; \alpha_1 .., \alpha_m; x_{b_{k+m/2+1}}, .. x_{b_n})$
    for $p \leftarrow m$ to 1 **do**
        GENERATE-TRANS-REGION$(\tilde{x}, k, p)$ (2)
    end for
    return $\tilde{x}$
end function

3.2 Generating New Samples

Using the frame interpolation model defined in the previous section, we want to generate intermediary frames for joining 2 brain regions belonging to different samples. A procedure that would generate qualitative frames would need to optimize the following 3 criteria:

1. *Spatial coherence* – we want the generated frames to ensure a smooth transition between the 2 brain regions. Models trained on smaller p values generate smoother transitions. This is achieved by recursively generating the sequence with increasingly smaller p values. (See Algorithm 1)
2. *Low noise accumulation from intermediary frames.* – In essence, this procedure will start with the original left and right brain regions and generate frames in between. In order to generate "spatially coherent" frames we will need to use models with smaller p values. This means that we will need to

make use of intermediary frames, generated by models with larger p values. However, these intermediary frames represent out-of-distribution data. This leads to noise, and using these frames to further generate new frames leads to the accumulation of noise. We, therefore, need to ensure a minimal chain between the input frames and the final generated frames. This is obtained by following a binary traversal of the generated frames, as can be seen in Algorithm 2.

3. *Include frame context* – The model defined in Eq (6) requires that the input frames from both the left and the right region each include 2 frames at distance p between them. This adds additional complexity to the region-generating procedure. We handled this by iteratively increasing the dilation between the regions, as can be seen in Algorithm 2.

With this procedure we generated 2 categories of samples:

- **BrainFuse Dataset:** Fusions of 2 different samples: each brain is created by fusing together two different samples at a randomly selected location on a randomly selected axis. For the resulting samples, we also generate a label by linearly combining the source labels as in eq 2. An example of this can be seen in Fig. 3a. Using this procedure we generate 9000 samples.
- **MultiBrainFuse Dataset:** Fusions of multiple different samples: each brain is created by fusing together a variable number of brains, selected uniformly between 4 and 20. An example of this can be seen in Fig. 3b. These samples will not have an associated label, because they will be used for self-supervised pretraining and consistency regularization. This will be detailed in the next section. Using this procedure we generate 30000 samples.

Algorithm 2. Generate Transition Region

---

function Generate-Trans-Region$(\tilde{x}, k, p)$
 $g \leftarrow frame\_interpolation\_model(\theta_p)$
 $\tilde{x}_k \leftarrow g((\tilde{x}_{k-p}, \tilde{x}_{k-\frac{p}{2}}); (\tilde{x}_{k+\frac{p}{2}}, \tilde{x}_{k+p}))$
 for $j \leftarrow 1$ to p **do**
  $p' \leftarrow p + j$
  $k' \leftarrow k + j$
  $k'' \leftarrow k - j$
  $g \leftarrow frame\_interpolation\_model(\theta_{p'})$
  $\tilde{x}_{k'} \leftarrow g((\tilde{x}_{k'-p'}, \tilde{x}_{k'-\frac{p'}{2}}); (\tilde{x}_{k'+\frac{p'}{2}}, \tilde{x}_{k'+p'}))$
  $\tilde{x}_{k''} \leftarrow g((\tilde{x}_{k''-p'}, \tilde{x}_{k''-\frac{p'}{2}}); (\tilde{x}_{k''+\frac{p'}{2}}, \tilde{x}_{k''+p'}))$
 end for
 GENERATE-BRAIN$(\tilde{x}, k - \frac{p}{2}, \frac{p}{2})$

 GENERATE-BRAIN$(\tilde{x}, k + \frac{p}{2}, \frac{p}{2})$
end function

---

4   Brain Age Prediction

We evaluate our method on the well-known IXI dataset[1] by predicting the age of the subjects which is made available under the Creative Commons CC BY-SA 3.0 license.

The dataset consists of nearly 600 MR images of healthy brains in multiple modalities of which we used the T1, T2, and PD-weighted images. We selected 520 samples by eliminating subjects with missing image modalities or age information.

4.1   Data Preparation

We followed the label preprocessing methods described in [13], we use 40 age bins and transform our bin labels by transforming the one-hot distribution in a Gaussian distribution with the mean in the original label and $\sigma = 1.5$. All images had their values clipped between -1000 and 800, then normalized to the $[0, 1]$ interval and the MRIs were scaled to a size of $64 \times 64x64$. We stacked the modalities together obtaining a final image with 3 channels.

4.2   Training Methodology

We used a 3D variant of ResNet-50 [14] as the backbone and each image had one of the following transformations applied from the TorchIO library with default parameters, selected with equal probabilities [15]:

– A random affine transformation.: scaling, rotation, translation;
– Random Gaussian noise;
– Random MRI motion artifact [16];
– Random dense elastic deformation;
– Random bias field;

We follow a standard training procedure, with a *batch size* of 16, a *learning rate* of $1e - 3$ and Adam optimizer [12]. On top of this training procedure, we run multiple experiments by adding one or more of the following techniques:

– *BarlowTwins*
    As mentioned in the previous section, **MultiBrainFuse Dataset** consists of 30000 samples. In order to make use of this large quantity of unlabeled data we applied the Barlow Twins [17] self-supervised pretraining method. We trained the model for 35 epochs with a batch size of 32 and a learning rate of 1e-3. The model with the smallest validation loss – which occurred on epoch 29 – will be fine-tuned on the age prediction task.
– *Brain Fuse*
    Instead of training on the original samples, we train on the 9000 images from the **BrainFuse Dataset** described in the previous section.

---

[1] Available at https://brain-development.org/ixi-dataset/.

– *Raw Brain Fuse*
  In order to fairly compare the efficacy of our method, we also compare it with a specially designed procedure that mimics the behavior of *BrainFuse* but without using the Frame Interpolation Model. To be more precise, we generate a dataset **Raw BrainFuse Dataset** that also consists of 9000 images. However, these samples will simply be a concatenation between 2 regions of different brains. This is summarized in the following equation:

$$\tilde{x} = (x_{a_1}, ..x_{a_k}; x_{b_{k+1}}, ..x_{b_n}), x_a, x_b \in \mathbb{R}^{\mathbb{D} \times \mathbb{C} \times \mathbb{W} \times \mathbb{D}} \tag{6}$$

$$\tilde{y} = \frac{k}{n} * y_a + (1 - \frac{k}{n}) * y_b \tag{7}$$

– *Consistency Regularization*
  Adding an auxiliary loss that enforces consistent prediction under different augmentation has been shown to be an effective semi-supervised technique for leveraging unlabeled data. Therefore, we apply this technique by adding this auxiliary loss with data sampled from the **MultiBrainFuse Dataset**.

In Table 1 we report the average top 1, top 3, and top 5 accuracy metrics obtained over three runs to compare the performance impact of adding each of these methods.

Table 1. Results for the different training procedures. Each procedure has been run 3 times.

Method	Top1 Acc	Top3 Acc	Top5 Acc
NT (Normal Training)	$32.1 \pm 0.27\%$	$53.8 \pm 0.18\%$	$64.21 \pm 0.32\%$
NT + BT (Barlow/Twins)	$40.1 \pm 0.77\%$	$62.8 \pm 0.11\%$	$73.01 \pm 0.1\%$
NT + BT + BrainFuse	$50.11 \pm 0.3\%$	$71.16 \pm 0.12\%$	$82.9 \pm 0.22\%$
NT + BT + RawBrainFuse	$45.1 \pm 0.94\%$	$67.5 \pm 0.41\%$	$80.01 \pm 0.1\%$
NT + BT + BrainFuse + Consistency Regularisation	$\mathbf{51.4 \pm 0.84\%}$	$\mathbf{72.1 \pm 0.61\%}$	$\mathbf{83.8 \pm 0.52\%}$
NT + BT + RawBrainFuse + Consistency Regularisation	$46.6 \pm 0.9\%$	$68.8 \pm 0.78\%$	$81.1 \pm 0.31\%$

5 Limitations

Although our method provides a boost for the age prediction task, there are a few drawbacks. First of all, you need to train the frame interpolation model. Because the distance between the frames needs to be increased iteratively, it can take up to several days to train the model on a single GPU. The total compute time required on an NVIDIA RTX 2080 Ti is 6 d. Apart from the computational overhead, storing the generated datasets needs to be taken into account. An alternative to this would be to generate the samples during training, but this would slow down the process.

Besides the hardware limitations, we also noticed that in some extreme cases, the brains that we fused together were simply incompatible. This was due to significantly different brain dimensions, and one such example can be seen in Fig. 3c.

6   Conclusion

In this paper, we have presented a highly effective data augmentation procedure for the brain age prediction task. We also showcased how a simple self-supervised technique can be used to generate new samples in an easy and controlled manner, opening the way for alternatives to GANs, which can sometimes be difficult to train and condition.

References

1. Henaff, O.: Data-efficient image recognition with contrastive predictive coding. International conference on machine learning, PMLR (2020)
2. Dong-Hyun, L.: Pseudo-label: the simple and efficient semi-supervised learning method for deep neural networks. Workshop Challenges Representation Learn. ICML **3**(2), 896 (2013)
3. Nalepa, J., Marcinkiewicz, M., Kawulok, M.: Data augmentation for brain-tumor segmentation: a review. Front. Comput. Neurosci. **13**, 83 (2019)
4. Changhee, H., et al.: GAN-based synthetic brain MR image generation. In: 2018 IEEE 15th International Symposium on Biomedical Imaging (ISBI 2018). IEEE (2018)
5. Sangdoo, Y., et al.: CutMix: regularization strategy to train strong classifiers with localizable features. In: Proceedings of the IEEE/CVF International Conference on Computer Vision (2019)
6. Zach, E.-R., et al.: Improving data augmentation for medical image segmentation (2018)
7. Simon, N., Mai, L., Liu, F.: Video frame interpolation via adaptive separable convolution. In: Proceedings of the IEEE International Conference on Computer Vision (2017)
8. Yoshua, B., et al.: Curriculum learning. In: Proceedings of the 26th Annual International Conference on Machine Learning (2009)
9. Ronneberger, O., Fischer, P., Brox, T.: U-Net: Convolutional Networks for Biomedical Image Segmentation. In: Navab, N., Hornegger, J., Wells, W.M., Frangi, A.F. (eds.) MICCAI 2015. LNCS, vol. 9351, pp. 234–241. Springer, Cham (2015). https://doi.org/10.1007/978-3-319-24574-4_28
10. Koch, Gregory, Richard Zemel, R., Ruslan Salakhutdinov, R.: Siamese neural networks for one-shot image recognition. ICML Deep Learning Workshop. Vol. 2. No. 1 (2015)
11. Tan, M., Le, Q.: Efficientnet: Rethinking model scaling for convolutional neural networks. International conference on machine learning, PMLR (2019)
12. Kingma, Diederik P., Jimmy B.: Adam: a method for stochastic optimization." arXiv preprint arXiv:1412.6980 (2014)
13. Han, P., et al.: Accurate brain age prediction with lightweight deep neural networks. Med. image Anal. **68**, 101871 (2021)
14. Kaiming, H., et al.: Deep residual learning for image recognition. In: Proceedings of the IEEE Conference on Computer Vision and Pattern Recognition (2016)
15. Pérez-García, F., Sparks, R., Ourselin, S.: TorchIO: a Python library for efficient loading, preprocessing, augmentation and patch-based sampling of medical images in deep learning. Comput. Methods Programs Biomed. **208**, 106236 (2021)

16. MRI k-Space Motion Artefact Augmentation: Model Robustness and Task-Specific Uncertainty
17. Jure, Z., et al.: Barlow twins: Self-supervised learning via redundancy reduction. In: International Conference on Machine Learning. PMLR (2021)

Robust Zero Watermarking Algorithm for Medical Images Based on BRISK-FREAK and DCT

Fangchun Dong[1], Jingbing Li[1(✉)], Jing Liu[2], and Yen-Wei Chen[3]

[1] School of Information and Communication Engineering, Hainan University, Haikou 570228, China
21220854000140@hainanu.edu.cn, Jingbingli2008@hotmail.com
[2] Research Center for Healthcare Data Science, Zhejiang Lab, Hangzhou, Zhejiang 311121, China
liujinglj@zhejianglab.com
[3] Graduate School of Information Science and Engineering, Ritsumeikan University, Shiga 525-8577, Japan
chen@is.ritsumei.ac.jp

Abstract. With the development of mobile Internet technology, the technology in the field of medical image processing is constantly updated and iterated. Digital watermarking technology plays an important role in the field of medical image processing, providing guarantee for the security of medical image information. Aiming at the poor robustness of medical image watermarking algorithms to geometric attacks, a robust zero-watermarking algorithm for medical images based on BRISK-FREAK and discrete cosine transform (DCT) is proposed. First, Binary Robust Invariant Scalable Kepoints (BRISK) was applied to extract the feature points of the medical image. Then, Fast Retina Keypoint (FREAK) was used to describe the extracted feature points and generate a feature descriptor matrix. Further, DCT was performed on the FREAK descriptor matrix, and the low-frequency part was processed via the perceptual hash algorithm to obtain a 32-bit binary feature vector. In order to enhance the security of the watermark information, the logistic mapping algorithm is utilized to encrypt the watermark before embedding the watermark. Finally, with the help of the zero watermarking technology, the proposed algorithm can be embedded and extract the watermark without changing any of the medical image information. Experimental results show that the algorithm has good robustness under some conventional attacks and geometric attacks. Especially under geometric attacks, the performance of the algorithm is excellent.

Keywords: BRISK algorithm · FREAK descriptor · DCT · Medical image · Zero watermark

1 Introduction

The development of Internet information technology has promoted the integration of modern information technology and medical care [1]. Digital life is gradually closely related to our life, which brings convenience to our life and also brings security risks. At present, most medical information requires multimedia data transmission, and the misuse or even tampering of the original digital content makes image security still challenging in the field of medical imaging [2]. Digital watermarking is a widely used digital data protection technology. Digital watermarking embeds secret data into actual information. It can be regarded as an information hiding technology [3]. Watermarking technology can be used without affecting the judgment of doctors, Better hide patient information, with features such as invisibility and robustness. Watermarking technology is used in many applications, such as ownership protection, compared with other applications, medical image watermarking technology is favored by more researchers [4]. At this stage, as many medical image algorithms have poor robustness and cannot achieve satisfactory results, especially in resistance to geometric attacks, many algorithms can only have strong robustness to individual geometric attacks. Hence, it is necessary to design a new robust watermarking algorithm that can resist more kinds of attacks.

The watermarking algorithm based on the change domain mainly embeds the watermark by modifying the texture, frequency domain and other attributes of the original image, which has good robustness to conventional attacks. Surekah Borra et al. [5] proposed a blind robust medical image watermarking technology based on finite ridgelet transform (FRT) and singular value decomposition (SVD). Singular value decomposition is performed on the data set, and the watermark is embedded into the U matrix. Zermi N. et al. [6] proposed a robust digital watermarking algorithm for medical images based on DWT-SVD, applying the SVD algorithm to the LL sub-band of the DWT transform, and finally integrating the watermark into the the least significant bit of the S component is obtained. The results show that the algorithm has good robustness to conventional attacks such as salt and pepper noise. Rohit Thanki et al. [7] proposed an image watermarking algorithm based on RDWT–NSCT, which inserts watermarks in the Contourlet Transform (NSCT) and Redundant Discrete Wavelet Transform (RDWT) regions, which has certain invisibility and robustness. Jing Liu. et al. [8] proposed a watermarking algorithm based on dual-tree complex wavelet transform and discrete cosine transform (DTCWT-DCT), which has a good effect on conventional attacks and geometric attacks, especially in geometric attacks.

Zero watermarking technology is a watermark technology that does not directly embed watermark in the image. Zero watermark does not modify the original image data. Generally, the zero watermark is constructed by extracting the characteristics of the original image from the original image [9–11]. The local feature extraction algorithm has a good effect in the field of image watermarking due to its good rotation invariance and scale invariance. The mainstream feature extraction algorithms mainly include SIFT, SURF [12, 13] and other algorithms. Binary feature extraction algorithms have a faster running speed, and mainstream algorithms include BRIEF, ORB, BRISK, FREAK and other algorithms [14–16]. Yangxiu Fang et al. [17] proposed a zero-watermarking algorithm for medical images based on bandelet and discrete cosine transform, and performed SIFT algorithm on the original medical image to extract picture features, and then used Bandelet-DCT to extract the features of medical images from the extracted features Vector, combined with zero watermark technology to realize the embedding and extraction of watermark, this algorithm has good robustness. A Soualmi et al. [18] proposed an imperceptible watermarking method for medical image tampering detection, combining SURF descriptors with Weber descriptor (WD) and Arnold algorithm, and applying SURF technology to the sensing of medical images region of interest (ROI), and then select the region around the SURF point to insert the watermark, using the Weber descriptor to embed and extract the watermark. Cheng Zeng et al. [19] proposed a medical image zero watermarking algorithm based on KAZE-DCT, using the KAZE feature extraction algorithm to extract the original image features, and then performing DCT transformation on the extracted features, using perceptual hashing to obtain the feature sequence of medical images, meanwhile, the zero-watermark technology is used to embed and extract the watermark, and the algorithm has good robustness to geometric attacks. Based on the above research, it can be found that the binary feature extraction algorithm is less studied in the field of medical image watermarking, and most watermarking algorithms still have problems such as slow running speed and poor robustness, especially resisting geometric attacks. Aiming at these problems, this paper proposes BRISK- FREAK and DCT watermarking algorithms.

2 Basic Theory

2.1 BRISK Feature Extraction Algorithm

The BRISK (Binary Robust Invariant Scalable Kepoints) algorithm is an image local feature extraction algorithm proposed by Stefan Leutenegge et al. [20]. The BRISK algorithm has scale invariance and rotation invariance. This algorithm reduces the computing cost and runs faster than SIFT and SURF algorithms. It mainly uses FAST for feature point detection and constructs an image pyramid for multi-scale expression.

(1) Construction of scale space pyramid. Construct N octave layers (denoted by c_i) and N intra-octave layers (denoted by d_i), octave layer: the c_0 layer represents the original image with a scale of 1, the c_1 layer is two times the down sampling of the c_0 layer, and the c_2 layer is two times the down sampling of the c_1 layer, and so on; intra-octave layer: The d_0 layer is obtained by down sampling the c_0 layer by 1.5 times, the d_1 layer is the down sampling of the d_0 layer by two times, the d_2 layer is the down sampling of the d_1 layer by two times, and so on. See Eq. (1) for the scale calculation formula of each layer.

$$\begin{cases} t_{c_i} = 2^i \\ t_{d_i} = 1.5 \times 2^i \end{cases} \tag{1}$$

where t_{c_i} represents the scale relationship between the octave layer and the original image, and t_{d_i} represents the scale relationship between the intra-octave layer and the original image.

(2) Feature point detection. FAST corner detection is performed at each level of the scale-space pyramid.

(3) Non-maximum suppression. By comparing the detected candidate feature points with their location space and their neighbor points in the upper and lower scale spaces, and eliminating candidate points with smaller response values than other points, the purpose of non-maximum value suppression is achieved.

(4) Obtain feature point information. In the layer where the extreme point is located and the positions corresponding to the upper and lower layers, the FAST score value is interpolated with a two-dimensional quadratic function to obtain the score extreme point with sub-pixel positioning accuracy and its precise coordinate position; then the scale One-dimensional interpolation is performed on the direction to obtain the scale corresponding to the extreme point with sub-pixel positioning accuracy. Get the location and scale information of the feature points.

2.2   FREAK Feature Descriptor

The FREAK (Fast Retina Keypoint) feature descriptor is a feature descriptor proposed by Alexandre Alahi [21]. After being inspired by the principle of human eye recognition of objects, it is proposed to introduce binary feature descriptors, which are interested in perifoveal regions. The position of the object is estimated, and then verified by the fovea area with more dense photoreceptor cells, and finally the information of the object is determined. The FREAK feature descriptor is an improvement of the BRISK descriptor. Due to the circular symmetrical sampling structure of the FREAK descriptor itself, And at the same time, as the distance between the sampling point and the feature point increases, the radius of the Gaussian function of the sampling point circle becomes larger, so FREAK has stronger rotation invariance and scale invariance than the traditional feature description algorithm. Schematic diagram of FREAK sampling mode is shown in Fig. 1.

Each point in the Fig. 1 represents a sampling point, each circle represents a response area, and the radius of each circle represents the standard deviation of gaussian blur.

The FREAK algorithm uses a binary string to describe the feature points, which is represented by F.

$$F = \sum_{0 \leq a < N} 2^a T(Pa) \tag{2}$$

$$T(Pa) = \begin{cases} 1 \; if \, (I(P_a^{r1}) - (I(P_a^{r2})) > 0 \\ 0 \; otherwise \end{cases} \tag{3}$$

In the Eq. (3), $I(P_a^{r1})$ is the gray value of the sampling point after Gaussian blurring, $T(Pa)$ is a piecewise function, Pa is a pair of sampling points, if $I(P_a^{r1}) > I(P_a^{r2})$, $T(Pa) = 1$, otherwise $T(Pa) = 0$.

There are a total of 43 sampling points in FREAK's sampling mode, which can generate approximately one thousand sampling point pairs. The encoding values of some sampling point pairs have no practical effect on feature description, but will cause feature redundancy, so the feature point pairs must be screened.

(1) Establish an L × N matrix H for L feature points, and each row of the matrix represents the binary descriptor of each feature point.
(2) Calculate the mean value of each column of the matrix H. In order to obtain representative features, the variance should be large, which requires that the average value of the column should be close to 0.5.

(3) According to the distance between the mean and 0.5 from small to large, and then reorder the columns in the matrix H in order of variance from large to small.

(4) Select the first k columns as the final binary descriptor.

The FREAK descriptor adopts a symmetrical sampling structure, and the FREAK algorithm uses 45 symmetrical and long-distance sampling points to calculate its gradient to add direction information to the feature points and realize the rotation invariance of the algorithm. The calculation formula is shown in Eq. (4). Direction the information is shown in Fig. 2 symbol.

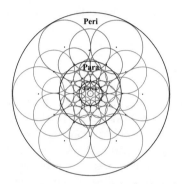
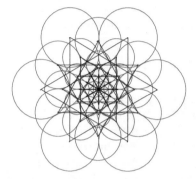

Fig. 1. Schematic diagram of FREAK sampling mode

Fig. 2. FREAK descriptor direction information

$$O = \frac{1}{M} \sum_{Po \in G} (I(P_o^{r1}) - I(P_o^{r2})) \frac{P_o^{r1} - P_o^{r2}}{||P_o^{r1} - P_o^{r2}||} \tag{4}$$

In the Eq. (4), O is local gradient information, M represents the number of sampling point pairs, P_o represents the position of sampling point pairs, G represents the set of sampling point pairs, and P_o^{ri} is a two-dimensional vector of the spatial coordinates of sampling points.

2.3 Discrete Cosine Transform (DCT)

DCT transform is often used for lossy data compression of images, which has separability and energy concentration. After DCT transforming images, most of the energy is concentrated in low-frequency regions. The two-dimensional DCT is shown in Eq. (5):

$$F(u, v) = C(u)C(v) \sum_{x=0}^{M-1} \sum_{y=0}^{N-1} f(x, y) \cos\left[\frac{(x + 0.5)u\pi}{M}\right] \cos\left[\frac{(y + 0.5)v\pi}{N}\right]$$

$$u = 0, 1, ..., M - 1; v = 0, 1, ..., N - 1 \tag{5}$$

$$C(u) = \begin{cases} \sqrt{\frac{1}{M}}, & u = 0 \\ \sqrt{\frac{2}{M}}, & u = 1, 2, ..., M - 1 \end{cases}, \quad C(v) = \begin{cases} \sqrt{\frac{1}{N}}, & v = 0 \\ \sqrt{\frac{2}{N}}, & v = 1, 2, ..., N - 1 \end{cases} \tag{6}$$

2.4 Logistic Mapping

The Logistic chaotic system produces complex irregular motion, which refers to a quasi-random process that occurs in a deterministic system, which is non-convergent and non-periodic. Among them, the logistic map is one of the most famous chaotic systems, the definition form of the Logistic map is as Eq. (7).

$$X_{K+1} = \mu \times X_K \times (1 - X_K) \, \mu \in [0, 4], X_K \in (0, 1) \tag{7}$$

where μ denotes the branch parameter. When $3.5699456 \le \mu \le 4$, the Logistic map enters the chaotic state, and the Logistic chaotic sequence can be used as an ideal key sequence. It is set in this paper, $\mu = 4, X_K = 0.2$.

3 Zero Watermarking Algorithm

This paper proposes a medical image digital watermarking algorithm based on BRISK-FREAK-DCT, which combines the BRISK feature extraction algorithm, FREAK feature description algorithm, DCT transformation and perceptual hash function. The watermark image encryption adopts logistic chaos encryption and zero watermark technology embedding and extracting watermarks have good robustness in geometric attacks and some traditional attacks, and meet the requirements of zero watermark and blind extraction. It mainly includes four steps: medical image feature extraction, watermark encryption, watermark embedding, watermark extraction and decryption.

3.1 Medical Image Feature Extraction

This paper randomly selects a brain CT image with a pixel size of 512 pixels × 512 pixels, uses the BRISK feature extraction algorithm to extract the feature points in the image, and then uses the FREAK feature description to describe the feature points, extract the feature vector $B(i, j)$ of the medical image, and analyze the extracted features. After DCT transformation of the vector, a characteristic matrix $D(i, j)$ is obtained, and the upper left corner of the characteristic matrix is selected to obtain a 2 pixels × 16 pixels low-frequency coefficient matrix $V(i, j)$, and the sign conversion is performed on the low-frequency coefficient matrix. The elements greater than 0 in the matrix are set to 1, and other elements are set to 0. Get the hash value $H(i, j)$, which is a sequence of binary features. The specific steps are shown in Fig. 3.

3.2 Watermark Encryption

In order to enhance the anti-interference and security of the watermark algorithm, the chaotic system of logistic mapping is used to displace the watermark image chaotically to obtain the encrypted watermark image, and the branch parameters are taken to enter the chaotic state, and then the watermark image is scrambled to obtain the encrypted watermark $L(i, j)$. The specific steps are shown in Fig. 4.

3.3 Embed Watermark

After the watermark is encrypted, we embed the watermark into the medical image: first, use BRISK-FREAK-DCT to extract the features of the original image, obtain the binary feature sequence $H(i,j)$, and then perform XOR operation on the binary feature sequence $H(i,j)$ and the encrypted watermark $L(i,j)$ to obtain The logical key $K(i,j)$ used to extract the watermark. This method of embedding watermark uses zero watermark embedding technology, which will not change the original image. The specific steps of embedding the watermark are shown in Fig. 5.

3.4 Watermark Extraction and Decryption

The extraction process of encrypted watermark is similar to the embedding of watermark. First, use BRISK-FREAK-DCT to extract features from the image to be tested, obtain a binary feature sequence $H'(i,j)$, $H'(i,j)$ perform an XOR operation with the logical key $K(i,j)$ to obtain the extracted encrypted watermark $L'(i,j)$, and restore the encrypted watermark $L'(i,j)$ to the original value through the initial value of the Logistic map. The specific watermark extraction steps are shown in Fig. 6.

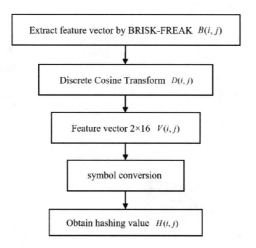

Fig. 3. Image feature extraction flowchart.

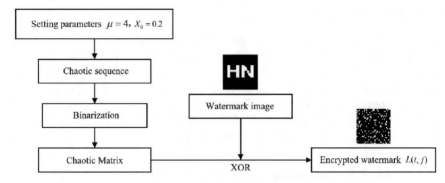

Fig. 4. Flowchart of watermark encryption.

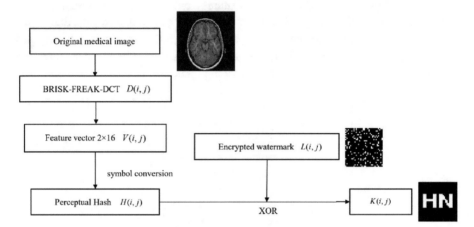

Fig. 5. Embed watermark flowchart.

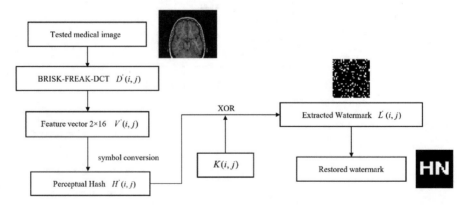

Fig.6. Flowchart of watermark extraction and decryption.

4 Experiments and Results

This paper uses the MATLAB 2022a platform to simulate and experiment on medical images, in which the medical image pixels are 512 pixels × 512 pixels, and the watermark image pixels are 32 × 32. The normalized correlation coefficient (NC) is used to compare the similarity between the original watermark and the watermark extracted from the image after the attack, so as to evaluate the ability of the algorithm to resist the attacks, and the quality of the image is represented by the peak signal-to-noise ratio (PSNR). In the case of medical images without any attacks, the NC values are all equals to 1.00.

4.1 Test Different Images

Before testing the anti-attack performance of medical images, we first use the proposed algorithm test ten different medical images, as shown in Fig. 7. We calculate their correlation coefficients to verify whether the algorithm can distinguish different medical images. The experimental results are shown in Table 1. The results show that the algorithm can distinguish different medical images.

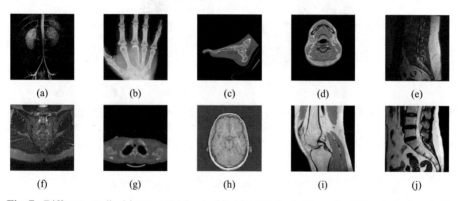

(a)   (b)   (c)   (d)   (e)

(f)   (g)   (h)   (i)   (j)

Fig. 7. Different medical images: (a) lung; (b) palm; (c) foot; (d) neck; (e) lumber spine 1; (f) sacroiliac; (g) chest; (h) brain; (i) knee; (j) lumber spine 2.

4.2 Conventional Attacks

The watermark is extracted after different degrees of JPEG compression and median filter attack on the medical image that already contains the encrypted watermark, as shown in Fig. 8. The experimental results are shown in Tables 2 and 3. The results show that the algorithm is robust against JPEG compression and median filtering attacks.

Table 1. Correlation coefficient of different medical image feature vectors (32 bits).

Image	(a)	(b)	(c)	(d)	(e)	(f)	(g)	(h)	(i)	(j)
(a)	1.00	0.29	0.11	0.12	0.14	0.04	0.20	−0.05	0.13	0.06
(b)	0.29	1.00	0.09	−0.07	0.13	0.01	0.28	0.13	0.23	0.25
(c)	0.11	0.09	1.00	0.31	0.25	0.43	0.08	0.27	0.30	0
(d)	0.12	−0.07	0.31	1.00	0.10	0.28	0.23	0.29	0.29	0.12
(e)	0.14	0.13	0.25	0.10	1.00	0.40	0.03	−0.11	0.27	0.25
(f)	0.04	0.01	0.43	0.28	0.40	1.00	0.01	0.25	0.49	0.34
(g)	0.20	0.28	0.08	0.23	0.03	0.01	1.00	0.12	0.01	0.15
(h)	-0.05	0.13	0.27	0.29	−0.11	0.25	0.12	1.00	0.29	−0.04
(i)	0.13	0.23	0.30	0.29	0.27	0.49	0.01	0.29	1.00	0.24
(j)	0.06	0.25	0	0.12	0.25	0.34	0.15	−0.04	0.24	1.00

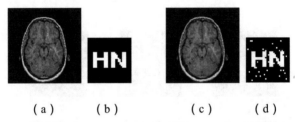

(a)   (b)   (c)   (d)

Fig.8. Medical Images under common attacks: (a) compression quality set to 15%. (b) the extracted watermark with compression quality set to 15%. (c) median filter [3 × 3], 20 times. (d) the extracted watermark under median filters [3 × 3], 20 times.

Table 2. Experimental results under JPEG compression attacks.

Compression quality (%)	5	10	15	20	25	30	35
PSNR (dB)	28.44	31.29	32.90	33.81	34.39	34.83	35.19
NC	0.63	0.71	1.00	1.00	1.00	1.00	1.00

Table 3. Experimental results under median filtering attacks.

Median filtering [3 × 3] (times)	5	10	15	20
PSNR (dB)	34.49	34.00	33.86	33.82
NC	0.72	0.72	0.80	0.89

4.3 Geometric Attacks

The watermark is extracted after performing different degrees of rotation, scaling, translation and cropping attacks on medical images that already contain encrypted watermarks, as shown in Fig. 9, and then observe the robustness of the algorithm against geometric attacks, and the experiments against rotation and scaling attacks The results are shown in Tables 4 and 5, and the experimental results of anti-translation and shear attacks are shown in Tables 6 and 7. The results can be seen: Even when the rotation angle is 60, the PSNR value of the picture is 13.55, the NC value is 0.80, and the overall NC value is close to 1, showing a strong ability to resist rotation attacks; When the zoom ratio is greater than or equal to 0.6 and less than or equal to 2.0, most of the NC values are greater than 0.8; when the encrypted medical image is moved to the right by 40%, the NC value is 0.79; when it is moved up by 35%, the NC value is 0.63; even if the encrypted medical image is cut by 40%, the NC value is 0.57; when the X-axis shears 40%, the NC value is 0.65. It is proved that the algorithm has good robustness against geometric attacks.

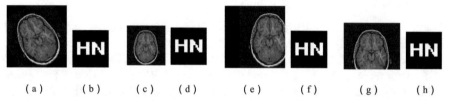

(a)   (b)   (c)   (d)   (e)   (f)   (g)   (h)

Fig. 9. Medical images under geometrical attacks: (a) rotate (counterclockwise) 45°; (b) the extracted watermark under rotation (counterclockwise) 45°; (c) scaling factor 0.8; (d) the extracted watermark under scaling factor 0.8; (e) right translation 20%; (f) the extracted watermark under right translation 20%; (g) Y-axis cropping 20%; (h) the extracted watermark under Y-axis cropping 20%.

Table 4. Experimental results under rotation attacks.

Angle (°)	5	15	30	45	60
PSNR (dB)	18.00	14.87	14.40	13.84	13.55
NC	1.00	0.89	1.00	1.00	0.80

Table 5. Experimental results under scaling attack.

Scaling	0.6	0.8	1	1.2	1.6	1.8	2.0
NC	0.71	0.79	1.00	0.89	1.00	0.89	1.00

Table 6. Experimental results under translation attacks.

Right translation					Up translation				
Scale (%)	5	15	25	40	Scale (%)	5	15	25	35
PSNR (dB)	14.51	12.90	11.30	10.08	PSNR (dB)	14.64	13.13	11.93	11.05
NC	1.00	1.00	1.00	0.79	NC	1.00	0.80	0.80	0.63

Table 7. Experimental results under cropping attacks.

Y-axis shear					X-axis shear				
Ratio (%)	10	20	30	40	Ratio (%)	10	20	30	40
NC	1.00	1.00	0.89	0.57	NC	1.00	1.00	0.71	0.65

4.4 Compare with Other Algorithms

To reflect the robustness of BRISK-FREAK-DCT, this algorithm is compared with DCT algorithm [22], DWT-DCT [23] and SIFT-DCT [17] algorithm in the face of different attacks, as shown in Fig. 10. The black in the figure represents DCT, blue represents DWT-DCT, green represents SIFT-DCT, and red represents BRISK-FREAK-DCT proposed in this paper. It can be seen from the experimental data that BRISK-FREAK-DCT has certain robustness in some conventional attacks, poor robustness in noise attacks, and better robustness in resistance to geometric attacks.

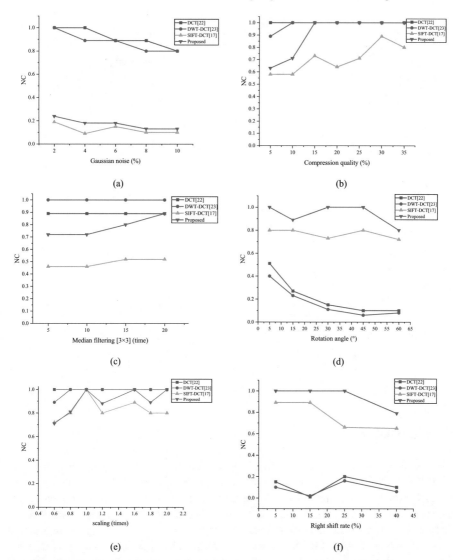

(a)

(b)

(c)

(d)

(e)

(f)

Fig. 10. Comparison of the results of different algorithms: (a) is the NC value comparison of different algorithms after Gaussian noise attack; (b) is the NC value comparison of different algorithms after JPEG compression attack; (c) is the NC value comparison of different algorithms after median filter attack; (d) is the NC value comparison of different algorithms after rotation attack; (e) is the NC value comparison of different algorithms after scaling attack; (f) is the NC value comparison of different algorithms after right shift attack; (g) is the NC value comparison of different algorithms after up shift attack; (h) is the NC value comparison of different algorithms after Y-axis shear attack; (i) is the NC value comparison of different algorithms after X-axis shear attack.

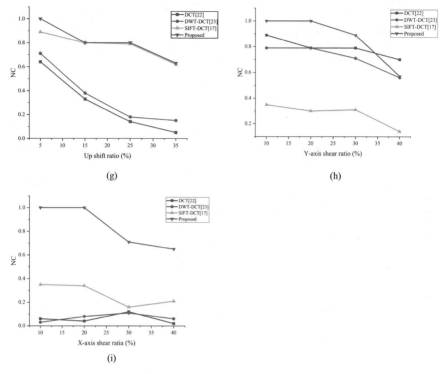

Fig. 10. (*continued*)

5   Conclusions

This paper proposed a zero-watermarking algorithm for medical images based on BRISK-FREAK and DCT. This algorithm used chaotic encryption technology, perceptual hashing algorithm and zero-watermarking technology to provide guarantee for the security of watermark information. Experimental results show that the algorithm has certain robustness to some conventional attacks, but is less robust to noise attacks, and performs well against geometric attacks. Therefore, this algorithm can be used in the field of medical images. In the next research, while improving the algorithm, we will also pursue an algorithm that can extract image features more effectively to deal with the problem of poor robustness of the algorithm to some attacks.

Acknowledgements. This work was supported in part by the Natural Science Foundation of China under Grants 62063004, the Key Research Project of Hainan Province under Grant ZDYF2021SHFZ093, the Hainan Provincial Natural Science Foundation of China under Grants 2019RC018 and 619QN246, and the postdoctor research from Zhejiang Province under Grant ZJ2021028.

References

1. Wu, H., et al.: The impact of internet development on the health of Chinese residents: Transmission mechanisms and empirical tests. Socioecon. Plann. Sci. **81**, 101178 (2022)
2. Menendez-Ortiz, A., Feregrino-Uribe, C., Hasimoto-Beltran, R., Garcia-Hernandez, J.J.: A survey on reversible watermarking for multimedia content: a robustness overview. IEEE Access. **7**, 132662–132681 (2019)
3. Mohanarathinam, A., Kamalraj, S., Venkatesan, G.K.D.P., Ravi, R.V., Manikandababu, C.S.: Digital watermarking techniques for image security: a review. J Ambient Intell. Human Comput. **11**(8), 3221–3229 (2020)
4. Alshoura, W.H., Zainol, Z., Teh, J.S., Alawida, M., Alabdulatif, A.: Hybrid SVD-based image watermarking schemes: a review. IEEE Access. **9**, 32931–32968 (2021)
5. Borra, S., Thanki, R.: A FRT - SVD based blind medical watermarking technique for telemedicine applications. IJDCF. **11**, 13–33 (2019)
6. Zermi, N., Khaldi, A., Kafi, R., Kahlessenane, F., Euschi, S.: A DWT-SVD based robust digital watermarking for medical image security. Forensic Sci. Int. **320**, 110691 (2021)
7. Thanki, R., Kothari, A., Borra, S.: Hybrid, blind and robust image watermarking: RDWT – NSCT based secure approach for telemedicine applications. Multimedia Tools Appl. **80**(18), 27593–27613 (2021). https://doi.org/10.1007/s11042-021-11064-y
8. Liu, J., et al.: A novel robust watermarking algorithm for encrypted medical image based on DTCWT-DCT and chaotic map. Computers, Materials Continua. **61**, 889–910 (2019)
9. Wang, X., Wen, M., Tan, X., Zhang, H., Hu, J., Qin, H.: A novel zero-watermarking algorithm based on robust statistical features for natural images. Vis Comput. **38**(9), 3175–3188 (2022)
10. Wang, H., Chen, Y., Zhao, T.: Modified Zernike moments and its application in geometrically resilient image zero-watermarking. Circuits Syst. Signal Process. **41**(12), 6844–6861 (2022)
11. Shi, S., Luo, T., Huang, J., Du, M.: A Novel HDR image zero-watermarking based on shift-invariant shearlet transform. Secur. Commun. Netw. **2021**, 1–12 (2021)
12. Bilik, S., Horak, K.: SIFT and SURF based feature extraction for the anomaly detection. http://arxiv.org/abs/2203.13068 (2022)
13. Zheng, Q., Gong, M., You, X., Tao, D.: A Unified B-spline framework for scale-invariant keypoint detection. Int. J. Comput. Vis. **130**(3), 777–799 (2022)
14. Zhang, L., Zhang, Y.: Improved feature point extraction method of ORB-SLAM2 dense map. Assem. Autom. **42**(4), 552–566 (2022)
15. Fatima, B., Ghafoor, A., Ali, S.S., Riaz, M.M.: FAST, BRIEF and SIFT based image copy-move forgery detection technique. Multimed Tools Appl. **81**(30), 43805–43819 (2022)
16. Shi, Q., Liu, Y., Xu, Y.: Image feature point matching method based on improved BRISK. Int. J. Wireless Mobile Comput. **20**(2), 132–138 (2021)
17. Fang, Y., et al.: Robust zero-watermarking algorithm for medical images based on SIFT and Bandelet-DCT. Multimedia Tools Appl. **81**, 1–17 (2022). https://doi.org/10.1007/s11042-022-12592-x
18. Soualmi, A., Alti, A., Laouamer, L.: An Imperceptible watermarking scheme for medical image tamper detection. IJISP. **16**(1), 1–18 (2022)
19. Zeng, C., et al.: Multi-watermarking algorithm for medical image based on KAZE-DCT. J. Ambient Intell. Human Comput. (2022). https://doi.org/10.1007/s12652-021-03539-5
20. Leutenegger, S., Chli, M., Siegwart, R.Y.: BRISK: binary Robust invariant scalable keypoints. In: 2011 International Conference on Computer Vision, pp. 2548–2555 (2011)
21. Alahi, A., Ortiz, R., Vandergheynst, P.: FREAK: fast Retina keypoint. In: 2012 IEEE Conference on Computer Vision and Pattern Recognition, pp. 510–517 (2012)
22. Liu, Y., Li, J.: DCT and logistic map based multiple robust watermarks for medical image. Appl. Res. Comput **30**(11), 3430–3433 (2013)

23. Liu, Y., Li, J.: The medical image watermarking algorithm using DWT-DCT and logistic. In: 2012 7th International Conference on Computing and Convergence Technology (ICCCT), pp. 599–603 (2012)

Robust Zero-Watermarking Algorithm
for Medical Images Based on SUSAN-DCT

Qinqing Zhang[1], Jingbing Li[1(✉)], Jing Liu[2], Uzair Aslam Bhatti[1], and Yen-Wei Chen[3]

[1] School of Information and Communication Engineering, Hainan University, Haikou 570228,
China
21220854000194@hainanu.edu.cn, Jingbingli2008@hotmail.com
[2] Research Center for Healthcare Data Science, Zhejiang Lab, Hangzhou 311121, Zhejiang,
China
liujinglj@zhejianglab.com
[3] Graduate School of Information Science and Engineering, Ritsumeikan University, Kusatsu,
Shiga 525-8577, Japan
chen@is.ritsumei.ac.jp

Abstract. With the digitization of medical systems, the information security of medical images faces great risks. In order to protect the personal information of patients contained in medical images, this paper proposes a robust medical image zero watermarking algorithm based on SUSAN-DCT. Firstly, SUSAN transform and block discrete cosine transform are processed on the original medical image. Then, calculate the Hu moment in blocks to obtain the feature matrix, and XOR it with the watermark image to construct a zero watermark. Before constructing the zero watermark, the original medical image is pre-processed using a logical encryption algorithm, and the reliability of the algorithm is improved. According to the simulation results, it can be seen that the algorithm has strong robustness under conventional and geometric attacks, and is a reliable and safe zero-watermarking algorithm.

Keywords: Zero watermark · Smallest Univalue Segment Assimilating Nucleus · Hu moments

1 Introduction

In the era of vigorous development of various communication technologies, the Internet is widely spread in our lives, and digital communication technologies are developing rapidly. However, as information becomes more transparent and widely disseminated, illegal phenomena such as digital multimedia objects being stolen and distributed freely have emerged, so issues such as digital media copyright and private information security have become urgent problems to be solved. Cryptography and digital watermarking [1, 2], as a branch of information hiding technology, play an important role in the protection of digital multimedia and become an important tool for copyright protection and information security. They not only prevent the loss of information leakage from the technical level, but also resist the attack on digital information in the transmission process, and ensure the integrity and security of information. Traditional digital watermarking usually combines the watermark with the spatial domain coefficients to change the value, which can hide the watermarked image in the carrier image. However, this operation will change the data of the carrier image to varying degrees, resulting in distortion. With the introduction of the concept of digital health care and the progress of the medical and information industries, image processing technology-assisted disease diagnosis has become an inevitable trend in the development of medical imaging. The misdiagnosis and subsequent collateral results caused by tampering with the original data will be incalculable. Therefore, traditional digital watermarking cannot meet the strict requirements for medical images in the medical field. Later, the zero watermarking [3] technique was proposed. Under the processing of this technology, the image features are extracted, and then combined with the watermarks. The algorithm can guarantee the originality of the carrier image data and embed the information contained in the watermark well.

Zero-watermarking at first usually combines different transform domains, which facilitates the embedding of the watermark. The literature [4] proposes blind watermarking algorithms based on RHFMs and DWT-DCT, which improves security but is less effective against geometric attacks. Literature [5] exploits the advantage of Gabor transform in scaling for feature extraction, which has better robustness against shear and rotation attacks. The literature [6] performs edge feature extraction based on Sobel operator and the algorithm has strong robustness but weak performance against scaling attacks. The literature [7] uses edge contour features for watermark embedding, which has better robustness against noise and compression attacks. Literature [8] proposes an efficient zero watermarking scheme based on quadratic generalized Fourier descriptors, which protects the maximum number of images through the selection of different parameters, but is weak against shearing attacks. Literature [9] designs a protection scheme based on the number of images, and applies LWT-QR decomposition to image fusion, which can protect multiple images simultaneously. Literature [10] proposes an algorithm based on region dissimilarity for the false alarm image problem, which is robust under multiple attacks and the algorithm has some scalability. Literature [11] introduces the concept of unconventional checkpoints to achieve robust watermarking and fragile watermarking with a relatively novel algorithm, but with poor robustness. The literature [12] uses the central pixel of the image as the center of the circle and extracts the image features by circular templates with different radii, and the algorithm is more resistant to rotation attacks. The literature [13] proposed an algorithm based on compressed sensing salient features, which reduces the complexity of the algorithm. The literature [14] divides circular regions by feature points and constructs image features by using singular value decomposition, and the algorithm has strong robustness.

However, the complexity of the above zero watermarking algorithms is high, and most of them are weak against rotation and clipping attacks, and their ability in distinguishing similar images needs to be enhanced, so to address these problems, this paper proposes a robust zero watermarking algorithm for medical images based on SUSAN-DCT. The watermark image is preprocessed before constructing the zero watermark, and applied logical mapping to chaos the watermark information. For original medical image, we first processed in blocks, utilized Smallest Univalue Segment Assimilating

Nucleus (SUSAN) and Discrete Cosine Transform (DCT) to obtain the transform coefficients. On the basis of the first step, a certain size of the low frequency coefficient region is selected. Then, the Hu invariant moment in the block is obtained by taking the block as the unit, and each Hu moment is selected as the effective signal. The judgment coefficient is obtained by data processing and taking the average sum of the maximum value and the median value, and the Hu moment of each block is compared with the judgment value. The size of each Hu moment is compared with the coefficient of determination, binarized to obtain a binary feature matrix, and finally the XOR operation is performed with the watermark image to obtain the key sequence, and the zero watermark construction process is completed.

2 Basic Theory

2.1 SUSAN Edge Detection

The advantages of the Smallest Univalue Segment Assimilating Nucleus (SUSAN) algorithm [15] are strong anti-noise, rotational invariance, and its detection principle does not depend on the results of the pre-image segmentation and avoids the gradient calculation.

The SUSAN algorithm is shown in Fig. 1. A circular template is used, and in practical applications, due to the digitization of images, a true prototype template cannot be realized, and an approximate circle is often used instead; the grayscale of each image pixel point inside the template is compared with the grayscale of the pixel at the center of the template, and given a threshold value, if the difference between the grayscale of a pixel inside the template and the grayscale of the pixel at the center of the template is less than the threshold value, the point is considered to have the same or similar grayscale as the kernel. The region consisting of pixels that satisfy such a condition is called the univalue segment assimilating nucleus.

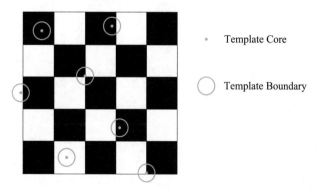

Fig. 1. Scan template for SUSAN algorithm

First established the size of the circular template, and then use this circular template to scan the entire image. The grayscale of each pixel inside the template is compared with the grayscale of the pixel in the center of the template, and then the difference between the two is compared with a threshold value to get USAN region. The formula for determining the USAN region is as follows.

$$c(r, r_0) = \begin{cases} 1 \, , |I(r) - I(r_0)| \leq t \\ 0 \, , |I(r) - I(r_0)| > t \end{cases} \tag{1}$$

$$c(r, r_0) = e^{-\frac{I(r) - I(r_0)}{t}} \tag{2}$$

where r_0 is the template center point, r is the template interior point, and t is the grayscale difference threshold. After obtaining the USAN area, its area size is calculated. The calculation formula is as follows.

$$n(r_0) = \sum c(r, r_0) \tag{3}$$

where $n(r_0)$ denotes the area of USAN with r_0 as the center of the circle. Finally, information extraction is performed. The USAN feature image is extracted by the following equation.

$$R(r_0) = \begin{cases} g - n(r_0) \, , n(r_0) < g \\ 0 \qquad , n(r_0) \geq g \end{cases} \tag{4}$$

where g denotes the geometric threshold, the smaller the value of USAN, the stronger the edge response.

2.2 Hu Moments

Origin moment:

$$m_{pq} = \sum_{x-1}^{M} \sum_{y-1}^{N} x^p y^q f(x, y) \tag{5}$$

Central moment.:

$$\mu_{pq} = \sum_{x-1}^{M} \sum_{y-1}^{N} (x - x_0)^p (y - y_0)^q f(x, y) \tag{6}$$

Normalized central moment:

$$\eta_{pq} = \frac{\mu_{pq}}{\mu_{00}^r} \tag{7}$$

where $r = \frac{p+q+2}{2}, p + q = 2, 3, \cdots$

Hu moment:

Seven invariant moments are constructed using second-order and third-order central moments [16], which can remain translational, rotational, and telescopic under continuous image conditions, with the following equations.

$$hu[0] = \mu_{20} + \mu_{02} \tag{8}$$

$$hu[1] = (\mu_{20} - \mu_{02})^2 + 4\mu_{11}^2 \tag{9}$$

$$hu[2] = (\mu_{30} - 3\mu_{12})^2 + (3\mu_{21} - \mu_{03})^2 \tag{10}$$

$$hu[3] = (\mu_{30} + \mu_{12})^2 + (\mu_{21} + \mu_{03})^2 \tag{11}$$

$$hu[4] = (\mu_{30} - 3\mu_{12})(\mu_{30} + \mu_{12})\left[(\mu_{30} + \mu_{12})^2 - 3(\mu_{21} + \mu_{03})^2\right]$$
$$+ (3\mu_{21} - \mu_{03})(\mu_{21} + \mu_{03})\left[3(\mu_{30} + \mu_{12})^2 - (\mu_{21} + \mu_{03})^2\right] \tag{12}$$

$$hu[5] = (\mu_{20} - \mu_{02})\left[(\mu_{30} + \mu_{12})^2 - (\mu_{21} + \mu_{03})^2\right] + 4\mu_{11}(\mu_{30} + \mu_{12})(\mu_{21} + \mu_{03}) \tag{13}$$

$$hu[6] = (3\mu_{21} - \mu_{03})(\mu_{30} + \mu_{12})\left[(\mu_{30} + \mu_{12})^2 - 3(\mu_{21} + \mu_{03})^2\right]$$
$$- (\mu_{30} - 3\mu_{12})(\mu_{21} + \mu_{03})\left[3(\mu_{30} + \mu_{12})^2 - (\mu_{21} + \mu_{03})^2\right] \tag{14}$$

2.3 Logical Mapping

In nonlinear dynamical systems, chaos is a type of stochastic process that is neither periodic nor convergent. The data in the chaotic region are characterized by iterative irreducibility, initial value sensitivity and parameter sensitivity. The logistic mapping, also known as the worm's mouth model, is a nonlinear dynamical system. This chaotic system is defined by the following equation.

$$X_{k+1} = \mu X_k (1 - X_k) , k = 0, 1, 2 \ldots, n \tag{15}$$

where μ is the bifurcation parameter, when $0 < X_0 < 1$ and $3.5699456 < \mu \leq 4$, the system works in a chaotic state [17].

The encrypted picture is resistant to image assaults because logical mapping may disorganize pixel values, alter the image's histogram, and preserve the gray value division information of the image's pixels.

3 Method

3.1 Watermark Encryption

Preprocessing the original watermark image before constructing the zero-watermark can effectively secure the information. We use the characteristics of the chaotic mapping of the logistics map to choas the image pixel positions, as shown in Fig. 2.

Step 1: Suppose the size of the watermark image is $m \times n$, the logistics map needs to set the initial value x_0 in advance, and then generate a one-dimensional chaotic sequence $X(j)$ with length $m \times n$ by iterating through Eqs. (15).

Step 2: A two-dimensional matrix $X(i, j)$ with size $m \times n$ is obtained by the dimensioning operation.

Step 3: The original watermark image $W(i, j)$ perform XOR operation with $X(i, j)$ to obtain the dislocated watermark image $XW(i, j)$. Without knowing the initial value x_0, the original watermark image cannot be recovered, thus ensuring the security of the watermark information.

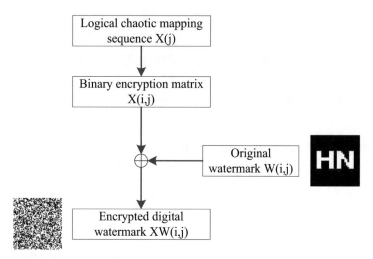

Fig. 2. Digital watermark encryption process

3.2 Watermark Embedding

The specific process of watermark embedding is shown in Fig. 3.

Step 1: The medical image $I(i, j)$ of size 512×512 is split into several small blocks of size 8×8, and SUSAN transform is applied to them. Then DCT transform is performed on SUSAN coefficients $S(i, j)$, and the low frequency coefficients are formed into matrix $IS(i, j)$ of size 64×64.

Step 2: The matrix $IS(i, j)$ is again split into small blocks of size 8×8, and the Hu invariant moment of each block is obtained in small blocks, and $Hu[0]$ is taken as the valid signal.

Step 3: Since the invariant moment is taught to be small, a 1×64 one-dimensional vector is obtained by scaling up its logarithmic value. The average of the sum of the maximum, minimum and median values in this one-dimensional vector is used as the discriminant A.

Step 4: Binarize the one-dimensional vector by comparing the magnitude of Hu of each image block with the discriminant A, and up-dimension the one-dimensional vector into a binary matrix $IF(i, j)$ of size 8×8 to obtain the feature matrix.

Step 5: Perform XOR operation on the binary matrix $IF(i, j)$ and the encrypted image $XW(i, j)$, and the obtained sequence is used as the secret key $Key(i, j)$ for extracting the watermark.

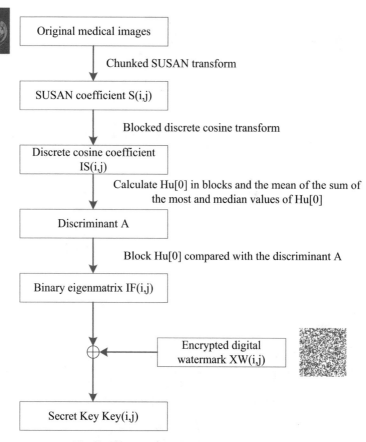

Fig. 3. Watermark embedding process

3.3 Extraction and Decryption of Watermark

After acquiring the feature matrix of the test medical picture, as illustrated in Fig. 4, the extraction and decryption are performed. The medical image may be attacked during transmission, so the test medical image is usually the medical image $I'(i, j)$ after being attacked, simulating the extraction of watermark in this case.

Step 1: Perform the processing of steps 1–4 in Sect. 3.2 on the test medical image $I'(i, j)$, i.e., perform SUSAN transform, DCT transform, calculate Hu moments and discriminant coefficients on $I'(i, j)$, compare the two sizes, and the binary matrix $IF'(i, j)$ by binarization is obtained.

Step 2: Perform XOR operation on the secret key $Key(i, j)$ and the binary matrix $IF'(i, j)$ to obtain the encrypted watermark $XW'(i, j)$ extracted from the test medical image.

Step 3: Use the matrix $X(i, j)$ obtained in 3.1 and perform XOR operation with the $XW'(i, j)$ to extract the watermark image $W'(i, j)$.

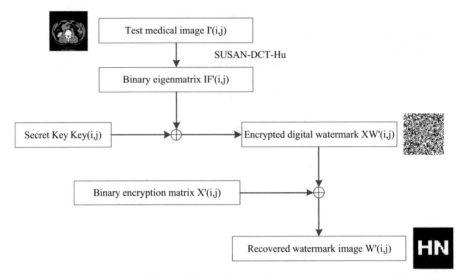

Fig. 4. Watermark extraction process

3.4   Watermark Evaluation

Peak signal-to-noise ratio and normalized correlation coefficient [18] are used as indicators of watermark quality. Image distortion is measured by PSNR, and as the attack intensity rises, the PSNR value falls. A higher NC value denotes a tighter resemblance between two photos. NC is a measure of similarity between two photographs.

$$NC = \frac{\sum_i \sum_j W(i,j) W'(i,j)}{\sum_i \sum_j [W(i,j)]^2} \tag{16}$$

$$PSNR = 10 \log_{10}[\frac{MN \max(I(i,j))^2}{\sum_i \sum_j [I(i,j) - I'(i,j)]^2}] \tag{17}$$

4   The Experimental Results

This paper's experimental setting is Matlab R2017b under Windows 10 operating system. In order to verify that this algorithm has the ability to distinguish different medical images, six medical images of different parts are prepared, any two images are selected for testing, two sets of feature data are obtained, and the correlation between the two is found. Figure 5 shows the six different medical images used in the experiment.

From Table 1, the correlation coefficients between medical images of different parts are less than 0.5, and the correlation coefficient obtained for the same image is 1.00, which indicates that the algorithm will not extract similar feature data for different images, thus reflecting the security of the algorithm.

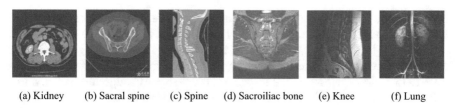

(a) Kidney   (b) Sacral spine   (c) Spine   (d) Sacroiliac bone   (e) Knee   (f) Lung

Fig. 5. Different medical images

Table 1. Correlation coefficient between the feature sequences of 6 test images (64 bits)

Image	Kidney	Sacral spine	Spine	Sacroiliac bone	Knee	Lung
Kidney	1.00	0.25	0.25	0.17	0.03	−0.17
Sacral spine	0.25	1.00	0.06	0.22	−0.17	0.44
Spine	0.25	0.06	1.00	0.04	0.02	0.02
Sacroiliac bone	0.17	0.22	0.04	1.00	−0.02	0.12
Knee	0.03	−0.17	0.02	−0.02	1.00	−0.09
Lung	−0.17	0.44	0.02	0.12	−0.09	1.00

4.1 Watermark Extraction Results After Attacks

To evaluate the algorithm's resistance to attacks, the original medical images was exposed to various assaults, the strength of the attacks was varied to produce different test medical images, as shown in Table 2 and Fig. 6.

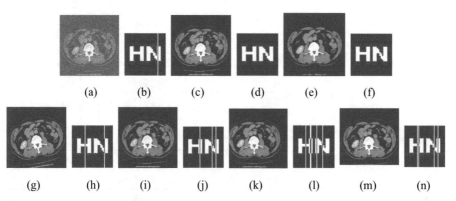

(a)   (b)   (c)   (d)   (e)   (f)

(g)   (h)   (i)   (j)   (k)   (l)   (m)   (n)

Fig. 6. The attacked image and the extracted watermark: (a) Gaussian noise 10%, (c) JPEG compression 9%, (e) Median filter 5 × 5, 5 times, (g) Rotation (counter clockwise) 10°, (i) Scale 0.8 times, (k) Translation (left) 7%, (m) Cropping (Y direction) 10%, (b), (d), (f), (h), (j), (l), (n) Extracted watermark

From Table 2, it can be analyzed that the PSNR of the test medical image decreases when the intensity of the attack gradually increases, indicating that the quality of the image after the attack becomes worse, but the NC is more than 0.5. Under the conventional attacks, when the intensity of Gaussian noise attack is in the range of 1% to 40%, the NC ranges from 0.91 to 1.00, which indicates that the algorithm has good resistance to Gaussian noise attack. When the intensity of JPEG compression attack is in the range of 1% to 15%, the NC is always higher than 0.5, which shows the algorithm still performs well in the face of JPEG compression. Boosting the window size of the median filter from 3 × 3 to 7 × 7, the NC obtained in this process is always 1.00, which indicates that the algorithm is better against median filtering. As a result, the algorithm still performs well under the high-intensity conventional attacks.

The algorithm also performs well against challenging geometrical assaults, particularly rotational attacks. When the original medical image is rotated from 1 degree to 50 degrees, the NC decreases from 1.00 to 0.55, still maintaining a value greater than 0.5. This result is analyzed from the principle thanks to the rotation invariance brought by the circular template of SUSAN algorithm. In the scaling attack, scaling down by 10% or scaling up by 120% can make the NC more than 0.5. The NC can also be in the range of 0.95 to 0.51 when the original medical image is panned to the left by 1%–20%. In the face of a 30% crop attack, it is possible to make the NC more than 0.5 and extract the watermark even if nearly one-third of the image information is lost, which shows that the algorithm's strong robustness against conventional and geometric attacks and can effectively resist the attacks.

Table 2. Test results under different attacks

Type of attacks	Parameters	PSNR	NC
Gaussian noise (%)	1	22.0129	1.00
	10	12.6096	0.95
	20	10.0669	0.95
	40	7.9866	0.91
JPEG Compression (%)	1	25.6408	0.95
	4	27.1824	0.95
	9	30.1652	1.00
	15	31.8064	1.00
Median Filter (5 times)	3 × 3	29.6279	1.00
	5 × 5	26.6607	1.00
	7 × 7	24.7441	1.00
Rotation (°) (counter clockwise)	1	24.3945	1.00
	10	16.6806	0.93
	20	15.3369	0.83

(continued)

Table 2. (*continued*)

Type of attacks	Parameters	PSNR	NC
	30	14.8963	0.72
	50	14.2766	0.55
Scaling	0.1	—	0.69
	0.5	—	0.74
	0.8	—	0.88
	1.2	—	0.61
Translation (%) (left)	1	19.0836	0.95
	5	14.8827	0.95
	10	13.9180	0.67
	20	12.6585	0.51
Cropping (%) (Y direction)	1	—	1.00
	5	—	0.93
	10	—	0.74
	20	—	0.69
	30	—	0.53

4.2 Algorithm Comparison

To verify the superiority of this algorithm, the Gabor-DCT algorithm [19], Curvelet-DCT [20] algorithm and the proposed algorithm were selected for performance comparison under the same experimental environment, and Fig. 5 (a) was selected as the original carrier image. The experimental data are shown in Table 3 and Fig. 7.

Table 3. Performance comparison between different algorithms

Type of attacks	Parameters	Gabor-DCT[19]	Curvelet-DCT[20]	Proposed
Gaussian noise (%)	1	1.00	1.00	1.00
	5	0.90	0.89	0.91
	10	0.64	0.89	0.95
	20	0.74	0.59	0.95
JPEG Compression (%)	1	1.00	0.89	0.95
	4	1.00	0.89	0.95
	9	1.00	1.00	1.00

(*continued*)

Table 3. (*continued*)

Type of attacks	Parameters	Gabor-DCT[19]	Curvelet-DCT[20]	Proposed
Median Filter (5 times)	3 × 3	0.79	1.00	1.00
	5 × 5	0.65	1.00	1.00
	7 × 7	0.65	1.00	1.00
Rotation (°) (counter clockwise)	10	0.88	0.72	0.93
	15	0.88	0.57	0.93
	20	0.54	0.50	0.83
Scaling	0.8	1.00	1.00	0.88
	1.2	1.00	1.00	0.61
Translation (%) (left)	3	1.00	0.71	0.95
	5	1.00	0.62	0.95
	7	1.00	0.49	0.81
Cropping (%) (Y direction)	5	0.89	0.89	0.93
	7	0.72	0.89	0.88
	10	0.57	0.89	0.74

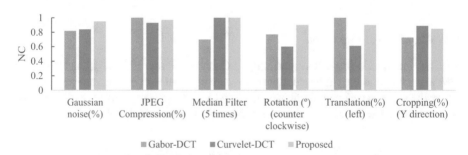

Fig. 7. Comparisons of the average NC

From Table 3, it can be seen that the proposed algorithm is better than the other two algorithms in combating Gaussian noise in the face of conventional attacks, and it is also more robust than Curvelet-DCT and Gabor-DCT in the face of JPEG compression as well as median filtering, respectively. In the case of geometric attacks, the anti-scaling performance of this algorithm is not as good as the other two algorithms. This result is due to the fact that the algorithm is based on chunking, while the other two algorithms process the data from the whole image, so the algorithm does not have an advantage for scaling attacks. However, the test results obtained by this algorithm are overall better than Gabor-DCT and Curvelet-DCT in the face of rotation and shear attacks. In the test against translation attacks, this algorithm outperforms Curvelet-DCT, which again shows that this algorithm has a strong resistance to attacks overall.

5 Conclusions

In this paper, a robust zero-watermarking algorithm for medical images based on SUSAN-DCT is proposed. Firstly, the SUSAN transform is performed on the original medical image, and the transformed image is processed by block discrete cosine transform. Then, the Hu moment calculated in each area is processed to obtain the discriminant coefficient, which is compared with the Hu moment of each block to construct a feature matrix. Furthermore, the feature matrix and the encrypted watermark are logically mapped, and then heteroskedasticity processing is performed to construct a zero watermark, which ensures the security of the algorithm. This algorithm combines the concepts of cryptography, watermarking technology and third parties to embed the information carried by the watermark without any modification to the original image and can be successfully extracted. Simulation experiments demonstrate that the proposed algorithm has strong robustness and good invisibility for both conventional attacks and geometric attacks.

Acknowledgements. This work was supported in part by the Natural Science Foundation of China under Grants 62063004, the Key Research Project of Hainan Province under Grant ZDYF2021SHFZ093, the Hainan Provincial Natural Science Foundation of China under Grants 2019RC018 and 619QN246, and the postdoctor research from Zhejiang Province under Grant ZJ2021028.

References

1. Xiang, S., He, J.: Database authentication watermarking scheme in encrypted domain. IET Inf. Secur. **12**(1), 42–51 (2018)
2. Xu, D., Su, S.: Separable reversible data hiding in encrypted images based on difference histogram modification. Secur. Commun. Netw. **2019** (2019)
3. Wen, Q., Sun, T.F., Wang, S.X.: Concept and application of zero-watermark. Acta Electron. Sin. **31**(2), 214–216 (2003)
4. Li, Z.Y., Zhang, H., Liu, X.L., Wang, C.P., Wang, X.Y.: Blind and safety-enhanced dual watermarking algorithm with chaotic system encryption based on RHFM and DWT-DCT. Digital Sig. Process. **115**, 103062 (2021)
5. Fan, D., Li, Y.Y., Gao, S., Chi, W.D., Lv, C.Z.: A novel zero watermark optimization algorithm based on Gabor transform and discrete cosine transform. Concurr. Comput.: Pract. Exp. **34**(14), e5689 (2022)
6. Xu, H.Y.: Digital media zero watermark copyright protection algorithm based on embedded intelligent edge computing detection. Math. Biosci. Eng. **18**(5), 6771–6789 (2021)
7. Li, D.X., Li, D., Jin, H.: Cartoon zero-watermark method based on edge contourlet feature and visual cryptography. Adv. Intell. Syst. Comput. **1304**, 984–990 (2021)
8. Wang, B.W., Wang, W.S., Zhao, P., Xiong, N.X.: A zero-watermark scheme based on quaternion generalized Fourier descriptor for multiple images. Comput. Mater. Continua **71**(2), 2633–2652 (2022)
9. Wang, B.W., Wang, W.S., Zhao, P.: A zero-watermark algorithm for multiple images based on visual cryptography and image fusion. J. Vis. Commun. Image Represent. **87**, 103569 (2022)
10. Wu, D.Y., Hu, S., Wang, M.M., Jin, H.B., Qu, C.B., Tang, Y.: Discriminative zero-watermarking algorithm based on region XOR and ternary quantization. J. Commun. **43**(2), 208–222 (2022)

11. Sharma, S., Zou, J.J., Fang, G.: A single watermark based scheme for both protection and authentication of identities. IET Image Proc. **16**(12), 3113–3132 (2022)
12. Yang, J.H., Hu, K., Wang, X.C., Wang, H.F., Liu, Q., Mao, Y.: An efficient and robust zero watermarking algorithm. Multimedia Tools Appl. **81**(14), 20127–20145 (2022)
13. Lang, J., Ma, C.L.: Novel zero-watermarking method using the compressed sensing significant feature. Multimedia Tools Appl. **82**(3), 4551–4567 (2023)
14. Wang, X.C., Wen, M.Z., Tan, X.D., Zhang, H.Y., Hu, J.P., Qin, H.: A novel zero-watermarking algorithm based on robust statistical features for natural images. Vis. Comput. **38**(9–10), 3175–3188 (2022)
15. Smith, S.M., Brady, J.M.: SUSAN - a new approach to low level image processing. Int. J. Comput. Vision **23**(1), 45–78 (1997)
16. Balakrishnan, S., Joseph, P.K.: Stratification of risk of atherosclerotic plaque using Hu's moment invariants of segmented ultrasonic images. Biomed. Tech. **67**(5), 391–402 (2022)
17. Zhang, Y., He, Y., Zhang, J., Liu, X.B.: Multiple digital image encryption algorithm based on Chaos algorithm. Mob. Netw. Appl. **27**(4), 1349–1358 (2022)
18. Zhu, T., Qu, W., Cao, W.: An optimized image watermarking algorithm based on SVD and IWT. J. Supercomput. **78**(1), 222–237 (2021). https://doi.org/10.1007/s11227-021-03886-2
19. Xiao, X., et al.: A zero-watermarking algorithm for medical images based on Gabor-DCT. In: Cheng, J., Tang, X., Liu, X. (eds.) CSS 2020. LNCS, vol. 12653, pp. 144–156. Springer, Cham (2021). https://doi.org/10.1007/978-3-030-73671-2_14
20. Qin, F.M., Li, J.B., Li, H., Liu, J., Nawaz, S.A., Liu, Y.L.: A robust zero-watermarking algorithm for medical images using curvelet-DCT and RSA pseudo-random sequences. In: Sun, X., Wang, J., Bertino, E. (eds.) ICAIS 2020. LNCS, vol. 12240, pp. 179–190. Springer, Cham (2020). https://doi.org/10.1007/978-3-030-57881-7_16

A Robust Watermarking Algorithm for Medical Images Based on DWT-Daisy and Discrete Cosine Transform

Yiyi Yuan[1], Jingbing Li[1(✉)], Jing Liu[2], Uzair Aslam Bhatti[1], and Yen-Wei Chen[3]

[1] School of Information and Communication Engineering, Hainan University, Haikou 570228, China
`21210810000036@hainanu.edu.cn`
[2] Research Center for Healthcare Data Science, Zhejiang Lab, Hangzhou, Zhejiang, People's Republic of China
`liujinglj@zhejianglab.com`
[3] Graduate School of Information Science and Engineering, Ritsumeikan University, Kusatsu 525-8577, Shiga, Japan
`chen@is.ritsumei.ac.jp`

Abstract. With the development of digital medical imaging technology, the transmission of medical data in the network is becoming more and more frequent. In order to protect patients' privacy information during transmission, a robust medical watermarking algorithm based on multilevel discrete wavelet transform (M-DWT), Daisy descriptor and discrete cosine transform (DCT) are proposed. The algorithm first performs a three-level DWT transform on the medical image, takes the center point of its low-frequency part LL3 sub-band as the center pixel point of Daisy descriptor, calculates the Daisy descriptor matrix of this point, and performs DCT transformation on it to obtain a 32-bit binary feature vector of the medical image. Then, we associate the feature vector with the watermark to complete the embedding and extraction of the medical watermark. In addition, in order to enhance the security of the watermark information without destroying the medical data information, the watermark is encrypted using the logical mapping, and the zero watermark technology is also adopted. The simulation results show that the proposed algorithm has strong robustness against traditional attacks and geometric attacks. In particular, the algorithm performs better under Gaussian noise attacks and rotation attacks. It also better balances the conflict between the robustness and invisibility of the image watermarking algorithm.

Keywords: DWT · Daisy descriptor · DCT · Medical image · Zero-watermarking

1 Introduction

Currently, although digital technology facilitates the collection, management, transmission, and storage of medical information, it also faces data security risks such as information loss, malicious attacks, and information leakage [1–3]. Different from general

Y.-W. Chen et al. (Eds.): KES InMed 2023, SIST 357, pp. 205–214, 2023.
https://doi.org/10.1007/978-981-99-3311-2_18

digital images, medical images, such as CT, MR, ultrasound and other medical images, as an important auxiliary means of disease diagnosis, contain a large number of patients' personal information. Once this information is leaked, it will cause huge security risks to patients and the society.

Digital watermarking can hide information without affecting the use value of the original medical image. Current work is focused on improving the robustness of watermarking schemes against geometric attacks [4, 5]. Existing solutions to resist geometric attacks can be broadly classified into [6, 7] invariant moment and transform-based algorithms, synchronization-based algorithms, and feature-based algorithms. (1) Application of invariant moments and transformations: For example, Zernike moments [8, 9], Legendre moments [10], tchebichef moments, Krawtchouk moments [11], complex moments (CMs) and polar harmonic transforms (PHTs) [12], quaternion polar coordinate harmonic transform (QPHT) [13], etc. Yamni et al. [14] proposed a new set of discrete orthogonal polynomials. This new set is called fractional discrete orthogonal Charlier moments (FrCM), and the algorithm achieves the embedding of the watermark by modifying the modulus of the coefficients of the real part of the FrCM moments. (2) Simultaneous-based watermarking algorithms. Wang et al. [12] used non-subsampling shear transform (NSST) to embed the watermark while using quaternion PHT and least squares support vector regression (LS-SVR) for simultaneous correction, which can accurately estimate the geometric distortion parameters. (3) Feature invariant-based method. Gong et al. [15] proposed a robust watermarking algorithm based on Harris, Speeded-up Robust Feature (SURF) and DCT. The algorithm first extracts the image corner points, then describes their corner points using the SURF algorithm, and finally the generated descriptor matrix and performs DCT transformation to extract the low-frequency part as feature vector, which has better robustness against geometric attacks. The current watermarking technology is not easy to overcome the problem of rotation attack, the existing algorithm has improved the ability of geometric attacks, but the effectiveness of the rotation attack is relatively weak.

To address the problem of robustness against rotation attacks in geometric attacks, this paper proposes to extract feature vectors from original images by combining Daisy descriptor, DWT and DCT and encrypt watermark by applying chaos technology to improve the security of watermarking information [16]. The experimental results show that the algorithm can accomplish the embedding and extraction of zero-watermarking. It is robust against conventional and geometric attacks, especially for Gaussian noise attacks and rotation attacks.

2 Related Basic Theory

2.1 Daisy Descriptor

Existing local descriptors, such as SIFT and SURF, have been applied in image watermarking algorithms and have proven successful in feature extraction via local descriptors. In this paper, Daisy local descriptor is used, which retains the robustness of SIFT and GLOH and can be computed quickly on each image pixel [17, 18].

Figure 1 shows the regional structure of the Daisy descriptor. As shown in the figure, the algorithm mainly uses a circular form, where each circle represents a region. This structure is characterized by the fact that the region around the center point does not change when a rotation occurs [15, 17], thus achieving a certain degree of rotational robustness.

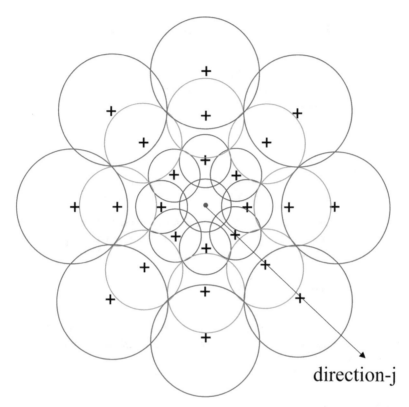

Fig. 1. Area structure of Daisy descriptor.

Suppose a point $p(u_0, v_0)$ on image I as the central pixel point of the Daisy descriptor. First, we take three circles with different and multiplicatively increasing radii centered on point p. The radius is proportional to the standard deviation of the Gaussian kernel. In addition, eight sampling points are obtained at 45° intervals on top of each circle. For this sampling point (u, v) the gradient value in direction i is expressed by $G_i(u, v)$ as follows, and the gradients in each of the eight directions of this sampling point are calculated.

$$G_i(u, v) = \left(\frac{\partial I}{\partial i}\right)^+, 1 \leqslant i \leqslant 8 \qquad (1)$$

$$\left(\frac{\partial I}{\partial i}\right)^+ = max\left(\frac{\partial I}{\partial i}, 0\right) \qquad (2)$$

Then the Gaussian kernel convolution is computed for the gradient map with different Σ values, and the Gaussian convolution values of the sampled points on different layers can be obtained by multiple Gaussian convolution computations [15]. For the point (u, v), its gradient histogram $h_\Sigma(u, v)$ can be expressed as follows.

$$G_i^\Sigma = G_\Sigma * G_i(u, v) \tag{3}$$

$$h_\Sigma(u, v) = [G_1^\Sigma(u, v), G_2^\Sigma(u, v), ..., G_8^\Sigma(u, v)]^T \tag{4}$$

where $G_1^\Sigma, G_2^\Sigma, ..., G_8^\Sigma$ represents the gradient histogram in 8 different directions.

Finally, the gradient histograms of the central pixel point p and the 24 sampled points on the circle are calculated. And use the vector of these 25 points together to represent the descriptor of the feature point p located at the center. Then the Daisy descriptor of point p is:

$$D(u_0, v_0) = \begin{bmatrix} h_{\Sigma_1}^T(u_0, v_0) \\ h_{\Sigma_1}^T(l_1(u_0, v_0, r_1)) \cdots h_{\Sigma_1}^T(l_8(u_0, v_0, r_1)) \\ h_{\Sigma_2}^T(l_1(u_0, v_0, r_2)) \ldots h_{\Sigma_2}^T(l_8(u_0, v_0, r_2)) \\ h_{\Sigma_3}^T(l_1(u_0, v_0, r_3)) \ldots h_{\Sigma_3}^T(l_8(u_0, v_0, r_3)) \end{bmatrix} \tag{5}$$

where $l_i(u_0, v_0, r_j)$ denotes the location of the i-th sampled point above the j-th concentric ring in the structure centered on pixel point (u_0, v_0). The Daisy descriptor $D(u_0, v_0)$ of the pixel point (u_0, v_0) is a matrix and the size of this matrix is 25×8.

2.2 Discrete Wavelet Transform (DWT)

In the same wavelet decomposition layer, the LL sub-band is the low-frequency part, which has better robustness [19] when the watermark information is embedded in this position and can resist the interference of most conventional digital image processing.

3 Proposed Algorithm

3.1 Watermark Embedding

In this paper, the watermark is firstly encrypted using Logistic chaotic mapping to obtain the encrypted watermark sequence $EW(i.j)$. Then extract the feature vectors of the medical image, the specific steps are as follows: Firstly, the original medical image $I(i, j)$ is subjected to a three-level DWT transform, and the centroid of the lowest level wavelet coefficients is selected as the central pixel point of the Daisy descriptor to obtain the Daisy descriptor matrix $D(i, j)$ of this point. Then, we apply DCT transformed to take a 8×4 low-frequency coefficient matrix $F(i, j)$, and use hash function to generate a 32-bit feature vector $V(i, j)$. The watermark can be embedded into the medical image by performing the element-wise XOR operation between the feature vector $V(i, j)$ and the encrypted watermark $EW(i, j)$, and the logical key $Key(i, j)$ can be obtained at the same time, which is operated as follows:

$$V(i, j) = sign \begin{cases} F(i, j) \geq 0, 1 \\ F(i, j) < 0, 0 \end{cases} \tag{6}$$

$$Key(i, j) = EW(i, j) \oplus V(i, j) \tag{7}$$

Figure 2 shows the embedding algorithm.

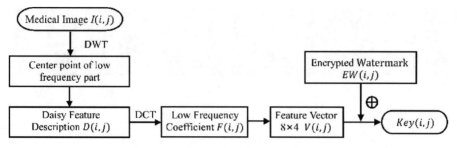

Fig. 2. Watermark embedding algorithm.

3.2 Watermark Extraction

Same as the steps above, the feature vector $V'(i,j)$ of the image under test $I'(i,j)$ is extracted by DWT-Daisy-DCT transform. The encrypted watermark $EW'(i,j)$ can be extracted by performing XOR operation between the feature vector $V'(i,j)$ of the image to be measured and the logical key $Key(i,j)$, which is operated as follows:

$$EW'(i,j) = Key(i,j) \oplus V'(i,j) \tag{8}$$

Figure 3 shows the watermark extraction process.

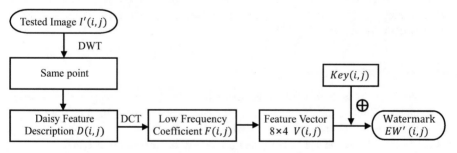

Fig. 3. Watermark extraction algorithm.

4 Experiments and Results

We select 6 different medical images to verify the distinguishability of the algorithm. Figure 4 and Table 1. show these 6 different medical images and the NC values between their 32-bit feature vectors. It can be seen from the data that the NC values between the different images are less than 0.5 and each has an NC value of 1.00. It is possible to distinguish between the different images, which is consistent with human visual characteristics.

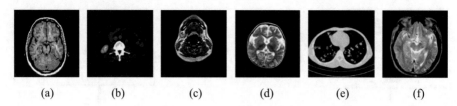

(a)   (b)   (c)   (d)   (e)   (f)

Fig. 4. Different tested images.

Table 1. Values of the correlation coefficients between different images (32 bit)

Image	(a)	(b)	(c)	(d)	(e)	(f)
(a)	**1.00**	0.09	0.24	0.38	0.23	0.38
(b)	0.09	**1.00**	0.01	0.26	0.22	0.39
(c)	0.24	0.01	**1.00**	0.12	-0.11	0.12
(d)	0.38	0.26	0.12	**1.00**	0.26	0.37
(e)	0.23	0.22	-0.11	0.26	**1.00**	0.26
(f)	0.38	0.39	0.12	0.37	0.26	**1.00**

In this experiment, we select a 512 pixel × 512 pixel CT image of the brain as the original image. A 32 pixel × 32 pixel binary image with 'HN' information is selected as the watermarked image (see Fig. 5(a)).

4.1 Conventional Attacks

Figure 5 shows the watermarked images extracted from the brain images under conventional attacks. Table 2. gives the results of the experiment. Observing these results, we found that when the Gaussian noise intensity is 30%, the NC value can still reach a high value of 0.93. When the JPEG compression quality is 10% of the original image, the NC value is 1.00. Hence, the experimental results show that the algorithm has strong robustness against conventional attacks.

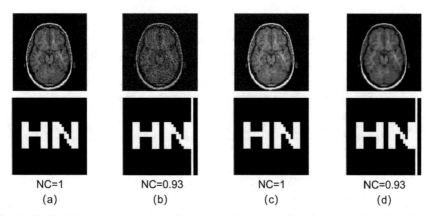

NC=1   NC=0.93   NC=1   NC=0.93
(a)   (b)   (c)   (d)

Fig. 5. Medical image and corresponding extracted watermark under conventional attack. (a) 'Brain' image; (b) Gaussian noise 10%; (c) JPEG Compression 10%; (d) Median Filtering (5 × 5, 10 times).

Table 2. Experimental data of conventional attacks

Conventional attack	Gaussian noise			JPEG compression			Median filtering (10 times)		
	5%	20%	30%	5	10	15	3 × 3	5 × 5	8 × 8
PSNR/dB	14.31	9.77	8.77	28.43	31.29	32.90	33.99	28.55	19.16
NC	1.00	0.91	0.93	0.93	1.00	1.00	1.00	0.93	0.89

4.2 Geometric Attack

Figure 6 shows the watermarked images extracted from the brain images under geometric attacks. Table 3. gives the experimental data of the brain image under geometric attack.

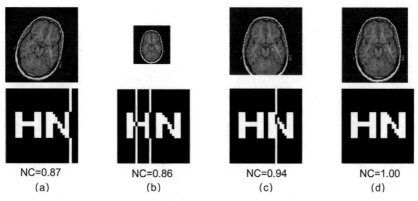

NC=0.87   NC=0.86   NC=0.94   NC=1.00
(a)   (b)   (c)   (d)

Fig. 6. Medical image and corresponding extracted watermark under geometric attack. (a) Rotation 20°; (b)Scaling (×1.5); (c) Cropping y-axis 10%; (d) Cropping x-axis 10%.

The experimental results show that the algorithm has significant advantages for resisting the rotation attack. The NC values all satisfy the requirement of greater than 0.5 when the rotation angle of the image to be tested is less than or equal to 70°.

Table 3. Experimental data of geometric attacks.

Attack	Intensity	PSNR	NC	Attack	Intensity	PSNR	NC
Rotation (clockwise)	20°	14.59	0.87	Cropping (Y axis)	10%	–	0.94
	50°	13.70	0.74		20%	–	0.81
	70°	13.43	0.52		30%	–	0.72
Scaling	0.5	–	0.85	Cropping (Y axis)	10%	–	1.00
	1.5	–	0.96		20%	–	0.91
	2	–	0.91		30%	–	0.63

4.3   Algorithm Comparison

The comparison of watermarking algorithms of DWT-DCT, KAZE-DCT, Daisy-DCT and DWT-Daisy-DCT are shown in Table 4., which demonstrate that the algorithm proposed in this paper is significantly better than the other algorithms in conventional attacks (Gaussian noise, JPEG compression and median filtering) and rotation attacks. The Daisy-DCT algorithm is also our proposed algorithm, and the difference between this algorithm and the algorithm proposed in this paper is the different selection of the central pixel point of the Daisy descriptor and the selection of the radius of the sampling point. The Daisy-DCT algorithm is Both the Daisy-DCT algorithm and DWT-Daisy-DCT algorithm can meet the attack of rotation angle within 70°. In conclusion, the anti-attack capability of the algorithm proposed in this paper is more comprehensive and balanced, and can resist conventional and geometric attacks well.

Table 4. Comparison with other algorithms.

Attack	Intensity	DWT-DCT	KAZE-DCT [16]	Daisy-DCT	DWT-Daisy-DCT
Gaussian noise	15%	0.80	0.53	0.58	**0.96**
	30%	0.78	0.53	0.52	**0.93**
JPEG compression	1%	**1.00**	0.81	0.95	0.82
	10%	1.00	0.81	0.96	**1.00**
Median filtering (10 time)	3 × 3	1.00	0.49	1.00	**1.00**
	8 × 8	0.95	0.52	0.92	**1.00**
Rotation (clockwise)	20°	0.42	0.65	**0.95**	0.87
	50°	0.50	0.59	**0.86**	0.74
	70°	0.30	0.21	**0.68**	0.52
Scaling	0.5	1.00	0.67	**1.00**	0.85
	2	1.00	0.51	**1.00**	0.91
Cropping (Y axis)	5%	0.82	1.00	0.90	**1.00**
	30%	0.39	**0.81**	0.64	0.72
Cropping (X axis)	15%	0.25	0.90	0.87	**1.00**
	30%	0.01	**0.81**	0.40	0.63

5 Conclusion

This paper proposed a robust watermarking algorithm for medical images based on DWT-Daisy and DCT. DWT-Daisy-DCT is first applied to extract image features, perceptual hashing then utilized to generate image feature sequences. By combining with zero watermarking technique, the proposed algorithm can easily embed and extract the watermark without changing any pixel values of the original image. Moreover, to enhance the security of watermark, logistic chaos mapping is introduced. Therefore, the proposed algorithm can be used in special cases such as medical images where image quality is strictly required, and shows good practicality in medical and other related fields. Experimental results show that the algorithm is robust to both conventional attacks and geometric attacks, especially in Gaussian noise attacks and rotation attacks.

Acknowledgements. This work was supported in part by the Natural Science Foundation of China under Grants 62063004, the Key Research Project of Hainan Province under Grant ZDYF2021SHFZ093, the Hainan Provincial Natural Science Foundation of China under Grants 2019RC018 and 619QN246, and the postdoctor research from Zhejiang Province under Grant ZJ2021028.

References

1. Khare, P., Srivastava, V.K.: A secured and robust medical image watermarking approach for protecting integrity of medical images. Trans. Emerging Telecommun. Technol. **32**(2), e3918 (2021)
2. Hemdan, E.-D.: An efficient and robust watermarking approach based on single value decompression, multi-level DWT, and wavelet fusion with scrambled medical images. Multimedia Tools Appl. **80**(2), 1749–1777 (2020). https://doi.org/10.1007/s11042-020-09769-7
3. Daham, A., Ouslim, M., Hafed, Y., et al.: Robust watermarking method to secure medical images applied to ehealth. In: 13th International Conference on Information and Communication Systems (ICICS), pp. 379–385 (2022)
4. Nazari, M., Mehrabian, M.: A novel chaotic IWT-LSB blind watermarking approach with flexible capacity for secure transmission of authenticated medical images. Multimedia Tools Appl. **80**(7), 10615–10655 (2020). https://doi.org/10.1007/s11042-020-10032-2
5. Liu, J., Li, J., Ma, J., et al.: A robust multi-watermarking algorithm for medical images based on DTCWT-DCT and Henon map. Appl. Sci. **9**(4), 700 (2019)
6. Zhang, H., Li, Z., Liu, X., et al.: Robust image watermarking algorithm based on QWT and QSVD using 2D Chebyshev-Logistic map. J. Franklin Inst. **359**(2), 1755–1781 (2022)
7. Evsutin, O., Dzhanashia, K.: Watermarking schemes for digital images: robustness overview. Sig. Process.: Image Commun. **100**, 116523 (2022)
8. Dwivedi, R., Srivastava, V.K.: Geometrically robust digital image watermarking based on Zernike moments and FAST technique. In: Advances in VLSI, Communication, and Signal Processing: Select Proceedings of VCAS 2021, pp. 671–680. Springer, Singapore (2022). https://doi.org/10.1007/978-981-19-2631-0_58
9. Wang, H., Chen, Y., Zhao, T.: Modified Zernike moments and its application in geometrically resilient image zero-watermarking. Circuits Syst. Sig. Process. **41**(12), 6844–6861 (2022)
10. Hosny, K.M., Darwish, M.M., Fouda, M.M.: New color image zero-watermarking using orthogonal multi-channel fractional-order legendre-fourier moments. IEEE Access **9**, 91209–91219 (2021)
11. Hassan, G., Hosny, K.M., Farouk, R.M., et al.: New set of invariant quaternion krawtchouk moments for color image representation and recognition. Int. J. Image Graph. **22**(04), 2250037 (2022)
12. Wang, X., Xu, H., Zhang, S., et al.: A color image watermarking approach based on synchronization correction. Fund. Inform. **158**(4), 385–407 (2018)
13. Niu, P.P., Wang, L., Wang, F., et al.: Fast quaternion log-polar radial harmonic fourier moments for color image zero-watermarking. J. Math. Imaging Vis. **64**(5), 537–568 (2022)
14. Yamni, M., Daoui, A., Karmouni, H., et al.: Fractional Charlier moments for image reconstruction and image watermarking. Sig. Process. **171**, 107509 (2020)
15. Gong, C., Li, J., Bhatti, U.A., et al.: Robust and secure zero-watermarking algorithm for medical images based on Harris-SURF-DCT and chaotic map. Secur. Commun. Netw. **2021**, 1–13 (2021)
16. Zeng C, Liu J, Li J, et al. Multi-watermarking algorithm for medical image based on KAZE-DCT. Journal of Ambient Intelligence and Humanized Computing, 1-9 (2022)
17. Yuan, X.C., Li, M.: Local multi-watermarking method based on robust and adaptive feature extraction. Sig. Process. **149**, 103–117 (2018)
18. Tola, E., Lepetit, V., Fua, P.: Daisy: an efficient dense descriptor applied to wide-baseline stereo. IEEE Trans. Pattern Anal. Mach. Intell. **32**(5), 815–830 (2009)
19. Abadi, R.Y., Moallem, P.: Robust and optimum color image watermarking method based on a combination of DWT and DCT. Optik **261**, 169146 (2022)

Robust Watermarking Algorithm for Medical Volume Data Based on PJFM and 3D-DCT

Lei Cao[1], Jingbing Li[1,2(✉)], Jing Liu[3], and Yen-Wei Chen[4]

[1] School of Information and Communication Engineering, Hainan University, Haikou 570228, China
21220854000132@hainanu.edu.cn, jingbingli2008@hotmail.com
[2] State Key Laboratory of Marine Resource Utilization in the South China Sea, Hainan University, Haikou 570228, China
[3] Research Center for Healthcare Data Science, Zhejiang Lab, Hangzhou 311121, Zhejiang, China
liujinglj@zhejianglab.com
[4] Graduate School of Information Science and Engineering, Ritsumeikan University, Kusatsu 525-8577, Shiga, Japan
chen@is.ritsumei.ac.jp

Abstract. With the rapid development of information technology and digital image processing, digital imaging technology is gradually mature and widely used in the field of medicine. The use of computed tomography (CT) and magnetic resonance imaging (MRI) for diagnosis has become an indispensable and effective auxiliary means of modern medical diagnosis. It not only facilitates the diagnosis of doctors and real-time information exchange, but also effectively solves the problem of uneven distribution of medical resources. However, medical data is vulnerable to various malicious attacks when spreading and sharing information on the network, and there is a risk of disclosure of patient privacy. To solve this problem, this paper proposes a robust watermarking algorithm for medical volume data based on deformed Jacobi-Fourier moments and 3D discrete cosine transform. The algorithm first used PJFM moment to extract the features of each slice of 3D medical volume data. Then the feature matrix was transformed by 3D-DCT to combine the contour information and detail information of each slice, and the visual feature vector was obtained by applying perceptual hash technology. In addition, the proposed algorithm used Logistic Map to preprocess and encrypt the original watermark image, and utilized zero watermarking technology to embed,, which further improved the security and practicability of the algorithm. Simulation results show that the proposed algorithm has good robustness against common and geometric attacks, especially resist rotation attacks, cropping attacks and compression attacks.

Keywords: PJFM · 3D-DCT · Volume data watermarking · Zero watermarking

1 Introduction

Under the trend of rapid development of multimedia technology and network application, digitalization is more and more popular. Applying computer technology and information technology to the whole medical process is a new modern medical way, which is the development direction and management goal of public medical treatment. New medical technologies such as digital medical detection technology, remote diagnosis and treatment, and medical digital imaging technology have developed rapidly and been widely used in the medical process, accelerating the process of medical digitalization [1]. Among them, medical digital imaging technology has been widely used in radiology and cardiovascular imaging, and has been increasingly widely applied in other medical fields such as ophthalmology and dentistry, which not only provides convenience for remote diagnosis and treatment and academic exchanges, but also effectively solves the problem of uneven distribution of medical resources [2].

While medical information can be transmitted quickly and efficiently on the public network, it also faces some security problems, such as the interception and tampering of medical information has become easier, and there is the risk of disclosure of patient privacy. Medical image digital watermarking technology is an effective method to solve this problem. Medical information is hidden in medical images as watermark information, which ensures the security of information transmission and protects the privacy of patients [3].

At present, most medical images are 3D volume data, such as Computed Tomography (CT), Magnetic Resonance Imaging (MRI), and Ultrasonography (US) and other imaging equipment, 80% of the digital images generated are 3D volume data. Compared with two-dimensional images, three-dimensional volume data can provide more intuitive and accurate diagnostic information, and serve as an important basis and guidance for medical diagnosis [4]. 3D volume data model is widely used. It has become an urgent problem to realize the security protection and perfection detection of 3D volume data information under the network environment. In recent years, the application of watermarking algorithm in medical volume data has developed rapidly, mainly based on transformation, feature point, dimensionality reduction and other directions. Literature [5] proposed a robust digital watermarking embedding algorithm for volume data based on three dimensional discrete cosine transform (3D-DCT) technology and spread spectrum communication technology. The binary image can be directly embedded through spread spectrum communication technology to generate watermark information. Then, the watermark information and the original volume data are divided into discrete cosine transform (DCT) to realize the watermark embedding in the transform domain, which can resist the common attacks such as cutting, noise, filtering, rotation, etc., but the original volume data is needed to extract the watermark information, and the algorithm cannot resist the high intensity geometric attacks. Literature [6] Based on dual-density dual-tree complex wavelet transform, DD-DT CWT is based on the scale invariant feature transform (SIFT) digital watermarking algorithm for volume data, which realizes blind extraction and can resist some common and geometric attacks. However, the experiment proves that it is difficult to resist the geometric attack of large strength. In order to improve the ability of the algorithm to resist geometric attack, people start to study the establishment of a domain invariant to geometric transformation, and then watermark embedding and extraction. The methods of building such a geometrically invariant domain are usually divided into three categories. The first category is to transform the attacked image to its original size and orientation, which is very difficult to implement. The second type uses the local feature points of the image to construct the geometric invariant domain, but the watermark capacity is limited. The third kind of method is to embed the watermark signal into the geometric invariant domain. The method based on invariant moments is one of them, which is also the object of this paper.

Moment invariants are a highly condensed image feature with invariance of translation, scale, rotation and gray level. Researches on introducing invariant moments into digital watermarking algorithm can enhance the robustness of the algorithm [7]. Pseudo-Zernike Moments (PZM) and image normalization are used in literature [8]. Firstly, geometric invariant space is constructed through image normalization, and then some low-order moments are selected to quantize embedded watermarks. When extracting watermarks, the phase information of pseudo-zernike moments is used to correct the host image. The geometric invariance of moments is improved, and the algorithm is robust to geometric attacks, especially rotational attacks. A digital watermarking algorithm based on jacobi-fourier moments (JFM) is proposed in literature [9]. The binary watermarking sequence is embedded into the amplitude of JFM moments by quantization method using the rotational invariance of JFM moment amplitude. The algorithm can effectively resist geometric attacks and common attacks.

However, the above moment invariant digital watermarking algorithm cannot resist strong common attacks, and the algorithm can embed the watermark by changing some coefficient values of the image, which affects the quality of the image, so it is not suitable for processing medical images. Meanwhile, the above algorithms are applied to two-dimensional images, for the current development of medical digitization, the research of three-dimensional volume data digital watermarking algorithm is of great significance. Aiming at the above problems, this paper proposed a robust watermarking algorithm for medical volume data based on pseudo jacobi-fourier moments (PJFM) and three dimensional discrete cosine transform, 3D-DCT). PJFM is a deformation of JFM, proposed by Amu G L et al., with fewer moments, low time consumption and good rotational invariance [10–12]. The proposed algorithm combined the good rotation invariance of PJFM and the good resistance of 3D-DCT to common attacks. The feature matrix is obtained by PJFM transformation and normalization, and then the feature vector of volume data is extracted by 3D-DCT. Then the binary watermark encrypted by Logistic chaotic map is associated with the feature vector of volume data, and the associated binary sequence is stored and embedded in the watermark. Similarly, PJFM transform and 3D-DCT are used to extract the feature vectors of the data to be tested, which are associated with the binary sequence key stored with the third party to extract the watermark.

2 The Fundamental Theory

2.1 Pseudo Jacobi-fourier Moment

In 2003, Amu.G.L et al., proposed the theory of Pseudo Jacobi-Fourier moment, which has multi-distortion invariance such as gray level, scale, translation and rotation, and is suitable for image feature extraction [13]. The radial Jacobi polynomial in the interval [0,1] can be defined as:

$$G_n(p, q, r) = \frac{\Gamma(q+n)}{\Gamma(p+2n)} \sum_{m=0}^{n} (-1)^m \binom{n}{m} \frac{\Gamma(p+2n-m)}{\Gamma(q+n-m)} r^{n-m} \tag{1}$$

Suppose $s = n\text{-}m$, and when $p = 4$ and $q = 3$, the Jacobi polynomial can be transformed into:

$$J_n(r) = a_n \sqrt{(1-r)r} \sum_{s=0}^{n} b_{ns} r^s \tag{2}$$

In this way,

$$a_n = (-1)^n \sqrt{\frac{(2n+4)}{(n+3)(n+1)}} \tag{3}$$

$$b_{ns} = (-1)^s \frac{(n+s+3)!}{(n-s)!s!(s+2)!} \tag{4}$$

where n and m are the order of polynomials, n denotes a non-negative integer, and the value range of m is $-n \le m \le n$. The range of s is $0 \le s \le n$.

The polynomial satisfies the orthogonal normalization condition:

$$\int_0^1 J_n(r) J_k(r) r dr = \delta_{nk} \tag{5}$$

So in polar coordinates (r, θ), we can define a system of functions $P_{nm}(r, \theta)$, It is composed of radial function $J_n(r)$ and angular function $\exp(jm\theta)$.

$$P_{nm}(r, \theta) = J_n(r) \exp(jm\theta) \tag{6}$$

Obviously, the function system $P_{nm}(r, \theta)$ also satisfies the orthogonal normalization condition.

$$\int_0^{2\pi} \int_0^1 P_{nm}(r, \theta) P_{kl}(r, \theta) r dr d\theta = \delta_{nmkl} \tag{7}$$

According to the orthogonality theory, when the function satisfies $f(r)$ the Dirichlet condition, it can be expanded into a generalized Fourier series according to the orthogonal normalized polynomial $\{p_n(r)\}$ of the weight function $p(r)$. Then $f(r, \theta)$ can be expanded as:

$$f(r, \theta) = \sum_{n=0}^{+\infty} \sum_{m=-\infty}^{+\infty} \Phi_{nm} J_n(r) \exp(jm\theta) \tag{8}$$

Therefore, the deformed Jacobian ($p = 4$, $q = 3$) -Fourier moment can be obtained:

$$\Phi_{nm} = \frac{1}{2\pi} \int_0^{2\pi} \int_0^1 f(r, \theta) J_n(r) \exp(-jm\theta) r dr d\theta \tag{9}$$

where $f(r, \theta)$, denotes the image function and the value range of r is [0,1] (which represents the scale of the target image in the polar coordinate system). In essence, the deformed Jacobi moment refers to the center distance with the centroid of the target image as the origin of coordinates.

2.2 3D-DCT and 3D-IDCT

For data blocks of the size is $n_x \times n_y \times n_z$, 3D-DCT transform calculation is performed using the Eq. 3:

$$F(u, v, w) = C(u)C(v)C(w)[\sum_{x=0}^{n_x-1} \sum_{y=0}^{n_y-1} \sum_{z=0}^{n_z-1} f(x, y, z) \cdot \frac{(2x+1)u\pi}{2n_x} \frac{(2y+1)v\pi}{2n_y} \frac{(2z+1)w\pi}{2n_z}] \tag{10}$$

Here,

$$C(u) = \begin{cases} \sqrt{1/n_x} u = 0 \\ \sqrt{2/n_x} u \neq 0 \end{cases}, C(v) = \begin{cases} \sqrt{1/n_y} v = 0 \\ \sqrt{2/n_y} v \neq 0 \end{cases}, C(w) = \begin{cases} \sqrt{1/n_z} w = 0 \\ \sqrt{2/n_z} w \neq 0 \end{cases} \tag{11}$$

where $f(x, y, z)$ denotes the volume metadata value of the volume data V at (x, y, z), and $F(u, v, w)$ is the corresponding 3D-DCT transformation coefficient of the volume metadata [14].

In addition, the size of the block is $n_x \times n_y \times n_z$ calculated by 3D-IDCT transform:

$$f(x, y, z) = \sum_{u=0}^{n_x-1} \sum_{v=0}^{n_y-1} \sum_{w=0}^{n_z-1} [C(u)C(v)C(w) \frac{(2x+1)u\pi}{2n_x} \cdot F(u, v, w) \frac{(2y+1)v\pi}{2n_y} \frac{(2z+1)w\pi}{2n_z}] \tag{12}$$

where $C(u)$, $C(v)$, and $C(w)$ are the same as those in 3D-DCT transform Eq. (3).

2.3 Logistic Mapping

Logistic mapping is a one-dimensional discrete chaotic system with fast operation speed and better chaotic sequences can be generated by repeated iteration of equations [15]. The resulting chaotic sequence is very sensitive to the initial state and system parameters. The Logistic mapping is defined as:

$$x_{k+1} = \mu x_k (1 - x_k) \tag{13}$$

where, $0 < \mu \leq 4$ denotes branch parameter, $x_k \in (0, 1)$ is the system variable, and the number of iterations is k. A large number of studies on Logistic mapping have shown that when u reaches the limit value, that is, u = 3.5699456, the steady-state solution period of the system is ∞. As shown in Fig. 1, when 3.5699456 < μ ≤ 4, Logistic mapping presents chaotic state. Therefore, in order to achieve chaotic state, the value range of μ should be set as:

$$3.5699456 < \mu \leq 4 \tag{14}$$

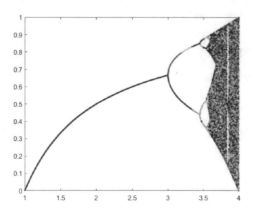

Fig. 1. Bifurcation plot of Logistic Map

3   Method

3.1   Feature Extraction

As the PJFM coefficient has good rotation invariance and satisfies the orthogonality characteristic, it is suitable for image feature description. We can use its characteristic to extract the feature vector of medical volume data [16]. The algorithm in this paper uses PJFM and 3D-DCT to extract perceptual hash values reflecting the features of medical Volume data. We select 128 pixel × 128 pixel × 27 pixel standard MRI brain volume data as the test object. Firstly, PJFM transformation was performed on each slice, and then PJFM normalization was performed to obtain the feature matrix. Finally, 3D-DCT transformation was performed on the reconstructed 3D feature matrix. Here, the perceptual hash threshold is the average coefficient value, and the length of the visual feature vector is selected as 32 bits. We further verify whether the feature vectors obtained from the volume data of various shapes after the algorithm processing are the effective features and whether the features are different due to the different contour shapes of the volume data. As shown in Fig. 2, we randomly selected 6 different volume data with different shapes to verify the discrimination between extracted visual feature vectors. According to the data in Table 1, the correlation coefficient between different volume data is low, which indicates that the algorithm can distinguish different volume data. Only when the shape is consistent, the NC value coefficient is 1, which further demonstrates the good performance of the algorithm for 3D contour feature extraction of medical volume data.

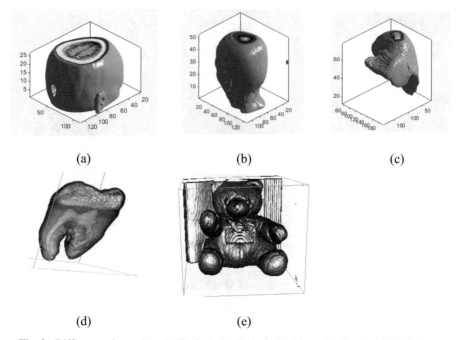

(a)   (b)   (c)

(d)   (e)

Fig. 2. Different volume data: (a) Brain 1; (b) Brain 2; (c) Liver; (d) Tooth; (e) Teddy bear.

Table 1. Correlation coefficients between perceptual hash values of different volume data (32bits).

	(a)	(b)	(c)	(d)	(e)
(a)	1	0.3266	0.2894	0.3671	0.2894
(b)	0.3266	1	0.1189	0.2218	0.3907
(c)	0.2894	0.1189	1	-0.1044	0.2000
(d)	0.3671	0.2218	-0.1044	1	0.3133
(e)	0.2894	0.2218	0.2000	0.3133	1

3.2 Watermark Encryption

Logistic Map scrambling algorithm is applied to the watermarking encryption process, as shown in Fig. 3. The initial value x_0 was used to generate chaotic sequence $X(j)$ by Logistic Map, and then the values in chaotic sequence $X(j)$ were sorted from small to large, and then the space of watermark pixels was scrambled according to the position changes before and after sorting of each value in $X(j)$, and finally chaotic chaotic watermark $BW(i, j)$ was obtained.

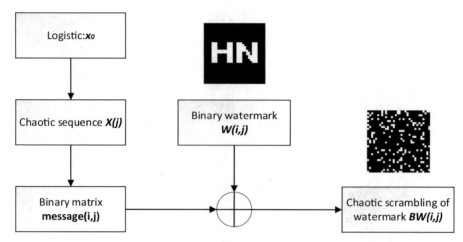

Fig. 3. The flow chart of watermark encryption.

3.3 The Embedding and Extraction of Watermark

The embedding process of robust watermark for medical volume data is as follows:

Firstly, PJFM and 3D-DCT transform were performed on the medical volume data, G(i, j, k) and the transformation coefficients F2(1:4,1:2,1:4) were selected for perceptual hash, the transformation rule is: when the coefficient is greater than or equal to the average value, the binary value is changed to "1", otherwise, the binary value is changed to "0", and the 32-bit visual feature vector V(j) is obtained. Then, the visual feature vector is XOR line by line with the encrypted watermark Scrambled(i, j) obtained by the Logistic chaotic scrambling algorithm to obtain the logical key Key(i, j), which is saved in the third party for watermark extraction (Fig. 4).

The extraction process of robust watermark for medical volume data is as follows:

The process of watermark extraction is the inverse process of watermark embedding. For example, the medical volume data G(i, j, k) is rotated 60° to obtain the medical volume data G'(i, j, k) under test, and then PJFM and 3D-DCT transform are performed on it. The transformation coefficient F2'(1:4,1:2,1:4) is selected for perceptual hash to obtain the 32-bit visual feature vector V'(j). Then the visual feature vector V'(j) is XOR line by line with the logical key Key(i, j) stored in the third party to extract the encryption watermark BW'(i, j) (Fig. 5).

3.4 Watermark Decryption

The decryption process of watermark by Logistic Map chaotic scrambling algorithm is shown in Fig. 6. Firstly, the binary feature sequence $X(j)$ is obtained by the same method as the watermark encryption, and the values of $X(j)$ are sorted according to the order from small to large. Then, the pixel position space in the watermark is restored according to the position change before and after the sorting of each value, and the restored watermark $W'(i, j)$ is obtained. By calculating the correlation coefficient NC value of original watermark $BW(i, j)$ and recovered watermark $W'(i, j)$, the attribution of medical volume data and embedded watermark information is determined.

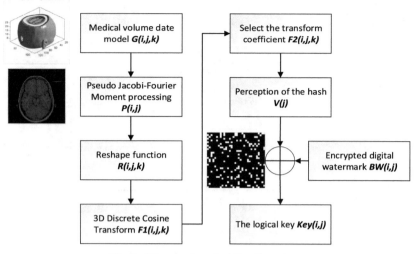

Fig. 4. Watermark embedding flow chart.

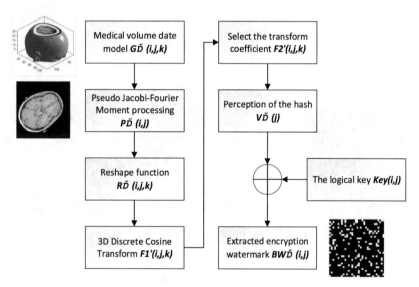

Fig. 5. The flow chart of watermark extraction.

4 The Experimental Results

4.1 Common Attacks

4.1.1 Gaussian Noise Attacks

The brain and volume data were attacked with Gaussian noise of different intensity. As shown in Table 2, the noise intensity ranges from 3% to 25%. From the observation, when the noise intensity is 10%, the brain volume data and corresponding slices have

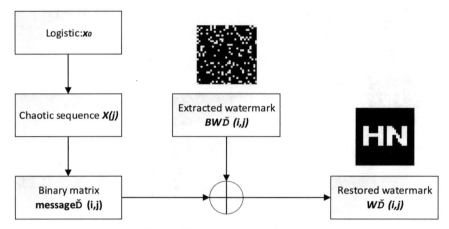

Fig. 6. The flow chart of recovery.

been seriously blurred, and the PSNR is 3.32 dB, only the blurred contour can be seen, but the extracted watermark NC value is still 0.80. When the noise intensity continues to increase by 25%, the PSNR is reduced to 0.09, and the NC value of the watermark is still 0.71. The implementation demonstrates that the proposed algorithm has good robustness to resist Gaussian noise attacks (Fig. 7).

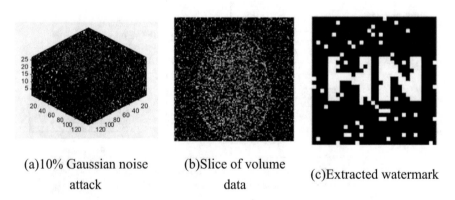

(a)10% Gaussian noise attack   (b)Slice of volume data   (c)Extracted watermark

Fig. 7. Gaussian noise attacks.

Table 2. Results of Gaussian noise attacks.

Noise intensity(%)	3	5	10	15	20	25
PSNR(dB)	8.03	6.02	3.32	1.81	0.79	0.09
NC	0.80	0.80	0.80	0.74	0.71	0.71

4.1.2 JPEG Compression Attacks

In the JPEG compression attack on brain volume data, it can be found in Table 3 that with the reduction of compression quality, the block effect becomes more and more obvious, and the distortion degree of volume data gradually increases. When the compression quality is 1%, the image has obvious block effect. However, the NC value of the extracted watermark is still as high as 1, and the NC value of the extracted watermark is all 1 for the attacks of different compression quality, such as 2%, 4%, 8%, 20%, 40%, etc., which shows that the watermark algorithm has very good robustness against JPEG compression attacks (Fig. 8).

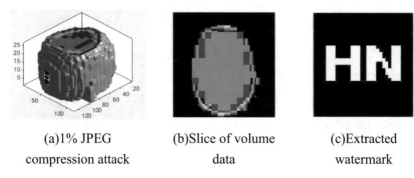

| (a)1% JPEG | (b)Slice of volume | (c)Extracted |
| compression attack | data | watermark |

Fig. 8. JPEG compression attacks.

Table 3. Results of JPEG compression attacks.

Compression quality(%)	1	2	4	8	20	40
PSNR(dB)	16.56	16.57	17.82	20.21	23.10	25.06
NC	1.00	1.00	1.00	1.00	1.00	1.00

4.1.3 Median Filtering Attacks

The brain and volume data are subjected to median filtering attacks with different window sizes and different filtering times. It can be found from Table 4 that with the increase of window size and filtering times, the PSNR value shows a gradual downward trend, and the surface contour of brain and volume data becomes gradually smooth, corresponding to the deterioration of slice quality. After [5 × 5] and [7 × 7] 20 times median filtering attacks, the extracted watermark NC value is still 1. Even after [15 × 15] 20 median filtering attacks, the extracted watermark NC value is still 0.89. It can be found that the algorithm has high robustness against median filtering attacks (Fig. 9).

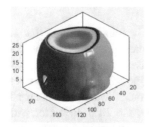

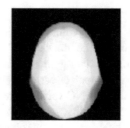

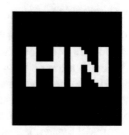

(a) [7x7] 20 Median filtering attack

(b)Slice of volume data

(c)Extracted watermark

Fig. 9. Median filtering attacks.

Table 4. Results of median filtering attacks.

Parameter	[5x5]			[7x7]			[15x15]		
Times	1	10	20	1	10	20	1	10	20
PSNR(dB)	21.14	18.69	18.07	18.91	16.98	16.58	15.48	13.06	11.80
NC	1.00	1.00	1.00	1.00	1.00	1.00	1.00	1.00	0.89

4.2 Geometric Attacks

4.2.1 Rotation Attacks

The brain and volume data were subjected to clockwise rotation attacks of 5° to 65° in order. The parameter values under each rotation Angle are shown in Table 5. It can be found in the table that even a very small rotation angle will have a great impact on the distortion of volume data. It can be seen from Table 5 that the NC value of the watermark extracted from volume data is 1 when the clockwise rotation ranges from 5° to 60°. From 60°, the NC value of the watermark extracted starts to decline. When the rotation reaches 65°, the PSNR value is only 10.00 dB, and the section image quality is already poor, but the NC value is still 0.72, which is larger than the dividing line 0.50. The information contained in the watermark is still legible. It is shown that the algorithm is very robust to rotation attack, and the good rotation invariance of PJFM moment is further verified (Fig. 10).

4.2.2 Scaling Attacks

The scaling attack was carried out on the brain and volume data. The parameter values under different scaling multiples are shown in Table 6. Since the size of the slice image was changed during the scaling, the PSNR value could not be calculated by the scaling operation, it was not marked in the table. As shown in Table 6, with the gradual increase of the scaling factor, the NC value gradually increases. When the magnification is 4 times, the NC value of the extracted watermark is still 1. When the size is reduced by 0.4 times, the watermark NC is still 0.72, which is higher than 0.50. Compared with

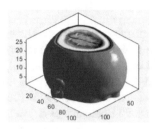 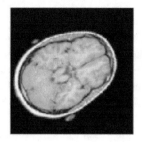 

(a)65° clockwise rotation attack   (b)Slice of volume data   (c)Extracted watermark

Fig. 10. Rotation attacks.

Table 5. Results of rotation attacks.

Rotate clockwise(°)	5	10	30	50	60	63	65
PSNR(dB)	16.54	13.97	11.68	10.52	10.17	10.07	10.00
NC	1.00	1.00	1.00	1.00	1.00	0.80	0.72

the original watermark, the watermark extracted by the watermark system has a strong correlation, which can be considered as a successful watermark extraction, indicating that the algorithm has good robustness against scaling attack (Fig. 11).

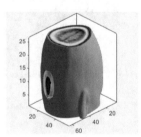 

(a)Scaling factor 0.4 attack   (b)Slice of volume data   (c)Extracted watermark

Fig. 11. Scaling attacks.

Table 6. Results of scaling attacks.

Zoom (×)	0.4	0.5	0.75	1	2	4
NC	0.72	0.80	0.89	1.00	1.00	1.00

4.2.3 Translation Attacks

Translation attack was carried out on brain and Volume data, and the results are shown in Table 7. It can be found that within the range of 2% to 12% translation to the left, with the increase of translation percentage, the black part of the right slice gradually increased, and the PSNR value gradually decreased. When the translation was 12% to the left, the NC value was 0.63. A vertical downward translation attack of 2% to 12% is applied to the volume data successively. When the translation percentage is 2% to 6%, the NC value remains 1, and when the translation percentage is greater than 6%, the NC value starts to decline slowly. As can be seen from section Fig. 12(e), when the downward translation is 12%, the details of the lower part of the brain have been lost, and the NC value is still 0.80, indicating that the algorithm has good robustness to the translation attacks.

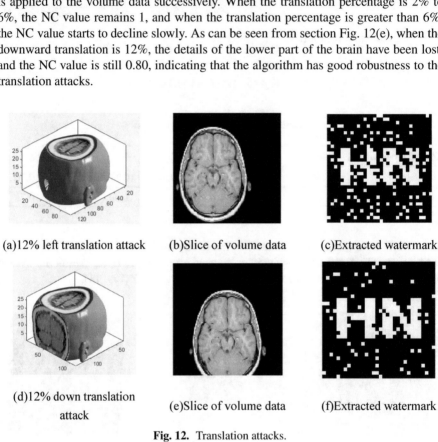

(a)12% left translation attack   (b)Slice of volume data   (c)Extracted watermark

(d)12% down translation attack   (e)Slice of volume data   (f)Extracted watermark

Fig. 12. Translation attacks.

Table 7. Results of translation attacks.

Direction	Left						Down					
%	2	4	6	8	10	12	2	4	6	8	10	12
PSNR(dB)	13.02	11.38	10.90	10.21	9.80	9.27	15.65	12.40	11.66	11.09	10.85	10.51
NC	1.00	1.00	1.00	0.79	0.63	0.63	1.00	1.00	1.00	0.89	0.89	0.80

4.2.4 Cropping Attacks

Brain volume data for cropping attacks, 5% to 60% range of Z-axis you can see from Fig. 13(a) when the cropping rate is 60%, the outline of brain volume data has taken place great changes, the upper data loss is severe, but even in this case, the extracted watermark NC value is still as high as 0.89, shows that the algorithm of Z axis cropping attacks robustness is very good.

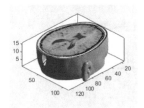   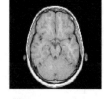   

(a)60% Z-axis cropping attack   (b)Slice of volume data   (c)Extracted watermark

Fig. 13. Cropping attacks (Table 8).

Table 8. Results of Z-axis cropping attacks.

Cropping (Z-axis %)	5	10	20	40	50	60
NC	1.00	1.00	1.00	1.00	1.00	0.89

4.3 Algorithms Comparison

To further verify the robustness of the proposed algorithm, we used the standard brain volume data (128 pixel × 128 pixel × 27 pixel) for quantitative analysis, and compared the robustness with other medical volume data digital watermarking algorithms. We combined this algorithm with the algorithm in "3D DWT-DCT and Logistic MAP Based Robust Watermarking for Medical Volume Data" proposed by Liu et al. [17]. And comparison of algorithms in "Medical Volume Data Watermarking Using Perceptual Hash 3D-DCT and Arnold Scrambling" proposed by Hu et al. [18], as shown in Table 9. Due to the excellent anti-common attacks performance of DCT transform, it can be seen that the NC value of the three algorithms is similar when the same intensity attack is applied in JPEG compression attack and median filtering attack, and the NC value of the proposed algorithm is slightly higher than the other two algorithms. Because deformed Jacobi-Fourier moments are sensitive to noise, Gaussian noise affects the feature description of pseudo Jacobi-Fourier moments on volume data slices, so the anti-Gaussian noise attack ability of the proposed algorithm is slightly lower than that of the two comparison algorithms. The proposed algorithm is superior to the two comparison algorithms in terms of rotation attack, downward translation attack and Z-axis cropping attack. It is worth mentioning that the excellent performance of the proposed algorithm in the aspect of anti-rotation attack, based on the good rotation invariance of the pseudo Jacobi-Fourier moments itself, the proposed algorithm can resist the attack of large rotation Angle. When the clockwise rotation degree is within the range of 5° to 40°, the NC value of the proposed algorithm is always 1, which is much higher than that of the two comparison algorithms. And the rotation to 40° reaches the limit of the two comparison algorithms, while the proposed algorithm can resist the attack of rotation to 65° after testing.

Table 9. Comparison results between different algorithms.

Type of attacks	parameter	3D-DCT [18]	DWT-DCT [17]	PJFM and 3D-DCT
Gaussian noise(%)	3	1.00	0.95	0.80
	15	1.00	0.88	0.74
	25	1.00	0.80	0.71
JPEG compression(%)	2	0.96	0.89	1.00
	10	1.00	0.94	1.00
Median fiter(20 times)	$[3 \times 3]$	0.96	0.95	1.00
	$[5 \times 5]$	0.94	0.95	1.00
	$[7 \times 7]$	0.93	0.95	1.00
Rotaion clockwise(°)	5	0.93	0.87	1.00
	20	0.80	0.87	1.00
	40	0.59	0.71	1.00
Scaling fator	0.5	0.96	1.00	0.79
	1.2	1.00	1.00	1.00
	4.0	1.00	1.00	1.00
Movement (down %)	2	0.97	1.00	1.00
	6	0.90	0.94	1.00
	12	0.75	0.61	0.79
Cropping(Z direction %)	4	0.97	1.00	1.00
	10	0.95	0.94	1.00
	20	0.94	0.88	1.00

5　Conclusions

This paper proposed a robust digital watermarking algorithm based on PJFM and 3D-DCT transform. The algorithm used the properties of logical mapping to scramble and encrypt the watermark in the frequency domain. Visual feature vectors are extracted by PJFM and 3D-DCT transform of medical volume data, and then the watermark is embedded by PJFM and 3D-DCT transform. The feature vectors of the medical data to be tested are extracted and associated with the binary sequences stored by the third party to extract the watermark. Using the concept of zero watermarking and third party, watermark embedding and extraction can be completed without affecting the quality of medical data, which ensures the security and accuracy of data. In addition, the binary watermark is encrypted by logistic chaotic map, which improved the security of the watermarking system. The experimental results show that the algorithm can effectively resist various common attacks and geometric attacks in the transmission process, especially in resist of rotation attacks, cropping attacks and translation attacks. In summary, the algorithm proposed in this paper can better protect the transmission security of medical volume data, and has robustness and invisibility.

Acknowledgements. This work was supported in part by the Natural Science Foundation of China under Grants 62063004, the Key Research Project of Hainan Province under Grant ZDYF2021SHFZ093, the Hainan Provincial Natural Science Foundation of China under Grants 2019RC018 and 619QN246, and the post doctor research from Zhejiang Province under Grant ZJ2021028.

References

1. Cao, Y.L., Zhang, K., Yi, M., Zhao, R.Q.: Medical digitization and digital medicine in the digital age. Soft Sci. Health **36**(10), 80–85 (2022)
2. Li, Y.J., Li, J.B.: Robust volume data watermarking based on perceptual hashing. Comput. Model. New Technol. **18**(11), 470–476 (2014)
3. Wang, L.: Application of digital watermarking technology to medical images. Comput. Inf. Technol. **30**(2), 18–12 (2022)
4. Liu, J., Ma, J.X., Li, J.B., Huang, M.X., Ai, Y.: Robust watermarking algorithm for medical volume data in internet of medical things. IEEE Access **8**, 93939–93961(2020)
5. Liu, W., Jiang, S.D., Sun, S.H.: Robust watermarking for volume data based on 3D-DCT. Acta Electronica Sinica **33**(12) (2005)
6. Han, H.G., Liu, J.X., Li, B.: Digital watermarking algorithm for volume data based on DD-DT CWT and SIFT. J. Graph. **36**(2), 145–151 (2015)
7. He, B., Wang, X., Zhao, J.: Robust image watermarking resisting to RST attacks based on invariant moments. Comput. Eng. Appl. **46**(1), 183–186 (2010)
8. Ke, T.T., Chen, Q.: A robust image Watermarking to geometric attacks based on Pseudo-Zernike moments. ShuJu TongXin, pp.43–46 (2017)
9. Sun, Y.X., Wang, X.W., Li, L.D., Li, S.S.: Image watermarking based on Jacobi-Fourier moment. Comput. Eng. Appl. **50**(4), 94–97 (2014)
10. Amu, G.L., Hasi, S.R., Yang, X.Y., Ping, Z.L.: Image analysis by Pseudo-Jacobi(p = 4, q = 3)-fourier moments. Appl. Opt. **43**(10), 2093–2101 (2004)
11. Zhu, H.Q., Yang, Y., Gui, Z., Chen, Z.: Image analysis by generalized Chebyshev-Fourier and generalized Pseudo-Jacobi-Fourier moments. Pattern Recogn. **51**, 1–11 (2016)
12. Shi, J.J., Amu, G.L., Hasi, S.R.: Analysis of invariant property for improved PJFM'S. Microcomput. Appl. **30**(8), 42–44 (2011)
13. Amu, G.L., Yang, X.Y., Ping, Z.L.: Describing image with pseudo-jacobi(p=4, q=3)-fourier moments. J. Optoelectron. Laser. **14**(9), 981–985 (2003)
14. Chen, Q., Wang, N.: Digital watermarking algorithm based on tchebichef moments and logistic chaotic encryption. Packaging Eng. **40**(21), 228–234 (2019)
15. Zhao, J., Yang, H.B., Li, Y.W., He, J.Q.: Digital watermarking algorithm based on shifted legendre moments. Syst. Simul. Technol. **16**(1), 37–39 (2020)
16. Liu, Y.R., Yang, W.L.: Hand gesture recognition based on kinect and pseudo-jacobi-fourier moments. Transducer Microsystem Technol. **35**(7), 48–50 (2016)

17. Liu, Y.L., Li, J.B., Zhong, J.L.:3D DWT-DCT and logistic MAP based robust watermarking for medical volume data. Comput. Eng. Design **8**, 131–141 (2014)
18. Hu, Y.F., Li, J.B.: Medical volume data watermarking using perceptual hash 3D-DCT and arnold scrambling. In: 2014 7th International Conference on Information Management, Innovation Management and Industrial Engineering (ICIII). IEEE (2014)

Machine/Deep Learning for Smart Medicine and Healthcare

Deep Neural Network-Based Classification of Focal Liver Lesions Using Phase-Shuffle Prediction Pre-training

Jian Song[1,2], Haohua Dong[2], Youwen Chen[1], Lanfen Lin[3], Hongjie Hu[4], and Yen-Wei Chen[2(✉)]

[1] School of Mathematical Sciences, Huaqiao University, Quanzhou, Fujian, China
[2] College of Information Science and Engineering, Ritsumeikan University Shiga, Kusatsu, Japan
chen@is.ritsumei.ac.jp
[3] Department of Computer Science and Technology, Zhejiang University, Hangzhou, China
[4] Department of Radiology, Sir Run Run Shaw Hospital, Hangzhou, China

Abstract. Computer-aided diagnosis plays an important role in focal liver lesion diagnosis (classification) which is one of the leading causes of death worldwide. Due to their superior performance, deep learning-based frameworks have been widely applied in medical imaging, including image classification. However, the data-hungry nature of deep learning frameworks poses a great challenge due to the limited available annotated data samples. In this paper, we propose a self-supervised deep learning method for classification of focal liver lesion in multi-phase CT images. Here, we introduce a novel phase shuffle prediction task as a pretext function of self-supervised learning for pre-training deep neural networks. The phase shuffle prediction pre-training of network significantly improves classification accuracy in comparison to using a conventional pretrainedmodel (using ImageNet) and other rotation prediction-based self-supervised methods.

Keywords: deep neural network · self-supervised learning · phase shuffle prediction · pretrain · multi-phase CT image · focal liver lesion (FLL)

1 Introduction

Liver cancer is one of the leading causes of death worldwide. Accurate diagnosis is crucial for the treatment of liver cancers [1]. Multi-phase computer tomography (CT) images also known as contrast-enhanced dynamic CT images, are widely used to detect, locate and diagnose focal liver lesions (FLLs). A multi-phase CT image consists of a Non Contrast enhanced (NC) phase image that is scanned before the contrast agent is injected, an Arterial (ART) phase image that is scanned 25–40 s after the contrast injection, and a Portal Venous (PV) phase image is scanned after 60–75 s. An example of different FLLs (i.e., Cyst, Focal Nodular Hyperplasia (FNH), Hepatocellular Carcinoma (HCC), and

---

J. Song and H. Dong—Contributed equally to this paper.

© The Author(s), under exclusive license to Springer Nature Singapore Pte Ltd. 2023
Y.-W. Chen et al. (Eds.): KES InMed 2023, SIST 357, pp. 235–243, 2023.
https://doi.org/10.1007/978-981-99-3311-2_20

Hemangioma (HEM)) in these multiphase CT scans (NC, ART and PV) is shown in the Fig. 1. As shown in Fig. 1, FLLs have different visual characteristics at different time points (phases) before/after intravenous contrast injection. Examination of multi-phase CT images for diagnosis of focal liver lesions is a time-consuming and subjective task. As the computer-aided diagnosis plays an important role in focal liver lesion diagnosis (classification).

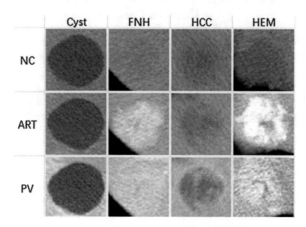

Fig. 1. Evolution patterns of four FLLs in three phases.

To date, several machine learning and deep learning-based methods have been proposed for classification of FLLs [2–8]. In the machine learning-based methods, low-level features such as density, texture features [2–4] and mid-level features such as bag-of-visual-words (BoVW) [5–8] are used for classification of FLLs. Deep learning techniques automatically extract high-level semantic features and outperform conventional machine learning-based methods, which rely on hand crafted low- and mid-level features. Recently, several deep learning-based networks have been introduced for focal liver lesion classification task. Frid-Arar et al. [9] proposed a multi-scale patch-based classification framework to detect focal liver lesions. Yasaka et al. [10] proposed a convolutional neural network with three channels corresponding to three phases (NC, ART and PV) for the classification of liver tumors in dynamic contrast-enhanced CT images. Liang et al. [11] proposed a method by combining a convolutional neural network with a recurrent neural network to extract temporal enhanced information. Though deep learning-based methods have achieved state-of-the-art results, the scarcity of annotated medical images hinders the classification accuracy. In our previous work, we have demonstrated that pretrained deep learning models with ImageNet [12] or self-supervised learning [13] can significantly improve the classification accuracy of focal liver lesions. In this paper, we propose a simple self-supervised learning method by shuffling the order of phase and predicting it. A simple yet useful approach is to pretrain feature extraction networks for phase sequence prediction with an unannotated multi-phase CT image dataset. We called our method Phase Shuffle Prediction.

This paper is organized in four sections. Section 2 gives a brief review of related work. The proposed approach is described in detail in Sect. 3. The experiments and results are shown in Sect. 4. The last part includes conclusion.

2 Related Work

2.1 Pre-trained ImageNet model

Transfer learning is a popular and useful technique for training a model with limited annotated data. It reuses a pre-trained model, which is pre-trained on ImageNet dataset, to other image classification tasks. Normally, the network's weights are updated using the limited annotated target dataset available, while retaining their original structure. The shape of Fully Connected (FC) layer, which serves as the classifier, is modified in accordance with the objective task classes and updated from scratch using the target dataset. Whereas in some other fine-tuning approaches, the target dataset is used to update the weights of deeper layers while keeping the weights of some shallower layers frozen. Wang et al. demonstrated that the pre-trained ImageNet models can improve the classification accuracy of FLLs [12]. However, the limitation of the pre-trained ImageNet model is that the domain of normal real-world images is different from that of medical images resulting in limited representations for the downstream medical images.

2.2 Self-supervised Learning

Self-supervised learning is a new paradigm of unsupervised learning for model pre-training. The self-supervised learning employs the target dataset for pre-training with a predefined task called as pretext task, in contrast to the pretrained ImageNet models, which use a different domain dataset for pre-training. The pipe line of the self-supervised learning has two steps:

(1) Pre-training a deep neural network model on a pretext task with unannotated dataset.
(2) Fine-tuning the pre-trained model for the target task with annotated dataset.

However, how to design the pretext task is a key issue in self-supervised learning. For this task, several self-supervised learning methods with different pretext tasks have been proposed such as context prediction [14], solving jigsaw puzzles [15], rotation prediction [16]. Whereas some other approaches such as Contrastive learning-based methods such as Moco [17] and SimCLR [18] are also proposed. We propose a multi-phase CT image-specific self-supervised learning approach that is inspired by rotation prediction [16], in which the phase order is shuffled and the pretext task is to predict the phase order. We called it Phase Shuffle Prediction.

3 Method'

3.1 Overview of the Proposed Method

The overview of the proposed method is shown in Fig. 2. It shows the multiphase CT images in their original order as well as an example of how CT images might be shuffled in order to train a network. Predicting the phase order is the pretext task this time. These weights are used to set up the model as a pretrained network at first, and it is then updated for the original task of classifying lesions using target labels, as depicted in the Figure. Each part of the proposed method is described in following sub-sections.

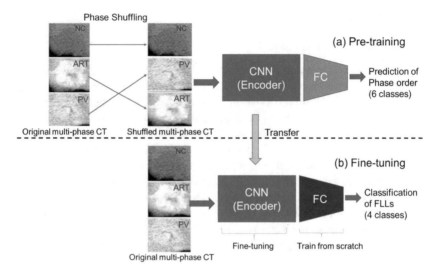

Fig. 2. Overview of the proposed method. (a) pretext task; (b) target task.

3.2   Phase Shuffling

The phase order of multi-phase CT images is randomly shuffled as shown in Fig. 2(a). The original order is NC, ART and PV. In case of Fig. 2(a), the phase order is shuffled to NC, PV and ART. The possible numbers of phase order are $M!$, where M is the number of phases. In this research, M is 3 and the total number of phase orders is $3! = 6$. In the proposed self-supervised learning, the pretext task is to predict the order of phases, which is a six-class classification problem (i.e., class 1: NC, ART, PV; class 2: NC, PV, ART; class 3: ART, NC, PV; class 4: ART, PV, NC; class 5: PV, NC, ART; class 6: PV, ART, NC).

3.3   Pre-training

These shuffled multi-phase CT images are used for pre-training as shown in Fig. 2(a). These shuffled images of three different CT phases are treated as a color image and are fed into the convolutional neural network (CNN). The input size is $3 \times 128 \times 128$. The CNN encoder is used to extract features. We use ResNet18 [19] as the CNN encoder, it has been widely used to perform image classification task in various previous work [12, 13]. The network architecture is shown in Fig. 3. The dimension of the output feature vector of ResNet18 is 512×1. We use a FC as a classifier. Since the pretext task is to predict the order of phases, which is a six-class classification problem, the output layer of FC has 6 neurons. Note that the FC will be replaced with a new FC in the downstream target task.

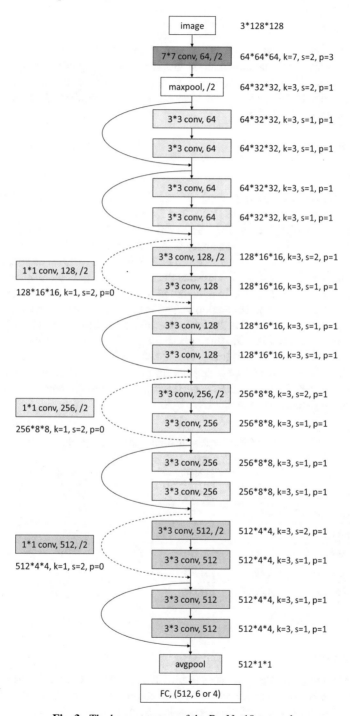

Fig. 3. The layer structure of the ResNet18 network.

3.4 Fine-Tuning

After pre-training weights of the pre-trained model (CNN encoder) are used as the initialization parameters and these weights are fine-tuned using original multi-phase CT images and their labels for the target task (i.e., classification of FLLs). Since the main task is to classify FLLs, which is a 4-class classification problem, the new FC has an output layer with four neurons.

4 Experiments

4.1 Data

The effectiveness of the proposed method was validated using our in house Multi-Phase CT dataset of Focal Liver Lesions (MPCT-FLLs) [20]. Four types of lesions (i.e., Cyst, FNH, HCC, and HEM) are used in our experiments, which are collected by Sir Run Run Shaw Hospital, Zhejiang University from 2015 to 2017. Totally, we have 85 CT volumes including 489 slice images (From each volume, a number of slices centered on the lesion center are selected). The slice thickness is 5–7 mm and in-plan resolution is 0.57–0.59 mm. The 2D slice image size is 512×512. Each CT image has three phases (i.e., NC, ART, PV). The region of interest (ROI) of each lesion was annotated by experienced radiologists. The 2D ROI slice images are used for experiments. Each ROI is resized to 128×128. The three phase images are treated as a color image with three channels. The size of input image is $3 \times 128 \times 128$.

The dataset is split into 5 groups to perform 5-fold cross validation. The data distribution is shown in Table 1. In each fold, we select one group as test dataset and remaining four groups are used as training dataset.

Table 1. Data distribution for 5-fold cross validation

Type	Cyst	FNH	HCC	HEM	Total
Group1:case (slice)	5(29)	4(15)	4(30)	4(21)	17(95)
Group2:case (slice)	6(31)	3(17)	4(29)	4(33)	17(110)
Group3:case (slice)	6(37)	3(7)	4(36)	4(17)	17(97)
Group4:case (slice)	6(24)	3(17)	4(35)	4(19)	17(95)
Group5:case (slice)	7(28)	3(20)	3(32)	4(12)	17(92)
Total:case (slice)	30(149)	16(76)	19(162)	20(102)	85(489)

4.2 Implementations

For the pre-training, we train our network for 1000 epochs using a batch size of 128. We use the Stochastic Gradient Descent with momentum as our optimizer with a learning rate of 0.01. For the training of the target task, we fine tune our network for 200 epochs using a batch size of 256. The learning rate is also 0.01. The training setup is shown in Table 2.

Table 2. Computation environment

GPU	NVIDIA GeForce RTX 3090
CPU	Intel(R) Xeon(R) Platinum 8358P
OS	Ubuntu 20.04
Deep Learning Framework	Pytorch

4.3 Results

We have compared the proposed training for phase shuffling prediction with other transfer learning methods including training from scratch, pre-train with ImageNet [12] and pre-train with rotation prediction (self-supervised learning) [16]. The comparison results are summarized in Table 3.

Table 3. Comparison with other transfer learning methods

Accuracy	Cyst	FNN	HCC	HEM	Avg
Train from scratch	94.71 ± 3.15	**91.79 ± 5.68**	82.66 ± 13.18	43.06 ± 20.92	80.84 ± 2.91
ImageNet [12]	95.56 ± 2.84	83.53 ± 13.62	80.99 ± 11.69	**72.38 ± 14.70**	82.78 ± 1.21
Rotation [16]	96.66 ± 2.89	88.44 ± 7.51	78.81 ± 13.81	60.30 ± 17.85	81.84 ± 1.72
proposed method	**98.27 ± 1.42**	86.22 ± 12.27	**82.90 ± 5.84**	63.72 ± 12.68	**84.82 ± 1.99**

As shown in Table 3, transfer learning methods achieve better results than training from scratch (without weights initialization using pretrained models). Both self-supervised learning methods achieve better results than pre-training model using ImageNet. The proposed phase shuffling prediction method outperforms the currently used rotation prediction method, providing better overall classification results for lesions.

5   Conclusion

In this paper, we propose a self-supervised deep learning method for classification of focal liver lesion in multi-phase CT images. We propose a novel phase shuffle prediction as a pretext task of self-supervised learning for pre-training the deep neural network. The phase shuffle prediction-based self-supervised learning significantly improves the classification accuracy compared with the conventional pre-training with ImageNet and existing rotation prediction-based self-supervised method.

Acknowledgement. Authors would like to thank Dr. Rahul Jain of Ritsumeikan University, Japan for his kind English proof. This research was supported in part by Natural Science Foundation of Xiamen City, Fujian Province, China under the Grant No. 3502Z20227199 and in part by the Grant-in Aid for Scientific Research from the Japanese Ministry for Education, Science, Culture and Sports (MEXT) under the Grant No. 20KK0234 and No. 21H03470.

References

1. Ryerson, A., Blythe, et al.: Annual report to the nation on the status of cancer, 1975-2012, featuring the increasing incidence of liver cancer. Cancer **12**, 1312–1337 (2016)
2. Roy, S., et al.: Three-dimensional spatiotemporal features for fast content-based retrieval of focal liver lesions. IEEE Trans. Biomed. Eng. **61**, 2768–2778 (2014)
3. Yu, M., et al.: Extraction of lesion-partitioned features and retrieval of contrast-enhanced liver images. Comput. Math. Meth. Med. **12** (2012)
4. Xu, Y., et al.: Combined density, texture and shape features of multi-phase contrast-enhanced CT images for CBIR of focal liver lesions: a preliminary study. In: Chen, Y.-W., et al. (eds.) Innovation in Medicine and Healthcare 2015, pp.215–224. Springer (2015)
5. Yang, W., et al.: Content-based retrieval of focal liver lesions using bag-of-visual-words representations of single-and multiphase contrast-enhanced CT images. J. Digital Imaging **25**, 708–719 (2012)
6. Diamant, I., et al.: Improved patch-based automated liver lesion classification by separate analysis of the interior and boundary regions. IEEE J. Biomed. Health Inform. **20**, 1585–1594 (2016)
7. Xu, Y., et al.: Bag of temporal co-occurrence words for retrieval of focal liver lesions using 3D multiphase contrast-enhanced CT images. In: Proceedings of 23rd International Conference on Pattern Recognition (ICPR 2016), pp. 2283–2288 (2016)
8. Xu, Y., et al.: Texture-specific bag of visual words model and spatial cone matching-based method for the retrieval of focal liver lesions using multiphase contrast-enhanced CT images. Int. J. Comput. Assist. Radiol. Surg. **13**(1), 151–164 (2017). https://doi.org/10.1007/s11548-017-1671-9
9. Frid-Adar, M., et al.: Modeling the intra-class variability for liver lesion detection using a multi-class patch-based CNN. In: Wu, G., Munsell, Brent C., Zhan, Y., Bai, W., Sanroma, G., Coupé, P. (eds.) Patch-MI 2017. LNCS, vol. 10530, pp. 129–137. Springer, Cham (2017)
10. Yasaka, K., et al.: Deep learning with convolutional neural network for differentiation of liver masses at dynamic contrast-enhanced CT: a preliminary study. Radiology **286**, 887–896 (2017)
11. Liang, D., et al.: Combining convolutional and recurrent neural networks for classification of focal liver lesions in multi-phase CT images. In: Frangi, A., Schnabel, J., Davatzikos, C., Alberola-López, C., Fichtinger, G. (eds.) MICCAI 2018. LNCS, vol. 7951, pp. 666–675. Springer, Cham (2018). https://doi.org/10.1007/978-3-030-00934-2_74
12. Wang, W., et al.: Classification of focal liver lesions using deep learning with fine-tuning. In: Proceedings of Digital Medicine and Image Processing (DMIP2018), pp.56–60 (2018)
13. Dong, H., et al.: Case discrimination: self-supervised feature learning for the classfication of focal liver lesions. In: Chen, Y.-W., et al. (eds.) Innovation in Medicine and Healthcare, Smart Innovation, Systems and Technologies (Proc. of InMed2021), pp. 241–249 (2021)
14. Doersch, C., et al.: Unsupervised visual representation learning by context prediction. In: Proceedings of the IEEE International Conference on Computer Vision, pp. 1422–1430 (2015)

15. Noroozi, M., et al.: Unsupervised learning of visual representations by solving jig-sawpuzzles. In: ECCV 2016. LNCS, vol. 9910, pp. 69–84. Springer, Cham (2016). https://doi.org/10.1007/978-3-319-46466-4_5
16. Spyros, G., et al.: Unsupervised representation learning by predicting image rotations. In: Proceedings of ICLR 2018 (2018)
17. He, K., et al.: Momentum Contrast for Unsupervised Visual Representation Learning. arXiv: 1911.05722 (2019)
18. Chen, T., et al.: A Simple Framework for Contrastive Learning of Visual Representations. arXiv:2002.05709 (2020)
19. He, K., et al.: Deep residual learning for image recognition. Proceedings of the IEEE Conference on Computer Vision and Pattern Recognition (2016)
20. Xu, Y., et al.: PA-ResSeg: a phase attention residual network for liver tumor segmentation from multi-phase CT images. Med. Phys. **48**(7), 3752–3766 (2021)

An Improved Multi-Instance Learning Model for Postoperative Early Recurrence Prediction of Hepatocellular Carcinoma Using Histopathological Images

Gan Zhan[1], Fang Wang[2], Weibin Wang[3], Yinhao Li[1],
Qingqing Chen[2], Hongjie Hu[2], and Yen-Wei Chen[1(✉)]

[1] College of Information Science and Engineering,
Ritsumeikan University, Kyoto, Japan
gr0502vs@ed.ritsumei.ac.jp,yin-li@fc.ritsumei.ac.jp,chen@is.ritsumei.ac.jp
[2] Department of Radiology, Sir Run Run Shaw Hospital,
Zhejiang University School of Medicine, Hangzhou, China
{wangfang11,qingqingchen,hongjiehu}@zju.edu.cn
[3] Research Center for Healthcare Data Science, Zhejiang Lab, Hangzhou, China
wangweibin@zhejianglab.com

Abstract. HCC(Hepatocellular carcinoma) is one of the primary liver cancer around the world, and it produces a high mortality rate in clinical. Surgical resection is the first-line treatment choice for patients with HCC, but the problem is patients will still have a great chance of recurrence after surgery. Therefore postoperative early recurrence prediction of HCC patients is necessary, which can guide physicians to manage the individualized follow-up so that we could increase the survival time of patients. MIL(multi-instance learning) model is mostly utilized in histopathological image analysis, and it has achieved promising results in most tasks, but it has one major limitation: the conventional MIL model loses the histopathological spatial structure information when generating the slide-level representation on flattened instance embeddings. In this light, we revisit the conventional MIL model and propose an improved MIL model to tackle the limitation. Our proposed method consists of three stages, the first stage is tissue patching, which is the same as the conventional MIL; the second stage is early recurrence probability heatmaps(ER-ProbMaps) generation, which is conducted by a well-trained patch-level prediction model on the tissue patches of the same slide; the final stage is to produce the slide-level recurrence prediction by a slide-level prediction model. We train the slide-level prediction model on obtained heatmaps to complete our postoperative early recurrence prediction task. Our experimental results show that our proposed improved MIL model can achieve superior performance than the conventional MIL model in our task.

G. Zhan and F. Wang—Frist authors with equal contributions.

Keywords: HCC postoperative early recurrence prediction ·
Histopathological images · MIL model · early recurrence probability
heatmaps · patch-level prediction model

1   Introduction

Hepatocellular carcinoma(HCC) is one of the primary liver cancer, it is the fifth
most common malignancy around the world. HCC produces a high mortality
rate in clinical and causes the second most common death related to cancer
worldwide [1]. For patients with HCC, there are many treatment choices, but
the first-line one is the surgical resection, and it is highly recommended by the
clinical practice guidelines if patients have a well-preserved liver function [2–
4]. However, patients with HCC would have a great chance of recurrence after
they had the tumor resection surgery, and the recurrence rate can reach about
$> 10\%$ in 1 year, 70–80% in 5 years after surgery [14]. Early recurrence(ER) was
defined as local tumor progression, intrahepatic distant recurrence, and extra-
hepatic metastasis within 2 years after liver resection. HCC patients with early
recurrence have a great chance to live longer than patients with non-early recurrence [15]. Therefore, if we have a method that could correctly predict HCC
patients at high risk of early recurrence after surgery, this could help the physician arrange the individualized follow-up, and increase the overall survival time
of HCC patients.

To this day, many methods have been proposed to solve the early recurrence
prediction for HCC patients. Existing methods based on clinical data mainly
use machine learning algorithms to complete the prediction task, for example,
Chuanli Liu et al. [5] compared the performance of 5 machine learning algorithms that project 37 quantitative and qualitative variables to the prediction
space, the result reveals that K-Nearest Neighbor is the optimal one for the
HCC early recurrence prediction task. The major limitation of the clinical data-
based method is it has no image modality information, so it could not effectively
show the tumor heterogeneity across HCC patients. Existing methods based on
CT(computed tomography) scans or MRIs(magnetic resonance imaging) could
be divided into two categories to solve the early recurrence prediction of HCC.
The first category is radiomics analysis [6]. Radiomics could be served as a
quantitative tool to extract features from medical images. For example, Ying
Zhao et al. [7] design a radiomics analysis pipeline, which first extracts 1146
radiomics features from each MRI phase, after feature selection on the features
of all phases, radiomics models are constructed by logistic regression algorithm
to complete the HCC early recurrence prediction task. The second category
is deep learning analysis [8], unlike radiomics analysis, deep learning analysis
doesn't have to do the feature selection to find the critical features related to
our task. Data-driven mechanism of deep learning models will automatically find
critical features that are related to our task. An example of deep learning analysis is the Deep Phase Attention prediction model proposed by Weibin Wang
et al. [10], which aims to complete the early recurrence prediction task of HCC

using multi-phase CT scans. The limitation of existing methods based on CT scans and MRIs is that they could not reflect enough tumor heterogeneity across HCC patients compared with histopathological images. CT scans or MRIs show the macroscopic structure of the tumor, while histopathological images show the microstructure of the tumor, such as cell morphology and tissue structure. Since cell morphology and tissue structure of histopathological images directly reflect the disease progression across patients, utilizing histopathological images has the advantage of image information over CT scans and MRIs in our prediction task.

WSI(whole-slide image) in histopathological images is a challenging computer vision domain. The main characteristic of WSI is the large image resolution, the resolution can reach as large as 120000×120000 pixels, thus it is hard to directly feed WSIs into deep learning models for analysis. Another characteristic of WSI is the hierarchical structure, each WSI contains plenty of tissue structures, and each tissue structure contains plenty of cell morphologies. Thus in histopathological image analysis, we need to consider the large resolution and hierarchical structure when designing a model to formulate the WSI representation. MIL(multi-instance learning) [13] is the most commonly used deep learning model in WSI classification or prediction tasks, it mainly uses the following three stages to formulate the WSI representation: 1) Select a single magnification objective, then do the tissue patching of every slide, normally the patch size is 256×256, 2) use the pre-trained feature extractor to project each patch in former step to a fixed length embedding, 3) global pooling(mean, max or attention) of all the patch embeddings in the same slide to construct the WSI representation, and then using an FC(fully connected) layer on WSI representation to finish prediction task. The MIL model has considered the large resolution in WSI, it utilized the patch-based late fusion architecture to formulate the WSI representation: patch-based model is first used to formulate the patch embedding, then late fusion design will combine all the patch embeddings to produce the WSI representation. However, the MIL model ignored the spatial layout of the hierarchical structure in WSI. When constructing the slide-level representation, since MIL will flatten all the patch embeddings in the same slide before pooling, the 2D spatial layout of tissue patches in WSI will be destroyed. Losing the unique organization of tissue structures inside every slide is not helpful to formulate the robust WSI representation for our prediction task.

With these observations, we revisit the conventional MIL model and propose an improved MIL model to tackle the limitation of the conventional MIL model for our early recurrence prediction task. Our task is a binary prediction task, in our research, HCC patients have recurrence in 2 years after surgery will be denoted as ER, and they will be denoted as Non-ER if they have recurrence after 2 years or no recurrence after sugery. Our proposed method has three stages to complete our task: 1) tissue patching, which is the same as the conventional MIL model; 2) ER-ProbMaps generation. We add a classifier in the conventional MIL pre-trained feature extractor to obtain our patch-level prediction model, and we finetune [9] it in our dataset, the patch label inherits from its slide-level recurrence label, thus we could obtain the ER-ProbMaps where each pixel

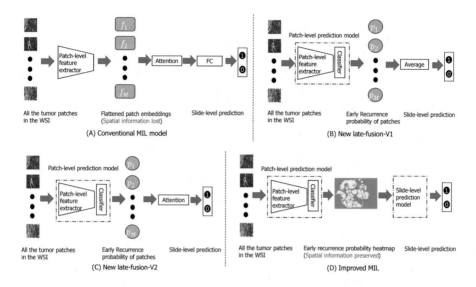

Fig. 1. The different patch-based late fusion designs for WSI analysis.

represents the corresponding patch in WSI, and each pixel value is the patch-level early recurrence probability; 3) unlike the slide representation in conventional MIL model, the heatmap could retain the patch spatial layout in WSI, thus we train the slide-level prediction model on the heatmaps to complete our early recurrence prediction task of HCC. Detailed experimental results show that our proposed method achieves superior performance to the conventional MIL model. To the best of our knowledge, we are the first to propose a deep learning model based on WSIs to tackle the postoperative early recurrence prediction task for HCC.

2   Proposed Method

As we described before, the large image resolution is one of the main characteristics of WSI, thus it is hard to directly feed the WSI into the deep learning model, and the patch-based late fusion architecture in conventional MIL is preferred for histopathological image analysis. In the section, we will first discuss different patch-base late fusion designs in our task, and then we will introduce our proposed method in detail.

2.1   Revisit the Late Fusion Design in MIL Model

Figure 1 shows different patch-based late fusion designs for WSI analysis, model A is the conventional MIL model [13], model B, C and D are the modified MIL models designed by us, and specifically model D is our proposed improved MIL model. Their main difference lies on the late fusion operation, the late fusion of conventional MIL model is conducted at the patch feature level, while the late fusion of models in B, C, and D are conducted at the patch decision level.

After we obtain tumor patches from WSI based on the corresponding tumor mask annotation, model A(MIL model) will first use the patch-level feature extractor to project each patch image to a fixed-length embedding, normally the feature extractor MIL used is the ResNet-50 [11] encoder pre-trained on ImageNet [12] (truncated after the 3rd residual block). Assuming the input slide is denoted as X, MIL commonly uses the 256×256 pixels as the patch size, thus tumor tissue patches we generated from slide X is $\{x_i\}_{i=1}^M$, where M is the number of tumor tissue patches, it is a variable depends on the image resolution of slide X. The x_i is the i-th patch in slide X, and the patch embedding for the corresponding i-th patch is denoted as f_i, so slide X is projected to be a collection of patch embeddings $\{f_i\}_{i=1}^M$ by the patch-level feature extractor. Then patch embeddings $\{f_i\}_{i=1}^M$ will be fed into the attention module, attention module will first calculate the attention score for each embedding as shown in formula 1: The V matrix and U matrix are the FC layer, the combination$(tanh(Vf_i^\top))$ of $tanh$ and V is to extract critical information from feature f_i, and the combination$(sigmoid(Uf_i^\top))$ of $sigmoid$ and U is to be served as a gate for $tanh(Vf_i^\top)$, the element-wise multiplication$(tanh(Vf_i^\top) \odot sigmoid(Uf_i^\top))$ is to obtain the filtered important information from f_i, and w is another FC layer, it will map the obtained information to the attention score for f_i, and we use softmax to normalize all the mapped attention scores as the ultimate attention score for each patch embedding. Suppose the ultimate attention score of i-th patch is a_i, each attention score will first multiply its corresponding patch embedding as $a_i * f_i$, after that, we combine all the weighted patch embeddings to produce the weighted-sum feature $\sum_{i=1}^M a_i * f_i$ as the formulated slide representation. Finally, we use an FC layer on the slide representation to complete our prediction task.

$$a_i = \frac{exp\left\{w^\top(tanh(Vf_i^\top) \odot sigmoid(Uf_i^\top))\right\}}{\sum_{k=1}^M exp\left\{w^\top(tanh(Vf_k^\top) \odot sigmoid(Uf_k^\top))\right\}} \tag{1}$$

2.2   Patch-level Prediction Model

For model B, instead of the patch-level feature extractor, we design a patch-level prediction model to produce the patch early recurrence prediction for each patch image. We add an FC layer as the classifier on the pre-trained ResNet-50 encoder of MIL to construct our patch-level prediction model. And we finetune the patch-level prediction model in our dataset. The early recurrence probability of the i-th patch in slide X produced by the patch-level prediction model is denoted as p_i. The process of our patch-level prediction model on the i-th tumor patch could be described in formula 2:

$$\{p_i, 1 - p_i\} = F_{patch}(x_i, \theta_{patch}) \tag{2}$$

The learning parameters of our patch-level prediction model are θ_{patch}, and each tumor patch in the same slide will inherit the slide recurrence label Y_i.

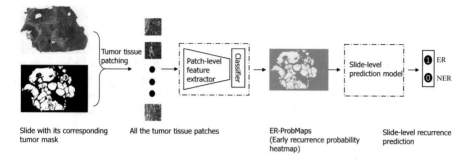

Slide with its corresponding tumor mask   All the tumor tissue patches   ER-ProbMaps
(Early recurrence probability heatmap)   Slide-level recurrence prediction

Fig. 2. The overall pipeline of our proposed improved MIL model for postoperative early recurrence prediction using histopathological WSI.

When we feed the i-th patch (x_i) of slide X into the model, it will generate the corresponding patch early recurrence prediction probability p_i. And we take the average of p_i as the slide-level early recurrence prediction probability P_{slide}, and $\{1 - P_{slide}\}$ will be the slide-level non-early recurrence prediction probability, hereby, we complete our prediction task with model B (Fig. 2).

For model C, we use the same patch-level prediction model to produce patch early recurrence prediction probability p_i for i-th tumor patch, but instead of averaging, we use the attention module of model A on patch probability p_i to calculate the slide-level weighted-sum early recurrence probability P_{slide} and $\{1 - P_{slide}\}$ will be the slide-level non-early recurrence prediction probability, hereby, we complete our prediction task with model C.

For model D, which is our proposed improved MIL model, we use the patch-level prediction model as well, but we not only obtain the patch early recurrence prediction probability p_i, we also record the coordinate of i-th tumor patch (x_i) in slide X, therefore we could obtain the ER-ProbMaps, where the spatial layout of patches in WSI is preserved. The motivation behind ER-ProbMaps is: Besides the large image resolution, the hierarchical structure is another important characteristic of the WSI. In this light, The MIL model in model A simply obtains slide-level representation by global pooling on flattened patch embeddings. However, the operation of flattening patch embeddings in MIL will lose the unique spatial layout of tissue structures in the WSI, which is not helpful for our task to learn a robust slide representation. And model B or C also didn't consider the spatial information of patches. Unlike them, in Model D, the ER-ProbMaps we generated from the patch-level prediction model could preserve the spatial layout of each patch in the WSI, thus we use the ER-ProbMaps to formulate the robust WSI representation in our task.

2.3 Slide-Level Prediction Model

The ER-ProbMaps preserves the spatial arrangement of each tumor patch in a WSI, thereby maintaining the unique connections among tumor patches in our specific task. By utilizing the deep learning model on ER-ProbMaps, as opposed to the slide representation or patch predictions where spatial information has been corrupted in model A, B and C, we can achieve a more generalized and meaningful outcome. Therefore, based on the generated ER-ProbMaps, we design the slide-level prediction model to complete our prediction task. Assuming the input ER-ProbMap of j-th slide(X_j) is denoted as z_j, considering the small dataset size in our research, we select ResNet18 as our slide-level prediction model. The process of the slide-level prediction model is described in formula 3:

$$\{P_j, 1 - P_j\} = F_{slide}(z_j, \theta_{slide}) \tag{3}$$

The learning parameters of our slide-level prediction model are θ_{slide}, slide recurrence label is Y_i. When we feed the j-th slide ER-ProbMaps z_j into the model, it will generate the corresponding slide early recurrence prediction probability P_j. Hereby, we complete our postoperative early recurrence prediction task of HCC patients.

3 Experiments

3.1 Patient Selection

This study protocol conforms to the ethical guidelines of the 1975 Declaration of Helsinki as refected in a priori approval by the institution's Human Research Committee. Informed consent was waived since this was a retrospective cohort study.

From 2012 to 2019, in the Sir Run Run Shaw Hospital Affiliated with the Medical College of Zhejiang University, 659 HCC patients who has undergone liver resection, pathologically confirmed as hepatocellular carcinoma were recruited in this retrospective study. Under the following exclusion criteria:(1) the patient received other anti-tumor treatments before surgery, such as TACE(trans-catheter arterial chemoembolization), RFA(radiofrequency ablation), (2) slides with poor staining quality or images with artifacts after scanning, and (3) less than 2 years of follow-up after surgery, 119 patients are included in our study, we collect 120 WSIs from the 119 HCC patients, each slide of the patient has the tumor annotations, which is made by the professional pathologist.

3.2 Dataset Preparation and Metrics

For the 120 WSIs of 119 patients in our histopathological datasets, we split 80% WSIs for the training set, 10% WSIs for the validation set, and 10% WSIs for the testing set, the two WSIs belong to the same patient are both in the training set. The slide from the early recurrence patient is denoted as the positive slide, and the slide from the non-early recurrence patient is denoted as the negative slide. The number of positive slides and negative slides in the training set, validation set, and testing set is shown in Table 1.

We select AUC(area under the ROC curve), and ACC(accuracy) to evaluate the model performance in our research. Cross-entropy loss is the loss function we used in both the patch-level prediction model and slide-level prediction model.

Table 1. Dataset Arrangement of WSIs.

	Training	Validation	Testing	Total
Positive slides	32	4	4	40
Negative slides	64	8	8	80

Table 2. Comparison of different late fusion designs.

Model	Slide AUC	Slide ACC
Model A(MIL-pre) [13]	0.750	0.667
Model A(MIL-ft) [13]	0.719	0.750
Model B	0.688	0.667
Model C	0.688	0.667
Model D(Improved MIL)	**0.781**	**0.833**

3.3 Comparison of Different Late Fusion Designs

We extract tumor patches at the 40× magnification objective. For patch-level prediction model training, the number of positive tumor tissue patches existing in positive WSIs of training set is 814067, and the number of negative tumor tissue patches existing in negative WSIs of training set is 1640262. To maintain the class-balanced training, we use all the positive patches and select half (8201117) of the negative patches, in total, we have 1634184 patches to train our patch-level prediction model. Since the feature extractor in the patch prediction model is already pre-trained in ImageNet, we finetune the model for 10 epochs in our dataset.

For model A(conventional MIL model), if it is utilized on patch embeddings pretrained from ImageNet, it will be denoted as MIL-pre, if MIL model is utilized on the patch embedding finetuned from our dataset, it will denoted as MIL-ft. We can tell from Table 2, MIL-ft can achieve slightly better performance than MIL-pre due to we finetuned the MIL patch feature extractor on our dataset. The performance comparison between model B and MIL-ft replies tumor tissue patch representation only is not well qualified for our HCC early recurrence prediction task. As for the comparison between model B and model C, they achieve the same result, that is because the patch prediction probability in each training WSI is close, thus it is hard for the attention module to explore meaningful differences across patch predictions. Based on the heatmap generated by the patch-level prediction model, when we further model the spatial tissue structure context using the slide-level prediction model, our proposed improved MIL model could achieve better performance than models B, C, and conventional MIL. Thus retaining the spatial layout of tissue structure is necessary to model the robust slide representation in our task.

4 Conclusion

In this paper, we revisit the conventional MIL model and construct our Improved MIL model on WSIs to tackle the postoperative early recurrence prediction of HCC patients. We take a deep analysis of the late fusion operation in the MIL model for WSI analysis, and we proposed the ER-ProbMaps generation to solve the spatial information corruption in the MIL model. Our proposed model consists of a patch-level prediction model and a slide-level prediction model. Detailed experiments reveal the effectiveness of our proposed method and it could achieve better performance than the most commonly used MIL model in our prediction task.

Acknowledgments. This work was supported in part by the Grant in Aid for Scientific Research from the Japanese Ministry for Education, Science, Culture and Sports (MEXT) under the Grant Nos. 20KK0234, 21H03470, and 20K21821, and in part by the Natural Science Foundation of Zhejiang Province (LZ22F020012), in part by Major Scientific Research Project of Zhejiang Lab (2020ND8AD01), and in part by the National Natural Science Foundation of China (82071988), the Key Research and Development Program of Zhejiang Province (2019C03064), the Program Co-sponsored by Province and Ministry (No. WKJ-ZJ-1926) and the Special Fund for Basic Scientific Research Business Expenses of Zhejiang University (No. 2021FZZX003-02-17).

References

1. Elsayes, K.M., Kielar, A.Z., Agrons, M.M.: Liver imaging reporting and data system: an expert consensus statement. J. Hepatocellular Carcinoma **4**, 29–39 (2017)
2. Thomas, M.B., Zhu, A.X.: Hepatocellular carcinoma: the need for progress. J. Clin. Oncol. **23**, 2892–2899 (2005)
3. Association, E.: Easl clinical practice guidelines: management of hepatocellular carcinoma. J. Hepatol. **69**, 182–236 (2018)
4. Marrero, J.A., et al.: Diagnosis, staging and management of hepatocellular carcinoma practice guidance by the American association for the study of liver diseases. Hepatology **68**(2018), 723–750 (2018)
5. Liu, C.: A k-nearest neighbor model to predict early recurrence of hepatocellular carcinoma after resection. J. Clin. Trans. Hepatol. **10**, 600–607 (2022)
6. Gillies, R.J., Kinahan, P.E., Hricak, H.: Radiomics: images are more than pictures, they are data radiology. Radiology **278**, 563–577 (2015)
7. Zhao, Y., et al.: Radiomics analysis based on multiparametric MRI for predicting early recurrence in hepatocellular carcinoma after partial hepatectomy. J. Magn. Reson. Imaging **53**, 1066–1079 (2020)
8. Krizhevsky, A., Sutskever, I., Hinton, G.E.: ImageNet classification with deep convolutional neural networks. Commun. ACM **60**, 84–90 (2017)
9. Kolesnikov, A., et al.: Big Transfer (BiT): general visual representation learning. In: Vedaldi, A., Bischof, H., Brox, T., Frahm, J.-M. (eds.) ECCV 2020. LNCS, vol. 12350, pp. 491–507. Springer, Cham (2020). https://doi.org/10.1007/978-3-030-58558-7_29
10. Wang, W., et al.: Phase attention model for prediction of early recurrence of hepatocellular carcinoma with multi-phase CT images and clinical data. Front. Radiol. 8, (2022)

11. He, K., Zhang, X., Ren, S., Sun, J.: Deep residual learning for image recognition. In: Proceedings of the IEEE Conference on Computer Vision and Pattern Recognition, pp. 770-778 (2016)
12. Deng, J., Dong, W., Socher, R., Li, L.-J., Li, K., Fei-Fei, L.: ImageNet: a large-scale hierarchical image database. In: IEEE Conference on Computer Vision and Pattern Recognition, pp. 248-255 (2009)
13. Ilse, M., Tomczak, J., Welling, M.: Attention-based deep multiple instance learning. In: International Conference on Machine Learning, pp. 2127-2136. PMLR (2018)
14. Bray, F., Ferlay, J., Soerjomataram, I., Siegel, R.L., Torre, L.A., Jemal, A.: Global cancer statistics: globocan estimates of incidence and mortality worldwide for 36 cancers in 185 countries. CA Cancer J. Clin. **68**(2018), 394–424 (2018)
15. Cheng, Z., et al.: Risk factors and management for early and late intrahepatic recurrence of solitary hepatocellular carcinoma after curative resection. HPB **17**, 422–427 (2015)

Teacher-Student Learning Using Focal and Global Distillation for Accurate Cephalometric Landmark Detection

Yu Song[1], Xu Qiao[2], Yinhao Li[1], and Yen-Wei Chen[1(✉)]

[1] Graduate School of Information Science and Eng, Ritsumeikan University, Shiga, Japan
chen@is.ritsumei.ac.jp
[2] Department of Biomedical Engineering, Shandong University, Jinan, China

Abstract. Cephalometric analysis is used frequently by dentists and orthodontists to analyze the role of the human skull in making a diagnosis and formulating treatment plans. To perform such analysis, cephalometric landmarks first need to be annotated manually. In recent years, various automatic cephalometric landmark detection methods, using deep learning, have been formulated and have achieved promising results. Previously, we proposed a teacher–student learning method based on composed ground truth images, and in this paper, we refine our previous methods using focal and global distillation during the teacher–student training process. We create a mask to distinguish the foreground and background areas of landmarks and perform knowledge distillation separately as the focal distillation. We also add a feature similarity penalty interceding between the teacher and student models as the global distillation. Our method achieves state-of-the-art performance on the in-house dataset provided by Shandong University.

Keywords: Cephalometric Landmark · Teacher–Student model · Knowledge Distillation · Focal and Global

1 Introduction

Cephalometric analysis aims to study the relationships between bony and soft tissue landmarks. It is used widely by dentists and orthodontists in the diagnosis and prognosis process [1]. There are many popular methods of analysis; among them, the Steiner and the Downs analyses are the most used [2]. To perform such analysis, lateral x-rays need to be taken first, then doctors will label the landmarks of bony and soft tissue based on different analysis methods. After that, the doctors will measure the relationships of different landmarks, such as the angles of and distances between different landmarks. The labeling work is time-consuming and labor-intensive considering the extremely high resolution produced by cephalometry x-rays. Also, the inter-variability between different doctors is hard to deal with. Under such circumstances, automatic cephalometric landmark detection methods are of significant salience.

Several benchmarks have largely pushed the research on automatic cephalometric landmark detection forward. In 2014 and 2015, the International Symposium on

Biomedical Imaging(ISBI) launched two grand challenges, aiming to recruit computer-aided methods to detect cephalometric landmarks automatically with high accuracy [3, 4]. In the ISBI's 2015 grand challenge, the best result was created by Lindner et al. [5]. Using a random-forest-based method, they achieved a 74.84% SDR) for a 2 mm precision range. Ibragimov et al. achieved the second-best results by using harr-like feature extraction with random-forest regression [6].

Deep learning has dominated this topic in recent years, and several methods have been proposed. The mainstream methods can be summarized as two types: either regressing landmarks' coordinates directly or producing heatmaps to locate landmarks' locations indirectly [7, 8]. In 2019, we proposed a two-step coarse-to-fine method to regress the coordinates; we undertook data augmentation to generate large patch samples for each landmark and achieved state-of-the-art performance at that time [9]. Payer et al. proposed a method that extracts spatial and local attention maps, along with learnable sigma, and their method regressed landmarks successfully with high accuracy [10]. In 2021, we proposed a teacher–student learning method for heatmap prediction. Conventional teacher-student models use large models to train a robust network and distill the knowledge to a small network for easier deployment. Different from conventional teacher-student model, we trained the teacher model using composed ground truth (GT) images and distilled the knowledge to the student model trained by original radiography, and our teacher–student learning strategy distilled knowledge from GT images boosted the performance [11].

In this paper, we make refinements based on our previous teacher–student learning work. We replace the previous distillation methods with focal and global distillation. We believe that the foreground and background have different levels of knowledge; therefore, they ought to be distilled separately with attention to different levels. Inspired by [12], we create a binary mask, where the foregrounds are the area of landmarks. We use this binary mask to perform foreground and background distillation loss calculations separately, which means we distill the focal knowledge of foreground and background with different levels of attention. We also add a global distillation loss to distill the global context information of the teacher's features, so that the global knowledge can also be distilled.

The rest of this paper will be arranged as follows: In Sect. 2, we introduce our proposed method in detail. In Sect. 3, we present our experiments and comparisons, and we provide a conclusion and discussion in Sect. 4.

2 Proposed Method

2.1 Overview

As shown in Fig. 1, there are three steps in general. In the first step, we trained a teacher model using composed GT images. We applied Gaussians to training images' labels and then concatenated them to the original images. In the second step, we froze the teacher model's encoder and trained the student model using focal and global distillation. For focal distillation, we used a binary mask to discriminate between the foreground and background. We believe that foreground information should be afforded more attention compared with the background. Therefore, we calculated the foreground distillation loss and background distillation loss separately. We not only distilled the knowledge focally but also added a global distillation loss to compensate for the continuity of the global context knowledge broken by the separation of foreground and background. In step 3, we fine-tuned the student model's decoder.

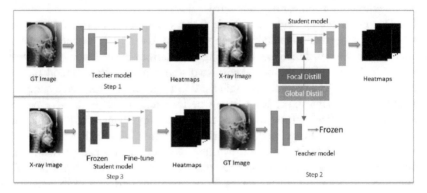

Fig. 1. Overview of proposed Focal and Global Teacher-Student distillation method.

2.2 Training of Teacher Model

For the training of the teacher model, we adopted the same pattern as our previously proposed teacher–student learning method. Here we will briefly reiterate the process. First, for landmarks of cephalometry, we apply Gaussian functions to all landmarks. We then add the Gaussians to the original cephalometry, as shown in Fig. 2. The teacher model is trained on such composed images. To let the teacher model learn the important features of landmarks instead of just copying the GT images' Gaussian regions, we also add random noise to the Gaussian regions of the GT images.

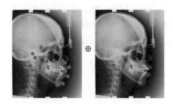

Fig. 2. Example of Composed GT images. We add Gaussians of landmarks on the original images (left) and concatenate with original images (right) as the GT images

Our motivation is that GT labels are usually only used in the calculation of loss functions, whereas we believe that it could be better used if we add this information directly to the original image to guide the training. Therefore, we trained a teacher model using composed images of GT labels, and we used this trained teacher model to guide the training of the student model.

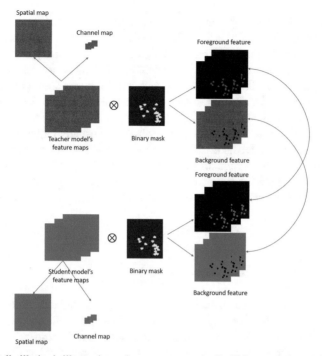

Fig. 3. Focal distillation's illustration, where we separately distill feature maps of foreground and background.

2.3   Focal and Global Distillation

In the second step, we aimed to train the student model by distilling the trained teacher model's knowledge. The input of the student model was the original x-ray cephalometry. Instead of distilling feature maps of the teacher model to the student model directly, we separated the distillation into focal distillation and global distillation. For focal distillation, we wanted to distill local important features. Specifically, we believe that the foreground and background areas should be addressed differently. More attention needs to be paid to the areas near landmarks (foreground). Therefore, we created a binary mask of landmark regions and applied this mask to the feature maps of the student and teacher. Thus, we could calculate the distillation loss of the foreground and background separately. As shown in Fig. 3, we also extracted the spatial attention maps and channel attention maps of the teacher model and applied this map to the calculation of distillation loss. The separated distillation loss is given as Eq. 1.

$$Loss_{fea} = \alpha \sum_{k=1}^{C} \sum_{i=1}^{H} \sum_{j=1}^{W} M_{i,j} A_{i,j}^{S} A_{k}^{C} (F_{k,i,j}^{T} - F_{k,i,j}^{S})^2$$

$$+ \beta \sum_{k=1}^{C} \sum_{i=1}^{H} \sum_{j=1}^{W} (1 - M_{i,j}) A_{i,j}^{S} A_{k}^{C} (F_{k,i,j}^{T} - F_{k,i,j}^{S})^2 \qquad (1)$$

In Eq. 1, C, H and W represent the channel, height, and weight of feature maps, respectively. M represents a binary mask of the foreground we created, and areas near landmarks are labeled as ones. Similarly, 1 − M represents a binary mask of the background we created, where areas which do not include landmarks are labeled as ones. A^S and A^C represent the spatial attention map and channel attention map of the teacher's feature map, respectively. F^T represents the teacher model's trained feature maps, F^S represents the student model's trainable feature maps. α and β are hyperparameters of foreground and background distillation loss, where α is usually larger than that of β.

Through Eq. 1, the focal distillation of the foreground and background are separated through binary masks. Each element makes the student model's features similar to that of the teacher's through the spatial and channel attention maps. For A^S and A^C, we simply take the absolute mean values of pixels and channels here, which are shown in Eq. 2.

$$A^S = H \cdot W \cdot softmax(\frac{1}{C} \cdot \sum\nolimits_{c=1}^{C} |F_C|)$$

$$A^C = C \cdot softmax(\frac{1}{HW} \cdot \sum\nolimits_{i=1}^{H} \sum\nolimits_{j=1}^{W} |F_{i,j}|) \tag{2}$$

Besides, we wanted to make the student's channel and spatial attention map similar to that of the teacher. Therefore, we also added an L1 feature similarity loss of the spatial and channel attention maps between the teacher's model and the student's model, which is given in Eq. 3, where γ is the hyper parameter, S and C represent spatial and channel attention maps and T and S represent the teacher's and student's maps, respectively.

$$Loss_{att} = \gamma \cdot \left(L1\left(A_S^T - A_S^S\right) + L1\left(A_C^T - A_C^S\right) \right) \tag{3}$$

The overall focal distillation loss is written as Eq. 4.

$$Loss_{focal} = Loss_{fea} + Loss_{att} \tag{4}$$

One of the drawbacks of focal distillation is that the global context information is cut out through the separation of the foreground and background. Therefore, we also added a global distillation loss to act as a compensation, which is given in Eq. 5, where δ is the hyperparameter, and f represents Cbam [13].

$$Loss_{global} = \delta \cdot \sum \left(f\left(F^T\right) - f\left(F^S\right) \right)^2 \tag{5}$$

The overall loss in the second step is shown as Eq. 6, where $Loss_{heatmap}$ is the mean squared error loss to predict landmarks' heatmaps.

$$Loss = Loss_{focal} + Loss_{global} + Loss_{heatmap} \tag{6}$$

2.4 Fine-Tune Student Model

Finally, after distilling knowledge focally and globally, we froze the student encoder and fine-tuned the decoder. Only the weight of the decoder was updated in this step.

3   Experiments

3.1   Datasets

We evaluated our method through the private dataset provided by Shandong University. In the dataset, we had a total of 100 images, and we chose to use ten-fold cross-validation to verify our method. Each cephalometry's resolution is 2136×1804 and each pixel is $0.1 \text{ mm} \times 0.1 \text{ mm}$, and we had a total of 19 bony landmarks annotated by professional doctors in Shandong University.

3.2   Implementation Details

We cropped and resized the images to two times smaller, with resolutions of 1000×900 for training and testing. We added random data augmentation with cropping, rotation, and affine transformation. The hyperparameters we used in the experiments of α, β, γ and δ are 0.005, 0.002, 0.002, 0.002. We created heatmaps for each landmark with a lambda of 8. We use U-Net as our backbone for both teacher and student model [14].

3.3   Evaluation Measurements

We used the mean radial error (MRE) and SDR to evaluate the performance, The MRE is given in Eq. 7:

$$MRE = \frac{\sum_{i=1}^{n} \sqrt{\Delta x_i^2 + \Delta y_i^2}}{n} \tag{7}$$

where Δx and Δy are the differences in the x-axis and y-axis between the predicted landmark location and GT, and n is the total number of test images. The definition of successful detection is as follows: If the radial error between the predicted landmark and the GT value is no greater than z mm (where $z = 2, 2.5, 3, 4$), the detection is considered successful (usually, a 2 mm range is acceptable in the medical field). The definition of SDR is given in Eq. 8:

$$SDR = \frac{N_a}{N} \times 100\% \tag{8}$$

where N_a indicates the number of successful detections and N indicates the number of total detections

3.4   Landmark Detection Results

We present the SDR and MRE results in Table 1. Our proposed method achieves 80.6% 2 mm detection accuracy and 1.395 MRE. One of the examples of our prediction result is given in Fig. 4.

Table 1. SDR and MRE Results of 2mm, 2.5mm, 3mm, 4mm range

Test result (Average of 10 fold cross-validation)

Anatomical Landmarks	2 mm (%)	2.5 mm (%)	3 mm (%)	4 mm (%)	MRE (mm)
1.naison	85.0	90.0	91.0	97.0	1.354
2.sella	97.0	97.0	98.0	99.0	0.702
3.orbitale	81.0	89.0	92.0	94.0	1.347
4.porion	67.0	75.0	80.0	89.0	1.883
5.ptm	78.0	80.0	88.0	92.0	1.521
6. Basion	71.0	82.0	84.0	92.0	1.820
7.bolton	66.0	72.0	78.0	82.0	1.967
8.ant.nasal spine	93.0	96.0	98.0	99.0	0.859
9. a point	58.0	66.0	74.0	81.0	2.126
10.post.nasal spine	93.0	96.0	97.0	97.0	0.823
11.upper 1 crown	65.0	72.0	84.0	90.0	1.726
12.lower incisor	82.0	90.0	97.0	97.0	1.463
13. Upper incisor	84.0	95.0	99.0	100.0	1.294
14. Gonion	68.0	75.0	83.0	89.0	1.765
15. Lower 1 crown	70.0	81.0	86.0	92.0	1.817
16. b point	83.0	88.0	90.0	93.0	1.626
17. Pogonion	97.0	97.0	98.0	99.0	0.803
18. Gnathion	98.0	98.0	98.0	98.0	0.787
19. Menton	95.0	96.0	98.0	98.0	0.830
Average:	80.6	86.0	90.2	93.6	1.395

3.5 Comparison

As shown in Table 2, we made a comparison with baseline methods and our previous teacher–student learning methods. From the table, we can conclude that our focal and global distillation method outperforms previous methods with higher accuracy, which also verifies the effectiveness of our proposed method.

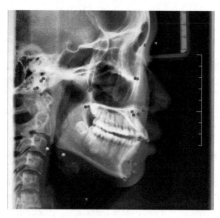

Fig. 4. An example of prediction result, where red dots represent ground-truth landmarks and blue dots represent predicted landmarks.

Table 2. SDR and MRE Results of 2 mm, 2.5 mm, 3 mm, 4 mm range

Method	2 mm (%)	2.5 mm (%)	3 mm (%)	4 mm (%)
Baseline:	77.8	81.4	86.2	90.6
[11]	80.3	85.8	90.1	**93.7**
Proposed	**80.6**	**86.0**	**90.2**	93.6

4   Conclusion and Discussion

In this paper, we proposed a refined teacher–student learning method for accurate landmark detection. We used a binary mask to separate foreground and background distillation; therefore, more foreground knowledge was focused during the training process. We also added a global distillation loss to our model to compensate for the discontinuity of cutting foreground and background; therefore, global context knowledge is also learned during the distillation process. We used a private cephalometric dataset and verified our thinking. Our proposed method achieved satisfactory results on automatic cephalometric landmark detection.

Acknowledgment. This work was supported in part by the National Natural Science Foundation of China under the Grant No. 61603218, in part by the Grant-in Aid for Scientific Research from the Japanese Ministry for Education, Science, Culture and Sports (MEXT) under the Grant No. 18H03267 and No. 17K00420, and in part by JST SPRING under the Grant No. JPMJSP2101.

References

1. Nijkamp, P., Habets, L., Aartman, I., Zentner, A.: The influence of cephalometrics on orthodontic treatment planning. Eur. J. Orthod. (2008). J. Clerk Maxwell, A Treatise on Electricity and Magnetism, 3rd ed., vol. 2. Oxford: Clarendon, 1892, pp.68–73

2. Oria, A., Schellino, E., Massaglia, M., Fornengo, B.: A comparative evaluation of Steiner's and McNamara's methods for determining the position of the bone bases. Minerva Stomatol. **40**(6), 381–385 (1991)

3. Wang, C.-W., et al.: T. Evaluation and comparison of anatomical landmark detection methods for cephalometric x-ray images: a grand challenge. IEEE Trans. Biomed. Eng. **53**, 1890–1900 (2015)

4. Wang, C., et al.: A benchmark for comparison of dental radiography analysis algorithms. IEEE Trans. Biomed. Eng. **31**, 63–76 (2016)

5. Bulat, I., Likar, B., Pernus, F., Vrtovec, T.: Computerized cephalometry by game theory with shape-and appearance-based landmark refinement. In: Proceedings of International Symposium on Biomedical imaging (ISBI) (2015). J. Clerk Maxwell, A Treatise on Electricity and Magnetism, 3rd ed., vol. 2. Oxford: Clarendon, 1892, pp.68–73

6. Arik Sercan, Ö., Ibragimov, B., Xing, L.: Fully automated quantitative cephalometry using convolutional neural networks. In: Proceedings of International Symposium on Biomedical imaging (ISBI) 2017, 4

7. Zhong, Z., Li, J., Zhang, Z., Jiao, Z., Gao, X.: An attention-guided deep regression model for landmark detection in cephalograms. In: Shen, D., Liu, T., Peters, T.M., Staib, L.H., Essert, C., Zhou, S., Yap, P.-T., Khan, Ai. (eds.) MICCAI 2019. LNCS, vol. 11769, pp. 540–548. Springer, Cham (2019). https://doi.org/10.1007/978-3-030-32226-7_60

8. Chen, R., Ma, Y., Chen, N., Lee, D., Wang, W.: cephalometric landmark detection by attentive feature pyramid fusion and regression-voting. In: Shen, D., et al. (eds.) MICCAI 2019. LNCS, vol. 11766, pp. 873–881. Springer, Cham (2019). https://doi.org/10.1007/978-3-030-32248-9_97

9. Song, Y., et al.: Automatic cephalometric landmark detection on x-ray images using a deep-learning method. Appl. Sci. **10**(7), 2547 (2020)

10. Payer, C., Štern, D., Bischof, H., Urschler, M.: Integrating spatial configuration into heatmap regression based CNNs for landmark localization. Med. Image Anal. **54**, 207–219 (2019)

11. Song, Y., Qiao, X., Iwmoto, Y., Chen, Y.-W.: A teacher-student learning based on composed ground-truth images for accurate cephalometric landmark detection. In: Proceedings of 2021 IEEE International Conference on Image Processing (IEEE ICIP 2021), Alaska, USA. September 19–22 2021

12. Yang, Z., et al.: Focal and global knowledge distillation for detectors. In: Proceedings of the IEEE/CVF Conference on Computer Vision and Pattern Recognition, pp. 4643–4652 (2022)

13. Woo, S., Park, J., Lee, J.-Y., Kweon, I.S.: CBAM: convolutional block attention module. In: Ferrari, V., Hebert, M., Sminchisescu, C., Weiss, Y. (eds.) ECCV 2018. LNCS, vol. 11211, pp. 3–19. Springer, Cham (2018). https://doi.org/10.1007/978-3-030-01234-2_1

14. Olaf, R., Fischer, P., Brox, T.: T.U-net: convolutional networks for biomedical image segmentation. In: International Conference on Medical Image Computing and Computer-Assisted Intervention, pp. 234–241 (2015)

Designing Deep Learning Architectures with Neuroevolution. Study Case: Fetal Morphology Scan

Smaranda Belciug[1]([✉]) [ID], Rodica Nagy[1,2] [ID], Sebastian Doru Popa[1] [ID],
Andrei Gabriel Nascu[1] [ID], and Dominic Gabriel Iliescu[1,2] [ID]

[1] Department of Computer Science, Faculty of Sciences, University of Craiova, Craiova,
Romania
sbelciug@inf.ucv.ro
[2] Department No. 2, University of Medicine and Pharmacy, Craiova, Romania

Abstract. The COVID-19 pandemic changed the way we practice medicine. The maternal-fetal care scenery has also been affected by the pandemic. Pregnancy complications, and even maternal of fetal death can be prevented if soon-to-be mothers are carefully monitored. Congenital anomalies are the most encountered cause of fetal death, infant mortality, and morbidity. A fast accurate diagnosis can be set if we merge the doctor's knowledge with Artificial Intelligence methods. The aim of this study is to statistically compare two neuroevolution methods (Differential evolution + Deep Learning and Evolutionary computation + Deep Learning) with two gradient based deep learning neural networks (DenseNet121 and InceptionV3), to see if they have the potential to revolutionize the healthcare system. We have applied and compared the four methods on second trimester morphology scan dataset. The experimental results showed that the two neuroevolution methods are comparable in terms of performance and outperform the gradient based methods.

Keywords: differential evolution · evolutionary computation · deep learning · statistical assessment · congenital anomalies

1 Introduction

In the year 2020, the COVID-19 pandemic forced us to change the way we practice medicine. Day by day, minute by minute, hospitals got more and more crowded with COVID-19 patients, disturbing the whole healthcare system landscape. No exception was made when it came to maternal-fetal care. Hence, changes in the routine of the maternal-fetal care were needed. The onset of the anxiety of being infected with Sars-COV-2, prevented soon to be mothers to seek medical care during their pregnancy. One of the most encountered issues in the pandemic was the outburst of long-lasting congenital anomalies, cause by either the actual infection with COVID-19, or by therapeutic procedures, [1]. Besides that, the number of caesarean sections has gone up, as a secondary aspect of the pandemic, [2].

Attending all scheduled morphology scans can detect possible problems of the fetus. If the ultrasound is interpreted correctly and the doctor identifies one or multiple congenital anomalies, then it gives the parents the possibility of knowing *a priori* the prognosis of their child's condition in terms of procedural risks, long-term mortality, morbidity, and quality of life. Unfortunately, reading the fetal morphology scan is acomplicated matter, and the current approaches are limited. The discrepancies between pre- and post-natal diagnosis obtained through a human interpreted ultrasound have a sensitivity between 27.5% and 96% [3]. These results are influenced by the experience level in performing ultrasounds, the time pressure, fetal involuntary movement, fatigue, and even maternal characteristics (i.e. obesity, [4]).

It is a fact that the COVID-19 pandemic represents a game changer when it comes to medicine. Medical care must be found at a faster pace. Using Artificial Intelligence can provide an early, fast, and accurate diagnosis. Deep learning (DL) diagnosis software was already given regulatory approval to be used in clinical practice, [5, 6]. Researchers all over the world are trying to optimize the design of the deep neural networks so that their performance in the medical field to improve, [7]. The aim of this study regards the maternal-fetal ultrasound image classification.

Two different pretrained convolutional neural networks (CNNs) and two non-DL algorithms have been applied on two sets of data containing maternal-fetal ultrasounds. The reported accuracies ranged between 54% and 93.6%, [8]. The fetal lungs and brain were segmented using DL and sequential forward feature selection technique and support vector machines on MRI (magnetic resonance images) and ultrasounds, [9]. The fetal brain was also segmented using a fully CNN applied on 3D images, [10]. The fetal cardiac function was assessed using a CNN applied on 4D B-mode ultrasound, [11]. In [12], the authors applied a mixture between differential evolution and DL to classify fetal view planes ultrasound images, while in [13] the authors used a merger between evolutionary computation and DL for the same purpose.

The race to finding the best architecture for a CNN has begun. There is no perfect solution that could be used in every problem. So, we need to determine the 'best-deal' between performance and computational effort when it comes to CNN applied in medicine. In recent years, the data scientists' effort has focused on automatically developing the CNN's architectures. Three directions can be pursued: progressive architecture search, [14], reinforcement learning [15–19], and evolutionary computation, [20, 21]. Different studies have shown that automated methods outperformed the manual tuned ones, [21–23].

The study focused on comparing two neuroevolution methods used for finding the best architecture of a CNN that can differentiate between the view planes in a second trimester morphology scan with two gradient based ones. The two neuroevolution methods focus on differential evolution and evolutionary computation. The remaining part of the paper is organized as follows: Sect. 2 presents the two neuroevolutionary algorithms, Sect. 3 deals with benchmarking dataset, while Sect. 4 details the results together with a statistical analysis of the performances. The paper ends with the conclusions and future work.

2   The Models

CNNs are a particular type of NNs. In a CNN we encounter three types of layers: the convolutional layer, the pooling layer, and the fully connected layer. The feature map is created by the convolutional layer, through the filters that scan the input and perform convolutions. The pooling layer is used to produce spatial invariance because it down samples the feature map obtained after a convolution. The network ends with the fully connected layer.

In a CNN there are multiple parameters that need to be tuned: the size of the filter, the stride (i.e. the number of pixels by which the filter is slide), and the zero-padding (i.e. the number of pixel that board the input).

As activation functions we can choose between the ones that induce non-linearities, and the one that takes a real vector score and transforms it into a probability vector. The functions that induce non-linearities are the: rectified linear unit layer (ReLU), Leaky ReLu, and Exponential linear unit (ELU). The other function is the generalized logistic function, the softmax.

Many CNNs have their architectures designed deterministic. In this paper we are going to compare two novel proposed neuroevolutionary algorithms, differential evolution/CNN, [12], and evolutionary computation/CNN, [13].

2.1   Differential Evolution / Convolutional Neural Network

Differential Evolution (DE) was developed in 1997, [24, 25]. This type of optimization algorithm is quite simple to apply and comprehend. It generates a temporary individual that has as starting inception the differences that exist in the given population and the evolutionary restructuration of the population. The algorithm reaches a good global convergence, and it is robust.

The mutation operation uses one-on-one competition. DE is capable to explore different solution in parallel, and to enable dynamic track of the existing search using its memory volume.

At each generation G, we have a population that consists of N candidates with M features per candidate. Each candidate is denoted through $X_{iG} = \left(x_{iG}^1, x_{iG}^2, \ldots, x_{iG}^M\right)$, $i = 1, 2 \ldots, N$. We initialize the population by randomly generating numbers between the upper and the lower bound of each features' search space for each feature.

$$X_i^n = X_i^{n,L} + rand() \cdot (X_i^{n,U} - X_i^{n,L})$$

where $i = 1, 2, \ldots, N$ and $n = 1, 2, \ldots, M$, $X_i^{n,L}$ is the lower bound of X_i^n, while $X_i^{n,U}$ is the upper one.

The mutation process involves three vectors $X_{r_1,G}, X_{r_2,G}, X_{r_3,G}$, whose values are used in the formula:

$$V_G^n = X_{r_1,G}^n + F \cdot \left(X_{r_2,G}^n - X_{r_3,G}^n\right),$$

where $X_{r_1,G}^n$ is the donor vector, F is the variation factor that takes values from [0, 1] and regulates the amplification degree of $X_{r_2,G}^n - X_{r_3,G}^n$.

The recombination process produces a trial vector, $U_{i,G+1}^n$, from the target and the donor vector, by applying the following equation:

$$U_{i,G+1}^n = \begin{cases} V_{i,G+1}^n, & \text{if } rand() > p_c \text{ or } i = I_{rand} \\ X_{i,G}^n, & \text{if } rand() < p_c \text{ and } i \neq I_{rand} \end{cases},$$

where $I_{rand} \in [1, M]$ is a random integer, and p_c is the recombination probability.

After the mutation and recombination operators had been applied, the selection operation starts. In this process, we compare the target vector to the trial one. The one that minimizes the fitness function is selected to form the next generation.

$$X_{i,G+1}^n = \begin{cases} U_{i,G+1}^n, & \text{if } f\left(U_{i,G+1}^n\right) < f\left(X_{i,G}^n\right) \\ X_{i,G}^n, & \text{otherwise} \end{cases}.$$

The DE algorithm is:

1. Randomly initialize the population.
2. Repeat:

   2.1. Apply mutation
   2.2. Apply recombination
   2.3. Apply selection

   Until the stopping criterion is reached.

In our study, the DE/CNN uses a population of fixed-length vectors that represent the CNNs architecture, $x_i = (\lambda, nH, fw, fh, pc, F)$, $i = 1, \ldots, q$, where q is the number of individuals in the population, λ is the number of convolutional layers, nH the number of neurons in a convolution, fw and fh are the filter's width and height, pc the crossover probability, and F the variation factor. After each convolution we have a pooling layer. We have selected the ReLU as the non-linear activation function, and softmax as the activation between the fully connected hidden layer and the output layer.

The DE/CNN algorithm can be summarized as follows:

1. Initialize the N candidate solutions randomly.
2. Built N CNNs having as architecture the candidate solutions.
3. Do:

   3.1. Train the CNNs and record their accuracies over the validation set.
   3.2. The loss of each CNN represents the fitness value of the respective candidate solution.
   3.3. Apply the mutation operator on each individual.
   3.4. Apply the recombination operator.
   3.5. Select the individuals for the next generation based on their validation loss.

   Until the stopping criterion is reached.
4. Return the best candidate solution that will give the network's architecture.

2.2 Evolutionary Computation/Convolutional Neural Network

The most used method of optimization is the evolutionary computation (EC). In this type of method, we deal with a population made of chromosomes, that are subjected to a number of different processes such as selection, recombination, and mutation. The chromosomes' structure resembles to the structure of the candidate solutions described in the previous section. The general scheme of an EC is, [26]:

1. Initialize the population randomly.
2. Compute the fitness score of each chromosome.
3. Repeat:

   3.1. Apply the selection operator for parent selection.
   3.2. Apply the recombination operator to produce offspring.
   3.3. Apply the mutation operator to generate diversity.
   3.4. Compute the fitness.
   3.5. Select the chromosomes that will form the next generation using the fitness.

   Until the stopping criterion is reached.

In our study, the EC/DL algorithm uses fixed-length integer arrays as chromosomes, $\mathbf{x}_i = (\lambda, nH, fw, fh, pc, pm)$, $i = 1, \ldots, q$, where q is the number of individuals in the population, λ is the number of convolutional layers, nH the number of neurons in a convolution, fw and fh are the filter's width and height, pc the crossover probability, and pm the mutation probability. We have chosen as the non-linear activation function the ReLU, and as the function between the fully connected layer and output layer the softmax function. The recombination operator was the total arithmetic crossover, while for mutation we have used the uniform operator.

The EC/DL algorithm has the following steps:

1. Generate randomly the N chromosomes.
2. Built N CNNs that have as architectures the structure of the respective chromosome.
3. Do:

   3.1. Train the CNNs and record their accuracies and loss values obtained on the validation set.
   3.2. Select the parents for recombination.
   3.3. Apply the recombination operator.
   3.4. Apply the mutation operator.
   3.5. Select the chromosomes that will form the next generation.

   Until the stopping criterion is met.
4. Return the best candidate solution that will give the network's architecture.

3 Application Case Study: Maternal-Fetal Ultrasound Planes

For our benchmarking process, we have used a dataset which contains maternal-fetal abdomen view-planes. The dataset is part of a prospective cohort study deployed at the maternity hospital University Emergency County Hospital of Craiova, Romania. All the participants were pregnant women that have admitted themselves for the second trimester morphology scan at the Prenatal Unit. The doctors informed them about the research project and invited them to take part of the study. All the patients were recruited consecutively. They gave a written consent and understood the study's implication.

The images regarded the abdomen and were acquired using Voluson 730 Pro (GE Medical Systems, Zipf, Austria) and Logic e (GE Healthcare, China US machines) with 2–5-MHz, 4–8 MHz, and 5–9 MHz curvilinear transducers. The dataset is split into 6 decision classes: 3-vessles plus bladder plane (253 images), gallbladder plane (123 images), transverse cord insertion plane (211 images), anteroposterior kidney plane (188 images), biometry plane (440 images), kidney longitudinal renal (326 images). All the images were anonymized and preprocessed so that the artifacts or text to be removed.

Because the sample size is too small, and because we wanted to avoid overfitting, we have used a data generator to enlarge the dataset's size. The following transformations have been applied to each image: rotation range = 20, width shift range = 0.1, height shift range = 0.1, brightness range $\in$ [0.7, 1.4], zoom range = 0.2, shear range = 0.2. Before training the models we have reshaped the images to 224 × 224 px.

Figure 1 presents a sample for every decision class.

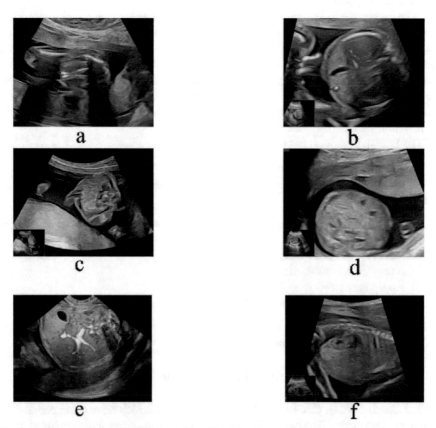

Fig. 1. (a) 3-vessels plus bladder plane; (b) gallbladder plane; (c) transverse cord insertion plane; (d) anteroposterior kidney plane; (e) biometry plane; (f) kidney sagittal plane.

4   Results

To complete our study, we have benchmarked the two neuroevolution models, DE/DL and EC/DL, with two gradient-based models (DenseNet121 and InceptionV3), when used to differentiate between different view planes in a maternal-fetal morphology scan. For all for four models we have applied the *10-fold cross-validation*. We have used power analysis to estimate the sample size (number of independent computer runs) needed to achieve a high statistical power. The estimated number was 50 runs (in a complete cross-validation cycle) for both models, in order to achieve a statistical power of 95% with type I error $\alpha = 0.05$. In Table 1, we present the average accuracy over 50 complete cross-validation cycles (ACC), together with the standard deviation (SD), precision, recall, and F1-score.

Table 1. Performance of DE/DL and EC/DL.

Model	ACC (%)	SD	Precision	Recall	F1-score
DE/DL	78.65	1.84	0.782	0.78	0.779
EC/DL	77.99	2.87	0.779	0.779	0.778
DenseNet121	63.97	2.23	0.643	0.637	0.633
InceptionV3	46.16	2.13	0.455	0.461	0.460

From Table 1 we can see that DE/DL outperforms EC/DL by a bit, in terms of average accuracy and also in terms of stability and robustness, DE/DL having a smaller SD. The neuroevolutionary methods outperform the gradient based ones. since the two novel methods outperform by far the gradient ones, we continued our statistical analysis with just these neural networks.

Our statistical analysis continued with the *data screening* process, which involved the *Kolmogorov-Smirnov & Lilliefors* test and *Shapiro-Wilk W* test for testing the normality of the sample data, and the *Levene* test and *Brown-Forythe* test for verifying the equality of variances. The data screening process checks whether the assumptions of the *t*-test are fulfilled or not. The results of the normality tests are presented in Table 2, whereas the results for the equality of variances are presented in Table 3.

Table 2. Normality tests results

Model	Kolmogorov-Smirnov		Shapiro-Wilk W	
	K-S max D	Lilliefors *p*	S-W W	*p*-level
DE/DL	0.073	0.2	0.987	0.83
EC/DL	0.082	0.2	0.984	0.79

Table 3. Equality of variances

Model	Levene F (1,df)/*p*-level	Brown-Forsythe (1,df)/*p*-level
DE/DL vs EC/DL	2. 567/0.113	2.345/0.122

Table 2 reveals that both samples that contain the 50 computer runs of the neuroevolutionary algorithms are normally distributed. Table 3 shows that the variances are equal. We can proceed with applying the *t*-test for independent samples, to see whether there exist significant statistical differences between the two methods' performances. We have applied the *t*-test with the Bonferroni correction. The results are depicted in Fig. 2 together with both models' accuracies shaped as boxplots and annotated with the corresponding *p-level*.

The results of the *t*-test shows that the performances of the DE/DL and EC/DL are comparable on this dataset.

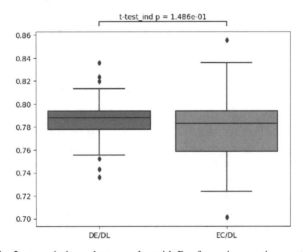

Fig. 2. *t*-test independent samples with Bonferonni correction results.

5 Conclusions

This study's aim was to provide a performance comparison between two neuroevolution methods and two gradient based deep learning neural networks when applied to differentiate between the abdomen view-planes of a maternal fetal morphology scan. We have benchmarked the models' performances using different statistical tests: power analysis, Kolmogorov-Smirnov & Lilliefors test, Levene test, Brown-Forsythe test, and *t*-test for independent samples with the Bonferonni correction. On this real-world dataset the two neuroevolutionary models performed the same, while outperforming the gradient based ones. The experiments must be deepened in terms of applying the two methods on other datasets, and also of adding other genes or features to the candidate solution vector.

Acknowledgement. This work was supported by a grant of the Ministry of Research Innovation and Digitization, CNCS – UEFISCDI, project number PN-III-P4-PCE-2021-0057, within PNCDI III.

References

1. Khan, M.S.I., et al.: Risk of congenital birth defects during COVID-19 pandemic: draw attention to the physicians and policymakers. J Glob. Health. **10**(2), 020378 (2020)
2. Dube, R., Kar, S.S.: COVID-19 in pregnancy: the foetal perspective – a systematic review. Neonatology **4**(1) (2020). https://doi.org/10.1136/bmjpo-2020-000859
3. Salomon, L., et al.: A score-based method for quality control of fetal images at routine second trimester ultrasound examination. Prenat Diag. **28**(9), 822–827 (2008)
4. Paladini, D.: Sonography in obese and overweight pregnant women: clinical, medico-legal, and technical issues. Ultrasound Obstet. Gynecol. **33**(6), 720–729 (2009)
5. Topol, E.J.: High performances medicine: the convergence of human and artificial intelligence. Nat. Med. **25**, 44–46 (2019)
6. Benjamens, S., Dhunno, P., Mesko, B.: The state of artificial intelligence-based FDA approved medical devices and algorithms: an online database. NPJ Digit. Med. **3**, 118 (2020)
7. Liu, X., et al.: A comparison of deep learning performances against healthcare professionals in detecting diseases from medical imaging: a systematic review and meta-analysis. Lancet Digit. Health **1**, e217-297 (2019)
8. Burgos-Artizzu, X.P., et al.: FETAL_PLANES_DB: common maternal-fetal ultrasound images. Nat. Sci. Rep. **19**, 10200 (2020)
9. Torrents-Barrena, J., et al.: Assessment of radiomics and deep learning for the segmentation of fetal and maternal anatomy in magnetic resonance imaging and ultrasound. Acad. Radiol. **19**, 30575–30576 (2019)
10. Namburete, A., et al.: Fully automated alignment of 3D fetal brain ultrasound to a canonical reference space using multi-task learning. Med. Image Anal. **46**, 1–14 (2018)
11. Phillip, M., et al.: Convolutional neural networks for automated fetal cardiac assessment using 4D B-Mode ultrasound. In: IEEE 16th International Symposium on Biomedical Imaging, pp. 824–828 (2019). https://doi.org/10.1109/ISBI.2019.8759377
12. Belciug, S.: Learning deep neural networks' architectures using differential evolution. case study: medical imaging processing. Comput. Biol. Med. **146**, 105623 (2022)
13. Ivanescu, R., et al.: Evolutionary computation paradigm to determine deep neural networks architectures. Int. J. Comput. Commun. Control **17**(5), 4886 (2022). https://doi.org/10.15837/ijccc.2022.5.4886
14. Liu, C., et al.: Progressive neural architecture search. In: Ferrari, V., Hebert, M., Sminchisescu, C., Weiss, Y. (eds.) ECCV 2018. LNCS, vol. 11205, pp. 19–35. Springer, Cham (2018). https://doi.org/10.1007/978-3-030-01246-5_2
15. Baker, B., et al.: Designing neural network architectures using reinforcement learning. In: International Conference on Learning Representations, ICRL, p. 2017 (2017)
16. Cai, H., et al.: Efficient architecture search by network transformation. In: Association for the Advancement of Artificial Intelligence, p. 2018 (2018)
17. Zhong, Z., Yan, J., Liu, C.L.: Practical network blocks design with Q-learning. In: International Conference on Learning Representations, 2017, ICLR, (2018)
18. Zoph, B., Le, Q.V.: Neural architecture search with reinforcement learning. In: International Conference on Learning Representations, 2017, ICLR (2017)
19. Zoph, B., Vasudevam V., Shlens, J., Le, Q.V.: Learning transferable architectures for scalable image recognition. In: Conference on Computer Vision and Pattern Recognition (2018)

20. Miikkulainen, R., et al.: Evolving deep neural networks, CoRR, abs/1703.00548 (2017)
21. Real, E., et al.: Large-scale evolution for image classifiers. In: Proceedings of 34th International Conference on Machine Learning, vol. 70, pp. 2902–2911 (2017)
22. Real, E., et al.: Regularized evolution for image classifier architecture search. In: 33rd AAAI 2019, IAAI 2019, EAAAI 2019, pp. 4780–4789 (2019)
23. Sun, Y., et al.: Evolving deep convolutional neural networks for image classification. IEEE Trans. Evol. Comput. **24**(2), 394–407 (2020)
24. Storn, R., Price, K.: Differential-evolution - a simple and efficient heuristic for global optimization over continuous spaces. J. Glob. Optim. **11**(4), 341–359 (1997)
25. Storn, R., Price, K.: Differential-evolution for multi-objective optimization. Evol. Comput. **4**, 8–12 (2003)
26. Gorunescu, F., et al.: An evolutionary computation approach to probabilistic neural networks with application to hepatic cancer diagnosis. In: 18th IEEE Symposium on Computer-Based Medical Systems, pp. 461–466 (2005)

PD-L1 Prediction of Lung Cancer by a Radiomics Method Using Rough Tumor Mask in CT Images

Xiang Lv[1], Huadong Liu[1], Rui Xu[1,2(✉)], Dingpin Huang[3], Yuan Tu[3], Fangyi Xu[3], Yi Gan[4], and Hongjie Hu[3(✉)]

[1] DUT-RU International School of Information Science and Engineering,
Dalian University of Technology, Dalian, China
[2] DUT-RU Co-Research Center of Advanced ICT for Active Life, Dalian, China
xurui@dlut.edu.cn
[3] Department of Radiology, Sir Run Run Shaw Hospital,
Zhejiang University School of Medicine, Hangzhou, China
hili@dlut.edu.cn
[4] Department of Pathology, Sir Run Run Shaw Hospital,
Zhejiang University School of Medicine, Hangzhou, China

Abstract. Programmed Death Ligand-1 (PD-L1) plays a key role in the success of immunotherapy for cancer treatment. However, immuno-histochemistry(IHC) based PD-L1 detection requires biopsy of patients ' tumor through surgery. In this paper, we discussed the possibility of predicting PD-L1 expression based on radiomics and rough tumor mask on CT images. We used various methods to obtain different rough tumor masks, and explored the radiomics feature based on these masks. Proved the feasibility of PD-L1 prediction based on rough tumor mask. The results of 5-fold cross validation experiment on our PD-L1 dataset shows that, the average AUC results of our method reached 0.8284 which outperformed the method based on precise delineation, provides a new paradigm for PD-L1 identification.

Keywords: Programmed Death Ligand-1 (PD-L1) · Lung Cancer · CT · Radiomics · Rough Cancer mask

1 Introduction

Lung cancer is one of the most lethal cancers in the world. Its treatment methods have always been the focus of medical research. Recently, with the development of immunotherapy, the mortality of lung cancer is decreasing year by year. Programmed death ligand 1 (PD-L1) is a key factor in immunotherapy, which determines the success of treatment [5]. It need patients to undergo immunohistochemistry (IHC) to test their tumor PD-L1 expression level to confirm whether themselves are suitable for immunotherapy. IHC requires biopsy of tumor tissue of patients. The results may vary due to different environments and sampling sites, resulting in missed and false detection [7]. Therefore, a non-invasive, high-precision and reproducible PD-L1 detection method is urgently needed. Computer tomography (CT) is a routine examination of lung cancer patients, which has the advantages of non-invasive and low-cost. It can reflect the growth state of tumor at the macro level, which provides the possibility to analyze tumor information through depth-learning or radiomics. Besides that, considering that tumor tissues with different PD-L1 expression levels may have different growth states. Therefore, it is feasible to predict PD-L1 expression level on CT images through radiomics.

By now, some experiments have proved that the expression level of PD-L1 in tumor tissue is related to its shape/texture. 1) Gouji et al. analyzed and compared the relationship between different PD-L1 expression levels and different tumor morphology [3]. 2) Sun Z. et al. analyzed the tumor texture feature of patients with different levels of PD-L1 expression by using radiomics [8]. Furthermore, 3) Tian P. et al. combined the radiomics features with deep learning to analyze the tumor morphology of patients with high expression level of PD-L1 on a larger dataset [1]. However, all of these methods are based on the internal feature of tumors, which required radiologist to label the tumor manually. This is time-consuming and expensive.

In this paper, we proposed that the PD-L1 prediction problem based on radiomics can be solved by rough tumor mask for following reasons: 1) Due to the different standards of different radiologist, there may exist deviations in the results of the tumor delineation. It is impossible to achieve accurate label to 1 pixel. 2) The feature calculation by radiomics depends on the image texture. A tiny mask difference will hardly affect the prediction accuracy. 3) The expression of PD-L1 may be related to its surrounding microenvironment. Therefore, a proper expansion of the mask area may benefit the prediction accuracy. For rough tumor mask, in this paper, we have tried a variety of methods to generate corresponding masks, including tightly-rounded, randomly-expanded and anisotropy-expanded. In addition, considering that extrapulmonary tissue may affect the feature extraction process, we also eliminated the interference of extrapulmonary tissue by introducing an additional whole-lung segmentation model. After that, we extracted and selected the radiomics features and put them into a machine-learning classifier for classification. According to the 5-fold crossover experiment on our private PD-L1 dataset, our average AUC reached 0.8284 which exceeded the carefully labeled ones.

In general, our contributions can be summarized as followed: 1. We have established a pipeline of lung cancer PD-L1 prediction based on rough tumor segmentation of CT images. 2. The performance of the proposed model was evaluated with a 5-fold cross-validation under our private PD-L1 data set, and its average AUC was 0.8284, which was equivalent to or even slightly improved by the radiomics method based on fine segmentation.

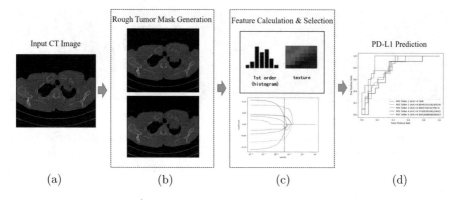

Fig. 1. Overview our proposed PD-L1 prediction method. (a), (b)represents the 2 different result of tumor rough mask. (c), (d) representative feature extraction and selection process respectively.

2 Rough Tumor Mask Based Radiomics Method for PD-L1 Prediction of Lung Cancer

In this paper, we propose a lung cancer PD-L1 prediction based on rough tumor mask on CT images, as shown in Fig. 1. Our data preparation involves original CT images, pulmonary segmentation and accurate tumor segmentation. Through a rough segmentation algorithm using the input data, we obtain a rough tumor mask result and extract features from the rough segmented areas. Next, we apply the LASSO regression algorithm [9] to select useful features and use the features to train our model using diverse widely used traditional Machine Learning classifiers. Finally, we evaluated the feasibility of our method by evaluating ROC curves. In this section, We will describe the rough mask of tumor and the selection of radiomics features in detail.

2.1 Rough Tumor Mask Generation

Mask is a critical operation in medical image processing that involves separating the region of interest (ROI) in an image from its surrounding background area. This technique allows for the extraction of diseased areas in an image, which can then be used to calculate the features of these areas. To achieve accurate tumor mask, Radiologists need to label CT images manually, which is time-consuming and expensive to obtain corresponding masks, as shown in Fig. 2.(a). In this paper, we propose two rough tumor masks based on precise labeling: tight bounding box and extended bounding box.

Tight bounding box can be automatically generated by external cube on the basis of accurate tumor mask, shown in Fig. 2.(b). Furthermore, through combining lung segmentation algorithm [10], we remove the extra-pulmonary part on the basis of preliminary rough segmentation results, which is shown in Fig. 2.(c).

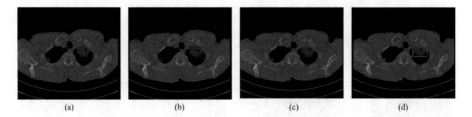

(a)   (b)   (c)   (d)

Fig. 2. Our proposed different rough mask methods. (a) represents accurate tumor mask, (b) represents tight bounding box mask with extra-pulmonary part, (c) represents tight bounding box mask without extra-pulmonary part, (d) represents extended bounding box mask.

However, radiologists may encounter difficulties in completely fitting the tight bounding box around a tumor during practical applications. To address this issue, we have extended the bounding box by a few pixels to simulate the approximate labeling results obtained by radiologists in real-world scenarios, as depicted in Fig. 2.(d). To demonstrate the use of rough masking, we have extended the bounding box using two approaches: fixed pixel value extension and random pixel value extension.

2.2 Feature Calculation and Selection

After getting the rough tumor mask, we use it and the accurate tumor mask as the mask to extract features on the CT images with pyradiomics [4]. Radiomics feature extraction typically yields abundant features (including Gray Level Co-occurrence Matrix (GLCM), Gray Level Run Length Matrix (GLRLM) Features, etc. It is noteworthy that considering the discrepancy between the accurate mask and the rough mask, we extract shape features solely from accurate mask, while disregarding shape features when employing rough mask). Thus, it is crucial to select useful features to train the classifier. In this paper, we employed the LASSO regression algorithm [9] to select useful features.

The LASSO (Least Absolute Shrinkage and Selection Operator) regression algorithm is a widely-used method for feature selection. It automatically identifies the most important features while filtering out the others. The following formula is typically used when employing the LASSO regression algorithm for feature selection:

$$\hat{\beta}_{lasso} = \arg\min \frac{1}{2N}(\mathbf{y} - \mathbf{X}\beta)^2 + \lambda||\beta||_1 \tag{1}$$

Here, $\hat{\beta}_{lasso}$ represents the coefficient vector solved by the LASSO regression algorithm, $\mathbf{y}$ is the target variable in the training set, $\mathbf{X}$ is the eigenmatrix of the training set, $||\beta||_1$ represents the L1 norm of the coefficient vector, which penalizes non-relevant features by making their coefficients become zero, N is the number of training samples, and λ is the regularization coefficient, which controls the complexity of the model.

In the feature selection process, we first use the LASSO regression algorithm to train all features and calculate the coefficient of each feature. Then, we select the features whose coefficients are non-zero as input for the classifier. Feature selection improves the generalization performance of the model, reduces model complexity, and enhances computational efficiency.

2.3 PD-L1 Prediction

The useful features selected with LASSO regression algorithm were used to train our classifiers. The input data for classifier training is composed of two parts: the feature matrix and the label vector. The feature matrix comprises extracted features, and each sample corresponds to a line of feature vectors. The label vector is used to indicate the category of each sample, such as whether it is malignant or benign. In this paper, we apply three traditional classifiers, Random Forest, K-Nearest Neighbor and Logistic Regression.

Random Forest (RF) [1] is a commonly used classifier in radiomics. As an ensemble learning algorithm, RF can build a powerful classifier by combining multiple decision trees. RF employs Bootstrap sampling and feature randomization to train each decision tree based on different data sets and random feature sets. During classification, each decision tree gives a classification result for the input sample and selects the final classification result by voting. RF has good robustness and generalization ability, and is not susceptible to overfitting, making it widely used in the classification and prediction of various cancer types such as lung cancer, liver cancer and breast cancer.

K-Nearest Neighbor (KNN) [2] is an instance-based classifier that classifies objects based on their similarity with samples of known categories. In classification, KNN first calculates the distance between the object to be classified and the known samples, then chooses K samples with the closest distance to vote, and assigns the object to be classified to the category with the most votes. KNN is simple and intuitive, and can be applied to multi-classification problems and nonlinear classification problems, so it can be used as a simple and effective classifier for prediction tasks in the field of radiomics.

Logistic Regression(LR) [6] is a supervised learning algorithm widely used in medical image classification. LR uses a specific linear regression method to divide the sample into two or more categories based on the different features in the sample that are assigned feature weights. It takes the eigenvalue as the input and its linearly weighted sum as the output. After processing by the sigmoid function, a probability value between 0 and 1 is obtained. When the probability value is greater than a certain threshold, the sample is classified as positive. When the probability value is less than the threshold, the sample is classified as a negative class. Currently, LR has been widely used in the diagnosis of lung cancer, breast cancer and other diseases, and has shown high diagnostic accuracy.

3   Experiments and Results

3.1   Data and Evaluation Protocols

All data involved in this study were provided by the Sir Run Run Shaw Hospital, Zhejiang Univerty. A total of 195 non-small cell lung cancer patients were enrolled. All their IHC slides were scanned and independently scored by two pathologists. According to the percentage($\geq 1\%$) of PD-L1 protein in both tumor and tumor infiltrating immune cells, the data are divided into positive and negative. After filter out 1) CT scans of poor quality, 2) lack of non-enhancement CT scans. Finally, 53 patients with PD-L1 positive expression and 124 with negative PD-L1 expression were involved. Informed consent was waived due to the retrospective nature of this study.

Initially, the input data is divided into a training set and a test set. The model is trained on the training set, and then the classifier is evaluated on the test set using metrics such as accuracy, recall rate, F1 value, ROC curve, etc. which are averaged over the 5 test subjects.

3.2   Experimental Results

Table 1. Comparison of proposed method with accurate mask and rough mask(RF represents Random Forest, KNN represents K-Nearest Neighbor, LR represents Logistic Regression).

Rough Mask	Extra-Pulmonary	AUC		
		RF	KNN	LR
×	×	0.8022	0.7658	0.7896
✓	✓	0.7172	0.7095	0.7810
✓	×	**0.8284**	0.7529	0.7974

Table 1 shows a comparative analysis of the differential diagnostic efficacy of radiomics methods utilizing accurate mask and rough mask in the ROC analysis. According to the 5-fold cross-validation, it is noteworthy that the rough mask of the external tumor cube not only yields comparable results to those obtained through the accurate mask, but also demonstrates superior predictive performance. This may be attributed to the reliance of radiomics feature computation on statistical analysis of image texture features, which renders small discrepancies resulting from imprecise mask insignificant in terms of feature computation. Moreover, it is challenging to attain complete accuracy in manual tumor region delineation. However, the performance of the predictive outcomes exhibited a marked decrease when the rough mask included extra-pulmonary part.

In order to investigate the impact of the extra-pulmonary part, we conducted a set of ablation experiments. To maximize the inclusion of the extra-pulmonary

Table 2. Ablation study of extra-pulmonary part on recognition accuracy.

Extra-Pulmonary	Extend Pixel	AUC		
		RF	KNN	LR
✓	0	0.7172	0.7095	0.7810
✗	0	**0.8284**	0.7529	0.7974
✓	5	0.7233	0.6304	0.7383
✗	5	0.7692	0.6322	0.7771
✓	10	0.6760	0.6486	0.6767
✗	10	0.7108	0.6708	0.7436

part in rough mask results, we extended the larger pixel value based on the outer cube of the tumor region, thereby accentuating the impact of the extra-pulmonary part on the experimental outcomes. The results in Table 2 clearly demonstrate a significant decrease in predictive performance with increasing extra-pulmonary part. This is likely due to the mixing of features extracted from the extra-pulmonary part with those from the tumor area, which can significantly impair the classification efficacy of the classifier.

Table 3. Experimental results of simulated rough mask using extended bounding box(0–1 represents random integer between 0 and 1).

Mask	Extend Pixel	AUC		
		RF	KNN	LR
accurate mask	–	0.8022	0.7658	0.7896
fixed extended mask	1	0.8299	0.7405	**0.8362**
	2	0.8072	0.7109	0.8165
	3	0.7953	0.7226	0.7971
	4	0.7808	0.7753	0.7942
	5	0.7692	0.6322	0.7771
random extended mask	0–1	0.7919	0.6869	**0.8177**
	0–2	0.7614	0.7454	0.8058
	0–3	0.7898	0.7199	0.7647
	0–4	0.7805	0.6928	0.7728
	0–5	0.7855	0.5847	0.7749

After mitigating the extra-pulmonary effects, we simulated the labeling process used by radiologists for rough mask. In practice, radiologists may not be able to accurately label the outer cube that fits tightly into the tumor area, and may instead expand the pixel value by several increments. To simulate this process, we extended the rough mask results of each training sample to a certain range of pixel values with two approaches. As shown in Table 3, better predictive performance can be achieved by randomly expanding the range of pixel values to 0–1. Simulated radiologists achieved better prediction, with accuracy of 75.81%, recall rate of 97.47 %, precision rate of 78.74%, and f1_score of 86.68 %compared to the accuracy of 74.15%, recall rate of 94.09%, precision rate of 77.21%, and f1_score of 85.83% obtained through accurate mask. This may be attributed to the fact that the region associated with PD-L1 prediction not only includes the tumor, but also its surrounding area, implying that using rough mask has a positive impact.

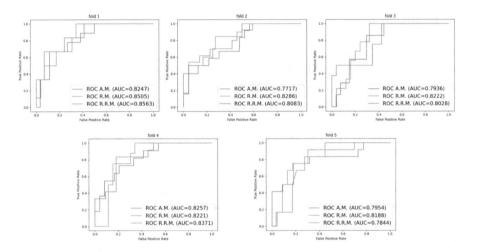

Fig. 3. 5-fold cross-validation AUC curve. (A.M. represents accurate mask, R.M. represents rough mask, R.R.M represents random rough mask).

Based on the experiments described above, we proceeded to predict the same group of 5-fold cross-validation using three methods: accurate mask, rough mask, and random rough mask simulating radiologists. The results are presented in Fig. 3. According to the ROC curve and AUC value obtained from the 5-fold cross-validation shown in the figure, it is evident that the rough mask can achieve results comparable to those of accurate mask, and may even yield better predictive performance in this problem.

4   Conclusion

In this paper, we propose a pipeline that uses tumor rough mask to predict PD-L1 expression. We have made a series of different kinds of tumor rough masks, and verified the influence of these different masks on the accuracy of PD-L1 prediction through the five-fold cross experiment. The experimental results show that our proposed rough mask feature extraction method is superior to the radiometric method based on fine segmentation.

Acknowledgment. This work was supported by National Natural Science Foundation of China (NSFC) under Grant 6177210, and by the Funda- mental Research Funds for the Central Universities of China.

References

1. Breiman, L.: Random Forests, Mach. Learn. **45**, 5–32 (2001). https://doi.org/10.1023/A:1010933404324
2. Goldberger, J., Roweis, S., Hinton, G., Salakhutdinov, R.: Neighbourhood components analysis. In: Advances in Neural Information Processing Systems, pp. 513–520 (2005)
3. Gouji, T., Kazuki, T., Tatsuro, O., Mototsugu, S., Yuka, K.: Computed tomography features of lung adenocarcinomas with programmed death ligand 1 expression. In: Clinical Lung Cancer (2017)
4. van Griethuysen, J.J.M., et al.: Computational radiomics system to decode the radiographic phenotype. Can. Res. **77**(21), 104–107 (2017)
5. He, J., Hu, Y., Hu, M., Li, B.: Development of pd-1/pd-l1 pathway in tumor immune microenvironment and treatment for non-small cell lung cancer. Sci. Rep. **5**, 13110 (2015)
6. Hosmer, D.W., Sturdivant, S.L.R.X.: Applied Logistic Regression. SAGE Publications, Inc. (2000)
7. Loughran, C.F., Keeling, C.R.: Seeding of tumour cells following breast biopsy: a literature review. Br. J. Radiol. **84**, 869–74 (2011)
8. Sun, Z., et al.: Radiomics study for predicting the expression of pd-l1 in non-small cell lung cancer based on Ct images and clinicopathologic features. J. Xray Sci. Technol. **28**, 449–459 (2020)
9. Tibshirani, R.: Regression shrinkage and selection via the lasso. J. Roy. Stat. Soc.: Ser. B (Methodol.) **58**, 267–288 (1996)
10. Xu, R., et al.: Bg-net: Boundary-guided network for lung segmentation on clinical CT images. In: International Conference on Pattern Recognition(ICPR) (2020)

Innovative Incremental K-Prototypes Based Feature Selection for Medicine and Healthcare Applications

Siwar Gorrab[(✉)], Fahmi Ben Rejab, and Kaouther Nouira

Université de Tunis, ISGT, LR99ES04 BESTMOD, Tunis, Tunisie
{siwarg9,fahmi.benrejab,kaouther.nouira}@gmail.com

Abstract. The real issue in healthcare systems is how to detect, gather, analyze and handle medical data to make people's lives advantageous and healthier. This is by contributing not only to understand recent diseases and therapies, but also to predict outcomes at earlier stages in order to make real-time decisions. Especially when raw data comes with missing values, redundancies, and/or inconsistencies, feature selection is required as a mandatory step to be applied before starting the learning process. Driven by the juxtaposition of big data and powerful machine learning techniques, this paper presents a medical application that improves the process of clinical care, advances medical research, and improves efficiency based on feature selection. This streaming feature application presents new solutions for helping in early detection of diseases, treatment recommendations, and clinical services to doctors. Experimental results show significant inertia results and efficient execution time compared to the batch k-prototypes and a proposed Incremental k-prototypes method.

Keywords: Big data · incremental attribute learning · feature selection · mixed features · k-prototypes · smart medical systems

1 Introduction

The application of big data methods and data mining techniques is growing quickly in the domain of clinical medicine and healthcare administration. Many of these exercises of big data analytic require advanced computational frameworks for high data volume and intensive data processing [1]. Actually, the huge amounts of healthcare and medical data, coupled with the need for data analysis and decision making tools has made data mining techniques interesting research areas. This is for the purpose of identifying meaningful information from huge data sets in medicine and healthcare fields. Specifically, the unsupervised clustering technique which helps to discover and understand hidden patterns in a healthcare data set. On a daily basis, large volumes of highly detailed healthcare data of mixed type are continuously forthcoming from multiple sources such as electronic health records, medical literature, clinical trials, insurance claims data, pharmacy records, and

© The Author(s), under exclusive license to Springer Nature Singapore Pte Ltd. 2023
Y.-W. Chen et al. (Eds.): KES InMed 2023, SIST 357, pp. 282–291, 2023.
https://doi.org/10.1007/978-981-99-3311-2_25

even information entered by patients into their smartphones or recorded on fitness trackers. These multiple data sources send sequences of data records, namely data streams, which further need to be analyzed and investigated. This data describes particulars about patients, their medical tests, and their treatments. Hence, the "curse of dimensionality" is a bottleneck in big data and artificial intelligence for medical and healthcare applications. It is a significant and challenging task to detect the informative features to carry out explainable analysis for high dimensional data. This is especially needed for medicine and healthcare applications. Considering that at anytime and all long the learning task, new instances including new incoming features, that further describe patients, might emerge. Doctors must deal with a streaming feature and object spaces when additionally new patients' parameters have to be tracked, new analysis have to be done, and new decisions have to be made to provide the best patient's followup [1]. However, not all added features are relevant for mining and decision making. This is due to the presence of inconsistent, redundant and irrelevant features in a higher amount. Hence, applying feature selection to remove these unwanted features, before modeling streaming data, decrease the computational complexity and speed the learning process [3].

In this paper, we address the problem of clustering mixed-type data based feature selection in a streaming feature and object environment for medicine and healthcare areas. It would be a smart medical and healthcare system, developed for the purpose of providing better insights into critical advances that can contribute to improve the efficiency and performance of health organizations and medical researchers. Into the bargain, we are looking for getting a picture of how reality mining, incremental attribute learning and selecting only relevant features among all incoming ones can improve healthcare systems and medical services. This work contributes in advancing medical research and improving the process of clinical care as well as their efficiency. Its intention is to enhance medicine with reducing cost and upgrading healthcare value and quality. It counts on k-prototypes algorithms and feature selection variance-threshold technique, created for incrementally grouping medical data streams with added features in order to make future predictions and healthcare recommendations. To sum up, the unique contribution that distinguish this proposed work from existing approaches are threefold: 1) a novel framework based on feature selection is proposed to manage streaming features for medical and healthcare applications; 2) our work advances the incremental attribute and object learning tasks in a streaming data and features environment; and 3) a new online streaming feature selection algorithm is proposed, with extensive experimental studies and comparisons between batch k-prototypes, Incremental Healthcare K-prototypes [1] and our proposal on four mixed medical healthcare data sets. The quality of the proposed method is validated based on run time value and similarity between and within clusters measures. The rest of the paper is organized as: the related work and the theoretical concepts of k-prototypes algorithm are discussed in Sect. 2. The proposed approach is detailed in Sect. 3. Section 4 presents the experimental study and discusses the corresponding results. Finally, Sect. 5 concludes the work.

2 K-Prototypes Method and Related Works

2.1 K-Prototypes Algorithm

The k-prototypes clustering algorithm was proposed in [4] to group mixed data set $X=\{x_1...x_n\}$ of n data points containing m_r numeric attributes and m_t categorical attributes into k different clusters (Fig. 1).

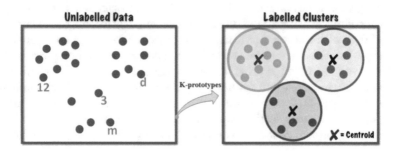

Fig. 1. K-prototypes clustering algorithm.

Algorithm 1: Conventional K-prototypes algorithm

1: **Data:** data set:X, number of clusters: k
2: **Result:** Cluster centers Q
3: **Begin**
4:    **Select** at random k primary cluster centres from X.
5:    **Repeat**
6:      **Assign** each data point in X to its closest cluster center.
7:      **Update** the cluster centres after each allocation.
8:    **Until** updated cluster centers are identical to the previous ones.
9: **End.**

2.2 Related Works

Medical and Healthcare Data Mining Applications. Big data in medicine and healthcare fields is driving big changes. Dhara et al. developed a Content-Based Image Retrieval System for Pulmonary Nodules [5] that helps radiologists to assist in self-learning and diagnosis of lung cancer. Aiming to deal with the high rate of false alarms generated by health monitoring systems in intensive care units, this work [6] puts forward a health monitoring system based on parallel-APPROX SVM. Also in [7], an artificial intelligence system capable of classifying skin cancer with a level of competence comparable to dermatologists has been proposed with a dermatologist-level classification of skin cancer using deep neural networks. Work proposed in [8] has successfully revealed predictive markers of depression from Instagram photos. Mehre et al. developed in [9] a content-based image retrieval system for pulmonary nodules through optimal feature sets and class membership-based retrieval. In [10], Zhong and Zhang have proposed an uncertainty-aware INVASE to quantify predictive confidence of healthcare problem and enhance breast cancer diagnosis based on feature selection. In [1], an advanced incremental attribute learning clustering method has been proposed as healthcare application to enhance patient's care and diseases assessment.

Unsupervised Feature Selection Methods. Despite its popularity and effectiveness with multiple supervised machine learning tasks, feature selection is still rarely used in unsupervised algorithms. Therefrom, work in [2] extends the k-mean clustering algorithm to provide an efficient unsupervised feature selection method for streaming features applications where the number of features increases while the number of instances remains fixed. A real-time k-prototypes method for incremental attribute and object learning tasks based on feature selection was proposed in [3]. Likewise, Bonacina et al. proposed in [11] a clustering approach, based on complex network analysis, for the unsupervised feature subset selection of time series in sensor networks. Also in [12] Shi, Dan, et al. have recently developed an unsupervised adaptive feature selection method with binary hashing model in order to exploit the discriminative information under the unsupervised scenarios. In this study [13], a Fuzzy C-Means (FCM) based feature selection mechanism for wireless intrusion detection is proposed.

Works provided in literature present a requirement to enhance clustering algorithms to deal with streaming data and mixed features environment in medicine and healthcare, specifically the k-prototypes method. Performing feature selection in such context is needed with reference to the few mentioned studies.

3   Proposed Approach

3.1   Definition and Approach Presentation

Here we shed light on a big data solution in medicine and healthcare fields, through IAL context. Since being proposed towards handling mixed data streams with newly joined features, FSIHK-prototypes method consists of extending the IHK-prototypes [1] method with a feature selection preprocessing technique. That is, to ensure the selection of relevant features before modeling the incoming mixed data streams. In actuality, our proposal covers the real challenge in healthcare systems: how to collect, analyze and manage the information to make people's lives healthier and easier. More to the point, our smart medical and healthcare system, FSIHK-prototypes, contributes not only to understand new diseases and therapies but also to predict outcomes at earlier stages and to make real-time decisions. It is an advanced incremental attribute and object learning k-prototypes algorithm based on feature selection preprocessing technique. It is founded on the proposed IHK-prototypes method [1], based on the Incremental K-prototypes algorithm [14]. But it precedes clustering these new emerging mixed data streams with applying feature selection as being a preprocessing technique that searches to pull out the most useful and pertinent features among all the incoming ones in a streaming objects and features environment. Actually, when you supply too many features to a model, it affects its performance and confuses the learning ability because they may not be all useful. Expressing differently, a row data may come with different forms of anomalies. This includes redundancy, inconsistency, irrelevance, imbalanced values and/or a large number of features. So, the core purpose of our proposed FSIHK-prototypes method involves their removal to attain appropriate features set. For example, a doctor is supposed to make a decision to group patients having similar type of diseases or health issues with a view to provide them with effective treatments. He asked if there were similar patients in the medical system hoping to gain insight into their disease progression or therapeutic outcomes. Thus, only relevant and important features should be selected for further analysis and appropriate decision making. Hence, feature selection can select pertinent features and remove irrelevant features, which helps to alleviate the curse of dimensionality and reduce the difficulty of learning tasks [15].

Here, we would like to investigate the impact of applying feature selection in a streaming features environment in order to check

1. Whether it can effectively eliminate irrelevant or redundant features without changing their semantics.
2. At what point this may improve the performance of learning and reduce the training time.

Glancing at Fig. 2, an overview of our proposal is presented as follows:

- First of all, medical or healthcare mixed data streams are continuously emerging from various sources and analysis. It contains new data rows, escorted with both categorical and numerical added features, describing patient's, diseases, treatments, etc. As a mandatory step, a feature selection preprocessing technique would be applied on these new incoming features. In our developed method, our feature selection module is based on the variance threshold technique that would be explained in the next subsection. Consequently, only consistent and useful patient's features are selected to carry out the upcoming learning steps.
- Once relevant streaming features are selected, we do inject them in the incremental learning module. This latter is based on the initially proposed IHK-prototypes algorithm [1], founded on the merge technique.

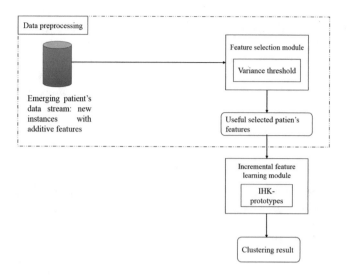

Fig. 2. An overview of the proposed FSIHK-prototypes approach through IAL context based on feature selection.

3.2 Feature Selection Module

Undoubtedly, numerous and various are the techniques used for feature selection implementation. However, feature selection is rarely used in unsupervised tasks (e.g. clustering), which makes it challenging to perform such study. So, in our study we are focusing on the efficiency of feature selection in IAL context rather then on the technique itself. Therewith, we have opted to use the variance threshold selector technique owing to the following facts:

- Its intention is to find out a subset of the most representative streaming features according to the variance criteria [3].
- It is a simple and effective baseline approach to feature selection.
- Variances of all added features are calculated in the whole data rows based on a feasible statistical computation.
- Systematically, features with zero variances are removed by default.

After calculating the variances of the recently joined streaming features, a variance threshold is fixed regarding the alteration of the calculated variances. Accordingly, the selected features are those present with a degree of variation higher then the fixed threshold.

3.3 Incremental Feature Learning Module

The IHK-prototypes [1] clusters continuously arriving mixed data, with newly joined attributes, within memory and time restrictions. It provides real-time results and performs well at the emergence of new healthcare streaming features. By way of illustration, healthcare data abounds in various forms. However, it is most conventionally found in the electronic health record, clinical diagnosis, human analysis, etc. Doctors need to deal with this dynamic scope of streaming features and data spaces so as to ensure the best patient's followup. To do so, the IHK-prototypes well performs as a healthcare/medical service provider for making suitable decisions regarding patient's health conditions.

4 Experiments and Results

4.1 Framework and Data Sets Description

The experiments have been performed on 4 real data sets containing numeric and categorical features ranging from 7 to 32. These benchmarking data sets belong to different applications in medicine and healthcare fields, and they are detailed in the following Table 1.

Table 1. Summary details of used real mixed healthcare data sets.

Data set	Number of objects	Number of attributes	Acronym
Stroke Prediction	5110	7 numeric, 5 categorical	SP
Pharmaceutical Drug Spending	1036	5 numeric, 2 categorical	PDS
Breast Cancer Wisconsin	569	31 numeric, 1 categorical	BCW
Personality Scale Analysis	315	6 numeric, 2 categorical	PSA

For a better understanding, we take for instance the BCW data set composed of 32 mixed features and 569 objects. Aiming to simulate the situation of streaming features in medicine and healthcare fields, we have firstly introduced an input data composed of 200 objects and 29 attributes. Hereafter, a new data stream with 369 instances and 32 attributes come to join the learning process. Likewise, we are familiar with 3 additional features.

4.2 Evaluation Measures

The experiments' results have been evaluated and discussed based on run time and indices that calculate the cluster cohesion and separation. Then combine them to compute the following quality measures: the Silhouette Coefficient [17] and the Sum of Squared Error [18]. An up and/ down arrow is assigned after each evaluation measure. The first means that a higher value is recommended and the second means exactly the opposite.

1. The run time (RT ↓): it reflects the time acquired to achieve the final clustering output, starting from the beginning of the learning procedure.
2. The Silhouette Coefficient [17] (SC ↑): it is adjacent to +1 in case of highly dense clustering, and -1 for incorrect clustering. As a consequence, high SC

values reflect a model with more coherent clusters. Composed of two scores a and b, SC is calculated using Equation (1):

$$s = \frac{b - a}{\max(a, b)} \tag{1}$$

Where a: is the mean distance between a sample and all other points in the same cluster; b: is the mean distance between a sample and all other points in the following closest cluster.

3. The Sum of Squared Error (SSE $\downarrow$): calculates the clusters inertia. SSE determines the dispersion of a cluster's elements regarding their cluster centers. So, clusters are better defined when their corresponding SSE value is closer to zero. SSE is calculated using Equation (2):

$$SSE_{x \in C} = \sum_{i=1}^{n} \sum_{j=1}^{m} (x_{kj} - c_j) \tag{2}$$

Knowing that c_j is the centre of the cluster j.

4.3   Results and Performance Analysis

Table 2 reveals experimental results in a comparison between the proposed FSIHK-prototypes method, the conventional k-prototypes and IHK-prototypes methods.

Table 2. Measured RT, SSE and SC scores of conventional k-prototypes vs. IHK-prototypes vs. FSIHK-prototypes methods per data set.

Data sets	K-prototypes			IHK-prototypes			FSIHK-prototypes		
	RT (second)	SSE	SC	RT (second)	SSE	SC	RT (second)	SSE	SC
SP	87.788	1.920	0.363	56.229	1.651	0.388	55.605	1.814	0.423
PDS	11.090	1.956	0.469	6.772	1.577	0.523	5.704	1.432	0.619
BCW	7.188	2.130	0.457	4.543	1.547	0.467	4.491	1.997	0.512
PSA	2.956	2.587	0.487	1.794	1.682	0.576	1,559	1.412	0.766

1. **Run Time Results Analysis:** the outcomes in Table 2 show that FSIHK-prototypes method has minimum execution time on the data sets whereas batch k-prototypes method has maximum execution time. We may also notice that the IHK-prototypes requires less time for its execution compared to the conventional k-prototypes. Despite that, the proposal of this study outperforms it with less by half time needed for its running.

2. **Sum Of Squared Error Results Analysis:** the results and comparisons in Table 2 conclude that both FSIHK-prototypes and IHK-prototypes outperform the batch k-prototypes method in terms of clusters' inertia. This is

explained with the acquisition of lower SSE values from respectively batch K-prototypes, IHK-prototypes and FSIHK-prototypes. Means that our proposed FSIHK-prototypes method leads to a better defined model with maximum similarity within clusters and minimum similarity between clusters.

3. **Silhouette Coefficient Results Analysis:** glancing at SC results for inspection of clusters, shown in Table 2, we validate that our proposal is the optimum feature learning method in a streaming medical feature's environment. This is because it achieves the highest SC scores for all used datasets.

The achieved results below confirm that incremental attribute and object learning form an interesting alternative. Our proposed FSIHK-prototypes method constitute one of the major concerns of big data in medicine and healthcare fields. As well, performing feature selection before modeling patient's emerging mixed data with supplementary features reduces execution time because less data leads to train faster. It also reduces over-fitting because it minimizes the possibility to make medical decisions based on noisy or inconsistent data. Besides, FSIHK-prototypes eases the learning process, speeds it up and defines a more coherent model that respects better basics of clustering. The capability of our streaming features method can be interpreted in understanding, classifying and predicting diseases at earlier stages, making real-time decisions, promoting patients' health, enhancing medicine. All by reducing cost and improving life expectancy and healthcare quality.

5   Conclusion

In this paper, we propose a smart incremental feature selection k-prototypes system for medicine and healthcare applications with streaming mixed data. This latter is continuously forthcoming with added features where the knowledge of the full feature space is unknown in advance. The goal here is to provide a scalable and real-time healthcare application, with the ability to select only relevant features among all coming ones. Our proposal may enhance advanced healthcare monitoring systems, innovative services and medical applications such as helping in early detection of diseases, treatment recommendations, and clinical services to doctors. Experiments and results emphasize the capability of our proposal when clustering big data in medicine and healthcare Fields. It outperforms the batch k-prototypes and the proposed IK-prototypes methods through various evaluation measures. We leave for future work to tackle the decremental attribute learning task. As well, we plan on directing our efforts towards handling the third dynamic space, namely the incremental class learning task.

References

1. Gorrab, S., Rejab, F.B., Nouira, K.: Advanced incremental attribute learning clustering algorithm for medical and healthcare applications. In: International Work-Conference on Bioinformatics and Biomedical Engineering, pp. 171–183. Springer, Cham (2022). https://doi.org/10.1007/978-3-031-07704-3_14

2. Almusallam, N., Tari, Z., Chan, J., Fahad, A., Alabdulatif, A., Al-Naeem, M.: Towards an Unsupervised Feature Selection Method for Effective Dynamic Features. IEEE Access **9**, 77149–77163 (2021)
3. Gorrab, S., Rejab, F.B., Nouira, K.: Real-Time K-prototypes for incremental attribute learning using feature selection. In: Alyoubi, B., Ben Ncir, CE., Alharbi, I., Jarboui, A. (eds.) Machine Learning and Data Analytics for Solving Business Problems, pp. 165–187. Springer, Cham (2022)
4. Huang, Z.: Extensions to the k-means algorithm for clustering large data sets with categorical values. Data Mining Knowl. Discovery **2**(3), 283–304 (1998)
5. Dhara, A. K., Mukhopadhyay, S., Dutta, A., Garg, M., Khandelwal, N.: Content-based image retrieval system for pulmonary nodules: assisting radiologists in self-learning and diagnosis of lung cancer. J. Digital Imaging **30**(1), 63–77 (2017)
6. Ben Rejab, F., Ksiaâ, W., Nouira, K.: Health monitoring system based on parallel-APPROX SVM. In: Rojas, I., Ortuño, F. (eds.) IWBBIO 2017. LNCS, vol. 10208, pp. 3–14. Springer, Cham (2017). https://doi.org/10.1007/978-3-319-56148-6_1
7. Esteva, A., et al.: Dermatologist-level classification of skin cancer with deep neural networks. Nature **542**(7639), 115–118 (2017)
8. Reece, A.G., Danforth, C.M.: Instagram photos reveal predictive markers of depression. In: EPJ Data Science, 6, pp. 1–12. Springer (2017)
9. Mehre, S.A., Dhara, A.K., Garg, M., Kalra, N., Khandelwal, N., Mukhopadhyay, S.: Content-based image retrieval system for pulmonary nodules using optimal feature sets and class membership-based retrieval. J. Digital Imaging **32**(3), 362–385 (2019)
10. Zhong, J.X., Zhang, H.: Uncertainty-aware INVASE: Enhanced Breast Cancer Diagnosis Feature Selection. In: arXiv preprint arXiv:2105.02693 (2021)
11. Bonacina, F., Miele, E.S., Corsini, A.: Time series clustering: a complex network-based approach for feature selection in multi-sensor data. Modelling **1**(1), 1–21 (2020)
12. Shi, D., Zhu, L., Li, J., Zhang, Z., Chang, X.: Unsupervised adaptive feature selection with binary hashing. IEEE Trans. Image Process. (2023)
13. Tseng, C.H., Tsaur, W.J.: Fuzzy C-means based feature selection mechanism for wireless intrusion detection. In: 2021 International Conference on Security and Information Technologies with AI. Internet Computing and Big-data Applications, pp. 143–152. Springer, Cham (2023). https://doi.org/10.1007/978-3-031-05491-4_15
14. Gorrab, S., Rejab, F.B.: IK-prototypes: incremental mixed attribute learning based on K-prototypes algorithm, a new method. In: Abraham, A., Piuri, V., Gandhi, N., Siarry, P., Kaklauskas, A., Madureira, A. (eds.) ISDA 2020. AISC, vol. 1351, pp. 880–890. Springer, Cham (2021). https://doi.org/10.1007/978-3-030-71187-0_81
15. Guo, Y., Hu, M., Tsang, E. C., Chen, D., Xu, W.: Feature selection based on min-redundancy and max-consistency. In: Advances in Computational Intelligence, 2(1), pp. 1–11 (2022)
16. Asuncion, A., Newman, D.: UCI machine learning repository (2007)
17. Rousseeuw, P. J.: Silhouettes: a graphical aid to the interpretation and validation of cluster analysis. J. Comput. Appl. Math. **20**, 53–65 (1987)
18. Kwedlo, W.: A clustering method combining differential evolution with the K-means algorithm. Pattern Recogn. Lett. **32**(12), 1613–1621 (2011)

Deep Learning in Medical Imaging

Prior Active Shape Model for Detecting Pelvic Landmarks

Chenyang Lu[1], Wei Chen[2], Xu Qiao[1(✉)], and Qingyun Zeng[3(✉)]

[1] Department of Biomedical Engineering, School of Control Science and Engineering,
Shandong University, Shandong 250061, Jinan, China
qiaoxu@sdu.edu.cn
[2] Department of Radiology, Shandong First Medical University and Shandong Academy of
Medical Sciences, Shandong 271000, Taian, China
[3] Affiliated Hospital of Shandong University of Traditional Chinese Medicine,
Shandong 250061, Jinan, China

Abstract. Measurement of pelvic landmarks is a standard analytical tool for diagnosis and treatment prognosis. The purpose of this study is to develop and verify an automatic detection system for detecting pelvic measurement landmarks on pelycograms. Pelycograms for 430 subjects were available. All images have 17 landmarks. In this paper, a deep neural network system with Active Shape Model (ASM) prior knowledge is proposed that can be used to automatically locate landmarks on pelycograms. The outline of the pelvis is obtained by ASM, and the landmarks are roughly detected. Then the landmarks are accurately detected by a depth neural network based on this prior knowledge. The system is evaluated by experiments, and the average radial error of the system is 4.159 mm and the standard deviation is 5.015 mm. 81.353% of the landmarks are within the clinically acceptable precision of 6 mm. At the same time, the integration of ASM prior knowledge also improves the detection accuracy by 1.007 mm. This method can quickly and accurately locate landmarks in pelycograms, and it is possible to significantly improve the clinical workflow of orthopedic treatment.

Keywords: Pelvic landmarks · ASM · Deep Neural Network

1 Introduction

Pelycograms are often used as a standard tool for orthopedic diagnosis, treatment planning, and correction. The detection of anatomical landmarks and surrounding soft tissues near the pelvis is a crucial first step in the diagnostic and prognostic treatment process. [1]. The landmarks for pelvic detection are used in many orthopedic analyses, such as the mid landmark of the first sacrum, the highest landmark of the femur, and the anterior superior iliac spine. Several distance and angle measurements are calculated from their positions, as shown in Fig. 1.

Accurate detection of pelvic markers in pelycograms is a challenging problem. The pelvis is a combination of highly complex bones. A 3D object that is projected onto a single 2D plane in a pelycogram, coupled with proximity to some organs, results in

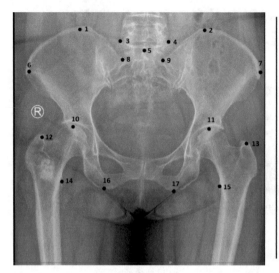

1 : Highest point of the right iliac crest
2 : Highest point of the left iliac crest
3 : Midpoint of the paraspinal sulcus of the
right superior sacrum
4 : Midpoint of the paraspinal sulcus of the
left superior sacrum
5 : Midpoint of the first sacrum
6: Right anterior superior iliac spine
7: Left anterior superior iliac spine
8: Right posterior superior iliac spine
9: Left posterior superior iliac spine
10: Highest point of right femur
11: Highest point of left femur
12: The greater trochanter of the right femur
13: The greater trochanter of the left femur
14: The lesser trochanter of the right femur
15: The lesser trochanter of the left femur
16: Right ischial tuberosity
17: Left ischial tuberosity

Fig. 1. Pelvic landmarks in an X-ray image

the structural overlap. In addition, with time, the pelvis will develop varying degrees of osteoporosis, hyperplasia, bone, and so on. Of course, because the data object is the patient, there will be varying degrees of pathological deformities. Coupled with the anatomical differences of the individual itself, it is very difficult to accurately locate the pelvic landmarks.

At the moment, the location of pelvic measurement landmarks is determined either by the traditional semi-automatic detection method [2–4] or solely by data from infants' and toddlers' pelycograms [5]. The disadvantages of the former are high algorithm complexity, low accuracy, and the need for pre-processing and post-processing for extensive data. The disadvantage of the latter is that the method is insensitive to pelvic x-ray data with a relatively irregular age span. Recently, Agomma et al. [6] applied CNN architecture to detect landmarks in front X-ray images of EOS through significance detection. Bastian Bier et al. [7] proposed a method to automatically detect landmarks in X-ray images independent of viewing direction and realized X-ray pose estimation in intraoperative landmark detection combined with preoperative CT. Feng-Yu Liu proposed a deep learning-based ROI detection framework that utilizes a single multi-box detector with a custom head structure based on the features of the obtained dataset [8]. Despite their use of neural networks, they still only processed standardized X-ray images of infants and toddlers.

Inspired by [9–11], we propose a method of pelvic landmark detection based on ASM. Based on ASM, this method roughly locates landmarks and bone edges, then embeds this information as prior knowledge into the deep neural network. To be more specific, we use ASM to detect a large number of landmark position information (including 17 landmarks) and segment bones, then use this part of position information to extract the region of interest of landmarks and input it into the deep neural network with the pyramid attention mechanism to finally get the precise coordinates of landmarks. The main contributions of this paper are as follows:

(1) A method that can directly embed the prior knowledge of ASM into the deep neural network is proposed.
(2) Experiments show that the overall detection framework proposed by us can accurately detect pelvic landmarks.

The remainder of this paper is organized as follows: Sect. 2 describes the construction method of the proposed model. Section 3 describes the experimental methodologies, and Sect. 4 presents the experimental results and discusses the observations. Finally, Sect. 5 concludes the paper, including suggestions for potential future work.

2 Methods

2.1 The Overall Framework

The overall framework of this method is shown in Fig. 2, which includes two parts: the first detection based on ASM and the second detection based on CNN. The second stage is the training depiction of one of the 17 landmarks in the first stage. A detailed explanation of each step is given below.

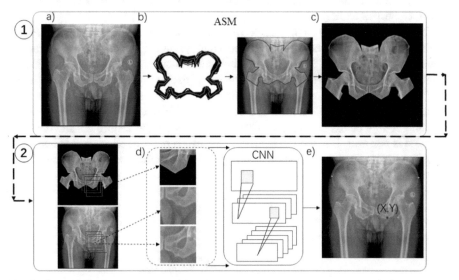

Fig. 2. Schematic of the overall detection framework. a) Input the original sample CT resize into the ASM part. b) Through normalization, principal component analysis, and other operations, the position information of landmarks is obtained. c) Output the ASM stage detection coordinates of 17 landmarks and obtain ROI accordingly. d) Obtain a large number of ROIs for the same landmark to train the second-stage detection CNN. e) Obtain the final predicted target position.

2.2 ASM for Pelycogram

Firstly, a pelycogram with 17 landmarks is given. However, these 17 points alone are not sufficient to use ASM. Select the edges of the target object with obvious corners, a "T" connection between edges, or easily located landmarks describing biological information. Between the 17 landmarks, more landmarks are added equidistantly along the boundary. The 49 key feature landmarks selected by us are shown in Fig. 3.a. Of course, the 17 landmarks that need to be detected at the end are among them.

For any picture in the training set, record the coordinate information of k = 49 key feature landmarks and save them in a text file. K key feature landmarks calibrated in a graph form a shape vector, as shown in Eq. 1.

$$\alpha_i = \left(x_1^i, y_1^i, x_2^i, y_2^i, \ldots, x_k^i, y_k^i\right), i = 1, 2, \ldots, n \tag{1}$$

In which $\left(x_j^i, y_j^i\right)$ represents the coordinates of the jth feature landmark on the ith training sample, and n represents the number of training samples. In this way, 330 training samples constitute n = 330 shape vectors. As shown in Fig. 3.b, the visualization of some input data shows a rather messy distribution.

Next, the Procrustes method is used to normalize $\pi = \{a_1, a_2, \ldots, a_n\}$ this training set. Specifically, 1: align all pelvic models in the training set to the first pelvic model, 2: calculate the average pelvic model α, 3: align all pelvic models to the average pelvic model α, 4: and repeat steps 2 and 3 until convergence. The result is shown in Fig. 3.c, 3.d is the confusion matrix.

Then we processed the aligned shape vector by principal component analysis (PCA), and the scale coefficient was 95%. The effect of multiplying PCA by adding or subtracting three standard deviations (STD) on the first model is shown in Fig. 3.e. On both sides of the ith feature landmark on the jth training image, m pixels are respectively selected along the direction perpendicular to the connecting line between the two feature landmarks before and after the landmark to form a vector with a length of $2m + 1$. The values of the pixels contained in the vector are derived to obtain a local texture g_{ij}, and the same operation is performed on the i th feature landmark on other training sample images in the training set to obtain n local textures $g_{i1}, g_{i2}, \ldots, g_{in}$ of the i feature landmark. Then, find the average of them,

$$\overline{g_i} = \frac{1}{n}\sum\nolimits_{j=1}^{n} g_{ij} \tag{2}$$

and variance,

$$S_i = \frac{1}{n}\sum\nolimits_{j=1}^{n} (g_{ij} - \overline{g_i})^T * (g_{ij} - \overline{g_i}) \tag{3}$$

In this way, the local feature of the ith feature landmark is obtained. By performing the same operation on all other feature landmarks, the local features of each feature landmark can be obtained. Thus, the Mahalanobis distance can be used to express the similarity measure between a feature landmark's new feature g and its trained local feature:

$$f_{sim} = (g - \overline{g_i})S_i^{-1}(g - \overline{g_i})^T \tag{4}$$

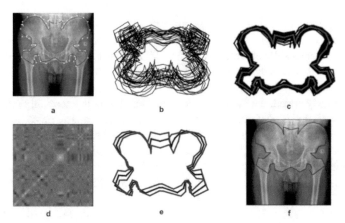

Fig. 3. ASM process of the pelvis. a) Landmarks for ASM. b) Partial input for visualization of ASM. c) Procrustes normalization results. d) Confusion Matrix. e) PCA analysis. f) ASM search results

In the ASM search phase, firstly, an initial model is obtained by an affine transformation of the average shape.

$$X = M(s, \theta)[a_i] + X_c \tag{5}$$

Find their new positions for all the feature landmarks and form their displacements into a vector $dX = (dX_1, dX_2, \ldots, dX_k)$. Through affine transformation and adjusting its parameters, the position X of the current feature landmark is closest to the corresponding new position $X + dX$. The variation of affine transformation parameters $d_s, d_\theta, d_{X_c}, d_{Y_c}$ can be obtained after an affine transformation.

$$M(s(1 + ds), (\theta + d\theta))[a_i + da_i] + (X_c + dX_c) = (X + dX) \tag{6}$$

Combined with the previous calculation, we can finally get

$$db = P^T da_i \tag{7}$$

Therefore, the updating process of the above parameters are as follows: $dX \rightarrow d_s, d_\theta, d_{X_c}, d_{Y_c} \rightarrow db$. The affine transformation parameters and b can be updated as follows: $X_C = X_C + \omega_t dX_c$, $Y_C = Y_C + \omega_t dY_c$, $\theta = \theta + \omega_\theta d\theta$, $s = s + \omega_s ds$, $b = b + \omega_b db$. In the above formula, $\omega_t, \omega_\theta, \omega_s, \omega_b$, are the weights used to control the change of parameters. In this way, a new shape can be obtained. As shown in Fig. 3.f, we cut up the bones according to the new shape we got.

2.3 Regression of Coordinates

The overall distribution of the landmarks to be detected in the pelycogram is scattered, while the overall pathological deformity is more serious, and most of the landmarks are only distributed in a local range of norms. Furthermore, because direct regression of multiple landmarks is a highly non-linear mapping that is difficult to learn [12–15], we choose to train a model with the same structure but different weights for 17 landmarks. On the basis of the results obtained by ASM, 300 regions of interest (ROI) with the size of 512 × 512 were extracted near each landmark, and the real labels were guaranteed in the ROI taken.

As previously stated, we intend to detect in a small patch where only one landmark can be detected, this is also our method of data augmentation. The patch size is derived from a thorough consideration of the ability to use global semantic information and the affordability of CNN and GPU. Its coordinates (x, y) in the ROI are taken out separately as the training label for the second detection part. Then we do data augmentation, as shown in Fig. 2.d, and we resize it to the 256 × 256 pixels that CNN and the GPU can handle. This means we will have 99000(300 × 330) images to train one model for landmark i ($i = 1, 2,...$ 17). The model we use at this stage is ResNet50 [16], in which the Pyramid Split Attention (PSA) [17] is added. The overall training process is shown in Fig. 4. ROI is extracted from 17 landmarks in the training data respectively, and then a CNN is trained for these 17 landmarks respectively. Finally, the X and Y coordinate information output by each model is combined to get the final result.

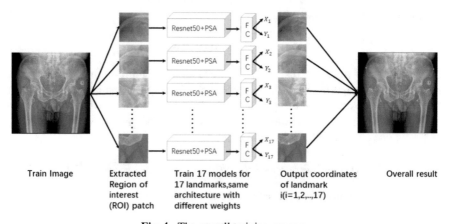

| Train Image | Extracted Region of interest (ROI) patch | Train 17 models for 17 landmarks,same architecture with different weights | Output coordinates of landmark i(i=1,2,..,17) | Overall result |

Fig. 4. The overall training process

3 Experiments

3.1 Datasets

Our data set collected pelvic X-rays from 430 patients. These patients span a wide age range, from 10 to 70 years old. All the X-rays were obtained in TIFF format, with resolutions ranging from 1670 × 2010 pixels to 3200 × 3200 pixels and a pixel spacing of 0.139 mm. We divided the data into a training set (330 images) and a test set (100 images). Each picture is marked by an experienced tagger as our landmark.

3.2 Evaluation Indices

In this paper, the detection performance is evaluated by the following indicators: according to the 2015 ISBI challenges on cephalometric landmark detection, we use the mean radial error (MRE) to make an evaluation. The mean radial error (MRE) is defined in Eq. (8):

$$MRE = \frac{\sum_{i=1}^{n} \sqrt{\Delta x^2 + \Delta y^2}_i}{n} \tag{8}$$

Δx and Δy are the absolute differences between the estimated and ground-truth coordinates of the x- and y-axes.

Because the predicted results have some differences from the ground truth. If the difference is within a certain range, we consider it correct within that range. In our experiment, we evaluate the range of z mm (where z = 4, 4.5, 5, and 6). For example, if the radial error is 3.5 mm, we consider it a 4 mm success. Equation (9) explains the meaning of successful detection rate (SDR):

$$SDR = \frac{N_a}{N} \times 100\% \tag{9}$$

where N_a indicates the number of accurate detections, and N indicates the total number of detections.

4 Result and Discussion

Our method can accurately detect the landmarks of the pelvis. The SDR, MRE, and STD at each landmark as shown in Table 1 on 100 images. With an accuracy of 71.294% (less than 4 mm), 74.176% (less than 4.5 mm), 76.529% (less than 5 mm), and 81.353% (less than 6 mm), there is a 4.159 mm MRE accuracy. Obviously, our method can accurately detect pelvic landmarks within the medically acceptable range.

However, the accuracy of several landmarks, such as points 1 and 2, is low. By analyzing the anatomical structure of the pelvis, we think that the reason for the low detection accuracy of these landmarks is that their positions are close to or even overlap with bones and soft tissues or internal organs, which leads to blurred X-ray images. At the same time, some places have bone spurs and osteoporosis.

In order to verify the accuracy improvement brought by the integration of the prior knowledge of ASM into the weights of the deep neural network, we compared the SDR with the STD for input data without an active shape pattern prior and for input data with an ASM prior. When the data is analyzed with ASM prior, the results are shown in Table 2. We can know that it is an effective way to integrate ASM into the weights of a deep neural network. We also compare the detection results of the current more popular U-net and CE-net, and the experimental results show that the method proposed in this article is efficient.

Even if our pelvic detection framework can improve detection accuracy and the integration of ASM prior knowledge can also improve accuracy, our method still has some defects. For example, while integrating the prior knowledge of ASM, it also inherits the errors of ASM steps, which means that there will be an error accumulation in the training process. At the same time, it is unavoidable that the amount of data is small and the labeling error is large. Because of the large pixel size of the pelvic X-ray data, even the trained annotator will have an error close to 3mm in the labeling process. However, we determine that the first error range for successful detection is 4mm, which means that it will have a great impact on our detection. It is worth noting that even if we train a model for each landmark, it is inevitable that when the ROI contains two or more landmarks in close proximity at the same time, it may have an impact on the detection results. However, because each feature point is at a different location, the local semantic information will be different. According to the distribution of 17 landmarks, only a small portion of this phenomenon will occur during the data enhancement, so the impact on the overall detection results is not great.

Table 1. Detection accuracy on 17 landmarks of the test

Test: 100 images

Anatomical Landmarks	SDR (Successful Detection Rate)				MRE mm	STD mm
	4 mm	4.5 mm	5 mm	6 mm		
1	51	53	55	60	6.595	6.366
2	34	36	41	52	7.861	6.960
3	93	95	95	95	2.242	4.802
4	88	88	89	89	3.577	6.393
5	76	79	81	83	4.982	8.439
6	75	77	78	81	4.124	4.659
7	72	74	75	79	3.752	4.449
8	63	67	71	74	5.137	5.685
9	49	57	63	76	5.248	5.654
10	81	82	86	91	2.809	2.713
11	55	61	64	74	4.194	2.942
12	93	93	95	97	1.937	2.516
13	89	91	91	92	3.025	4.939
14	87	89	90	91	2.987	4.724
15	67	71	75	83	3.892	3.728
16	70	75	78	86	3.914	4.923
17	69	73	74	80	4.432	5.365
Average:	*71.294*	*74.176*	*76.529*	*81.353*	*4.159*	*5.015*

Table 2. Accuracy of different methods

Ways	MRE (mm)	STD (mm)
CE-net	6.528	16.006
U-net	5.963	12.311
Resnet50 + PSA	5.166	6.289
Resnet50 + PSA + ASM	**4.159**	**5.015**

5 Conclusion

In this paper, a pelvic landmark detection framework is proposed that integrates ASM prior knowledge into the weight of a deep neural network. During model training, the rough landmark position and skeleton mask are obtained by ASM. This part of the a priori information is learned as a weight by the CNN in the form of partial ROI during the data augmentation. So that the prior information of ASM can fully benefit the detection accuracy of the model. With an accuracy of 71.294% (less than 4 mm), 74.176% (less than 4.5 mm), 76.529% (less than 5 mm), and 81.353% (less than 6 mm), there is a 4.159 mm MRE accuracy. The experimental results show that our overall framework has good detection performance, and the integration of ASM prior knowledge can also improve detection performance. In the future, we hope that our strategy can be widely applied to landmark detection in various fields.

Acknowledgments. Thanks to Fangwei Xu and his team numbers from Shandong Hospital of Traditional Chinese Medicine and her team members for providing the pelvis X-ray test data set. Thanks to Haifeng Wei from Shandong Hospital of Traditional Chinese Medicine for providing the pelvis X-ray training data set.

Funding. This work was supported by the Shandong Provincial Natural Science Foundation (Grant No. ZR202103030517) and the National Natural Science Foundation of China (Grant No. U1806202 and 82071148).

References

1. Torosdagli, N., Liberton, D.K., Verma, P., Sincan, M., Lee, J.S., Bagci, U.: Deep geodesic learning for segmentation and anatomical landmarking. IEEE Trans. Med. Imag **38**(4), 919–931 (2019)
2. Al-Bashir, A.K., Al-Abed, M., Abu Sharkh, F.M., Kordeya, M.N., Rousan, F.M.: Algorithm for automatic angles measurement and screening for developmental dysplasia of the hip (DDH). In: Proceedings of 37th Annual International Conference on IEEE Engineering in Medicine and Biology Society (EMBC), August 2015, pp. 6386–6389 (2015)
3. Wu, J., Davuluri, P., Ward, K.R., Cockrell, C., Hobson, R.S., Najarian, K.: Fracture detection in traumatic pelvic CT images. Int. J. Biomed. Imaging (2012)
4. Sahin, S., Akata, E., Sahin, O., Tuncay, C., Özkan, H.: A novel computer-based method for measuring the acetabular angle on hip radiographs. Acta Orthop. Traumatol. Turc. **51**(2), 155–159 (2017)

5. Liu, C., Xie, H., Zhang, S., Mao, Z., Sun, J., Zhang, Y.: Misshapen pelvis landmark detection with local-global feature learning for diagnosing developmental dysplasia of the hip. IEEE Trans. Med. Imaging (2020)

6. Agomma, R.O., Vázquez, C., Cresson, T., de Guise, J.A.: Automatic detection of anatomical regions in frontal X-ray images: comparing convolutional neural networks to random forest. In: Proceedings of Medical Imaging, Computer-Aided Diagnosis, Houston, TX, USA, February 2018, Art. no. 105753E (2018). https://doi.org/10.1117/12.2295214

7. Bier, B., et al.: X-ray-transform Invariant Anatomical Landmark Detection for Pelvic Trauma Surgery. In: Frangi, A.F., Schnabel, J.A., Davatzikos, C., AlberolaLópez, C., Fichtinger, G. (eds.) MICCAI 2018. LNCS, vol. 11073, pp. 55–63. Springer, Cham (2018). https://doi.org/10.1007/978-3-030-00937-3_7

8. Liu, F.-Y., et al.: automatic hip detection in anteroposterior pelvic radiographs - a labelless practical framework. J. Personal. Med. (2021)

9. Lindner, C., Wang, C.-W., Huang, C.-T., Li, C.H., Chang, S.-W., Cootes, T.F.: Fully automatic system for accurate localisation and analysis of cephalometric landmarks in lateral cephalograms. Sci. Rep. (2016)

10. Song, Y., Qiao, X., Iwamoto, Y., Chen, Y.-W.: Automatic cephalometric landmark detection on x-ray images using a deep-learning method. Appl. Sci. (2020)

11. Cootes, T.F., Taylor, C.J., Cooper, D.H., Graham, J.: Active shape models—their training and application. Comput. Vision Image Underst. (1995)

12. Pfister, T., Charles, J., Zisserman, A.: Flowing convnets for human pose estimation in videos. In: Proceedings of the IEEE International Conference on Computer Vision (ICCV), Santiago, Chile, 13–16 December 2015

13. Payer, C., Štern, D., Bischof, H., Urschler, M.: Regressing heatmaps for multiple landmark localization using CNNs. In: Ourselin, S., Joskowicz, L., Sabuncu, M.R., Unal, G., Wells, W. (eds.) MICCAI 2016. LNCS, vol. 9901, pp. 230–238. Springer, Cham (2016). https://doi.org/10.1007/978-3-319-46723-8_27

14. Davison, A.K., Lindner, C., Perry, D.C., Luo, W., Cootes, T.F.: Landmark localisation in radiographs using weighted heatmap displacement voting. In: Proceedings of the International Workshop on Computational Methods and Clinical Applications in Musculoskeletal Imaging (MSKI), Granada, Spain, 16 September 2018, pp. 73–85 (2018)

15. Tompson, J.J., Jain, A., LeCun, Y., Bregler, C.: Joint training of a convolutional network and a graphical model for human pose estimation. In: Proceedings of the Advances in Neural Information Processing (2014)

16. He, K., Zhang, X., Ren, S., Sun, J.: Deep residual learning for image recognition. arXiv: Comput. Vision Pattern Recogn. (2015)

17. Zhang, H., Zu, K., Lu, J., Zou, Y., Meng, D.: EPSANet: an efficient pyramid split attention block on convolutional neural network. arXiv: Comput. Vision Pattern Recogn. (2021)

Deep Learning System for Automatic Diagnosis of Ocular Diseases in Infants

Baochen Fu[1], Fabao Xu[2], Wei Chen[3], Chunyu Kao[4], Jianqiao Li[2(✉)], and Xu Qiao[1(✉)]

[1] Department of Biomedical Engineering, School of Control Science and Engineering, Shandong University, Jinan 250061, Shandong, China
qiaoxu@sdu.edu.cn
[2] Department of Ophthalmology, Qilu Hospital, Cheeloo College of Medicine, Shandong University, Jinan 250012, Shandong, China
[3] Department of Radiology, Shandong First Medical University and Shandong Academy of Medical Sciences, Taian 271000, Shandong, China
[4] Department of Statistics, Zhongtai Securities Institute for Financial Studies, Shandong University, Jinan 250100, Shandong, China

Abstract. Ocular disorders are common in infants. Eyesight vision damage may become permanent if an early diagnosis is not given. Therefore, early detection of ocular abnormalities can effectively improve vision health in infants. Here, we present a deep learning model to automatically diagnose eye diseases to address the lack of medical resources and availability of pediatric ophthalmologist professionals. To effectively detect ocular disorder, we propose using the ResNet50 feature extraction network containing a channel attention module. Additionally, we localize pathological structure employing the Gradient-Weighted activation maps (Grad-CAM) to visual the feature maps. The proposed CNNs framework aids in clinical diagnosis and achieves an F1-score of 0.987 and an area under the receiver operating characteristic (AUC curve) of 0.9998.

Keywords: deep Learning · retinal fundus images · artificial intelligence

1 Introduction

In infants, the visual nervous system expands rapidly. Vision can be permanently affected during this time by retinopathy of prematurity (ROP), retinoblastoma (RB), persistent fetal vascular disease (PFV) and other ocular diseases. Every year, ROP is believed to be the cause of blindness or severe visual problems in 30,000 premature infants globally [1]. Most ROP cases are mild and just go away on their own without needing any kind of treatment. However, a more severe stage may develop in 5–10% of ROP patients. This may result in retinal detachment or distortion and eventual irreversible blindness due to lack of treatment [2]. Newborns are generally unable to express their visual deficit because they are physically and cognitive immature and have limited visual experience. Misdiagnosis is common mainly due to the lack of pediatric ophthalmologists and the subjectivity of manual diagnosis. Therefore, it is essential to develop automated diagnostic tools to reduce visual impairment in infants.

© The Author(s), under exclusive license to Springer Nature Singapore Pte Ltd. 2023
Y.-W. Chen et al. (Eds.): KES InMed 2023, SIST 357, pp. 305–314, 2023.
https://doi.org/10.1007/978-981-99-3311-2_27

With the advancement of computer technology, artificial intelligence (AI) is now widely used in the medical sector [3]. An essential technique for building AI is machine learning (ML). ML extracts patterns from large amount of data samples and automatically learns the parameters required for algorithms [4]. ML has advanced due to the advancement of deep learning (DL), which is an essential subfield of machine learning. DL frameworks can handle input data without the need for manual feature engineering with a projection of high-dimensional data onto a lower-dimensional feature space [5]. Recently, Convolutional Neural Networks (CNNs), a commonly used DL method for image classification, has been employed in medical fields to automatic recognition of various diseases, including several eyes related disorders such diabetic retinopathy, glaucoma, and cataract [6]. Automated analysis and diagnosis of fundus images using CNN to build an intelligent diagnostic model for fundus diseases in infants can help in reducing the workload of doctors and improving the prognosis of infants and resource availability. Recently, some studies have been presented for this task. Li et al. [7] proposed a multi-label classification model for fundus diseases based on binocular fundus images, BFPC-Net, which takes binocular fundus images as input and adds an attention mechanism to classify diseases in a global and multi-label manner. Classification, achieved an accuracy rate of 94.23%. Mateen et al. [8] combined Gaussian Mixture Model (GMM), Visual Geometric Group Network (VGGNet), Singular Value Decomposition (SVD) and Principal Component Analysis (PCA) and softmax for region segmentation, high-dimensional feature extraction, feature selection and fundus image classification, respectively. Utilization of PCA and SVD feature selection with fully connected (FC) layers demonstrated the classification accuracies of 92.21%, 98.34%, 97.96%, and 98.13% for FC7-PCA, FC7-SVD, FC8-PCA, and FC8-SVD, respectively. Alyoubi et al. [9] developed a computer-aided screening system (CASS) based on two deep learning models. The first model (CNN512) uses the entire image as input to a CNN model that classifies it into one of five DR stages. The second model uses the YOLOv3 model for the detection and localization of DR lesions. Finally, the two proposed structures CNN512 and YOLOv3 are fused together to classify DR images and localize DR lesions, obtaining 89% accuracy, 89% sensitivity, and 97.3 specificity. Brown et al. [10] proposed the ROP-DL system to collect and extract retinal blood vessels classifying the segmented blood vessel maps as Plus, pre-Plus, or normal. Wang et al. [11] proposed the DeepROP automatic diagnosis system and developed two models for disease identification and severity grading. Convolutional neural networks were utilized by Durai et al. [12] to segment retinal tumor cells and classify tumors according to their malignancy. Zhang et al. [13] developed a DLA-RB using ResNet50 feature extraction network to automatically monitor the contralateral eye of a retinoblastoma patient and the offspring of a retinoblastoma survivor.

In this study, we present a deep learning algorithm to classify fundus images into four categories. We address the problems of data imbalance and enhance model performance and visualize output features to investigate and localize pathological structure.

2 Materials and Methods

2.1 Dataset

The study was approved by the Ethical Committee of Qilu Hospital in Jinan, Shandong Province, China (No. 2019095) and individual consent for this retrospective analysis was waived. In this study, a dataset of 3101 retinal fundus images from the ophthalmology center of Qilu Hospital is used. These fundus can be categorized into 4 groups, i. e., ROP, RB, PFV and Other. The 'Other' group includes Coats disease, pulse insufficiency, morning glory syndrome, post-vitrectomy, retinal detachment, fundus squeeze bleeding, and acupressure syndrome. Table 1 gives the number of samples for each group.

Table 1. Class distribution in dataset.

Category	Name	Number
0	ROP	2114
1	RB	533
2	PFV	286
3	Other	168

2.2 Image Preprocessing

Preprocessing is required for images in order to improve features, reduce noise, and ensure consistency. In the first step, we carefully review the images to look for any abnormality, such as overexposed, too dark, or too blurry. In the second step, we resize the spatial of the image to 224×224 to reduce the computational cost of the deep network.

2.3 Dataset Splitting

We split data into 80% training and 20% test samples for the experiments. Table 2 displays the number of samples for each category.

2.4 Evaluation Metrics

The performance of the model is evaluated by using four different metrics.

$$Recall = TP/(TP + FN) \tag{1}$$

$$Precision = TP/(TP + FP) \tag{2}$$

$$F1 - Score = (2 * Precision * Recall)/(Precision + Recall) \tag{3}$$

Table 2. The number of training and test set samples.

Category	Name	Training Set	Testing Set
0	ROP	1692	422
1	RB	427	106
2	PFV	229	57
3	Other	135	33

$$Accuracy = (TP + TN)/(TP + TN + FP + FN) \tag{4}$$

TP, FP, TN, and FN represent the number of True Positives, False Positives, True Negatives, and False Negatives, respectively [14]. We determine the evaluation indexes for each category and average the results to determine the final value.

The classification model can be assessed using the area under the curve (AUC) and receiver operating characteristic (ROC) curves. The True Positive rate and False Positive rate are described by the ROC curve. The macro-average AUC value can be calculated using the ROC curve. The model performs better in classification when the AUC is larger.

2.5 Network Architecture

Convolutional neural networks (CNN) have shown excellent performance in the field of computer vision. The ResNet50 model, which achieved first place in the 2015 ILSVRC imagenet competition, served as the baseline for this study [15]. Later, a squeeze and excitation (SE) channel attention block is introduced in to improve the efficiency of ResNet50 network. The SE channel module performs feature recalibration technique to enhance the quality of feature representations [16].

The residual learning-based ResNet block, which can efficiently use shallow features to acquire additional crucial feature information, is a key feature extraction network in image classification and recognition applications. Therefore, we use ResNet50 as the baseline network for the feature extraction in this study. Further, the combination of SE module with ResNet50 network enhances the model performance [17]. The network design of SE-ResNet50 model is shown in Fig. 1.

The SE channel attention modules are added to the convolution and identity block to weight the important feature information in the SE-ResNet50 model. The convolution block uses three convolution layers to extract visual features from the input images. To calculate the weight value of each channel, the SE module employs a global average pooling (GAP) operation followed by the fully connected layers (FC) and applies a sigmoid activation to determine the weight value of each channel. Unlike from convolutional blocks, identity blocks add their extracted feature outputs directly to the other features.

2.6 Experimental Setting

In the experiments, the Adam optimizer is used to optimize the network while the cross-entropy loss is employed to error corrections. The 224 x 224 spatial dimension of input image is used. The initial learning is set to the 0.00005 and a cosine annealing process is used with a minimum value of 0.00000005 to change it during training. Early stopping is used to avoid the model from over fitting. The batch size is 64. The entire experiment is built on the PyTorch learning framework and is trained on the Ubuntu 16.04 operating system. The system contains an Intel(R) Xeon(R) Silver 4210 CPU @ 2.20GHz, 256 GB RAM, and an NVIDIA Tesla V100-PCIe 32GB GPU for training and testing.

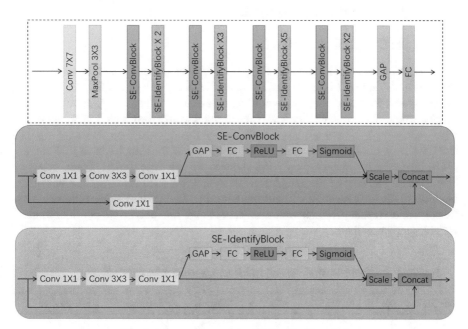

Fig. 1. The structure of the SE-ResNet50 model.

2.7 Dataset Imbalancing

The use of an unbalanced dataset can result in classification errors since the model will be biased toward the dominant class. To mitigate the adverse affects of unbalanced datasets, weight samplers, a preprocessing technique, can be used to balance classes by oversampling the minority class (category with few samples) and under sampling the majority class [18]. We add weights to each sample using the weighted random sampler that PyTorch has officially adopted. The probability of selecting each category of samples is determined by the its weight, the higher the weight of the sample, the greater the probability. Table 3 displays the weights utilized for training. The weight is obtained by calculating the reciprocal of the proportion of the number of samples in each category to the total number of samples.

Table3. Weight of each category.

Category	Name	Weights
0	ROP	1.4675
1	RB	5.8150
2	PFV	10.8428
3	Other	18.3926

3   Results Analysis and Discussion

3.1   Results Using Imbalance Data

The evaluation results for the Se-ResNet50 and ResNet50 models using imbalance data are shown in Table 4 using the test set data. Table 5 displays the Recall, Precision, and F1 scores for each category. According to the results the recall rates for PFV and 'Other' categories are generally low. Due to the unequal distribution of the data, the recall values for ROP and RB is 1.0 while for PFV and 'Other' Recall values are 0.89 and 0.94, respectively. As given in the Table 1, most of the samples have ROP disease (2114 images) while there are only 168 samples are available for the 'Other' category. Due to the imbalance of the categories, the model is biased towards class which has majority of data samples (ROP), and the minority class ("Other") has relatively poor categorization results. To improve the disease recognition ability, we consider to use a weight sampler method.

Table 4. Model classification results using imbalance data.

Model	AUC	ACC	Recall	Precision	F1-Score
Se-ResNet 50	0.9992	0.984	0.956	0.977	0.966
ResNet 50	0.9984	0.976	0.941	0.963	0.951

Table 5. Se-ResNet50 classification results of each category using imbalance data.

Category	Recall	Precision	F1-Score
0	1.00	0.99	0.99
1	1.00	0.99	1.00
2	0.89	0.96	0.93
3	0.94	0.97	0.95

3.2 Result Using Data Balanced Technique

Table 6 shows the overall classification results of the model using the Recall, Precision and F1-scores metrics for each category with the Weight Sampler technique. Table 7 gives the results for each category. Se-ResNet50 shows a improvement in performance. The Recall, Precision, and F1-Score are increased from 0.956 to 0.984, 0.977 to 0.989, and 0.966 to 0.987, while AUC increased from 0.9992 to 0.9998. The Recall of PFV is increased from 0.89 to 0.95 and the Recall of Other category has been increased from 0.94 to 1.0, indicating an improvement in model capability for categories with few samples.

Table 6. Model classification results using data balance technique.

Model	AUC	ACC	Recall	Precision	F1-Score
Se-Resnet 50	0.9998	0.992	0.984	0.989	0.987
Resnet 50	0.9997	0.990	0.971	0.984	0.977

Table 7. Se-ResNet50 classification results of each category using data balance technique.

Category	Recall	Precision	F1-Score
0	1.00	0.99	1.00
1	0.99	1.00	1.00
2	0.95	0.96	0.96
3	1.00	1.00	1.00

Confusion Matrix. We calculated confusion matrix using SE-Resnet50 model using data balanced technique. Each row of the matrix represents a specific occurrence of a predicted value, while the column displays the ground truth value [19], as shown in Fig. 2. The confusion matrix illustrates a quick analysis of each category's misclassification. The numbers along the main diagonal indicate the proportion of correctly predicted events in each category. The confusion matrix indicates that the model we train has a good accuracy as it has just one image prediction error for ROP and RB categories, three error cases for PFV, but none for 'Other'.

Class Activation Map. In addition to analyzing quantitative performance of model, we also investigate which model components are more important to the results. We produced class activation maps (CAM) to demonstrate the contribution of different regions to the final classification prediction [20]. This is useful in enhancing our understanding of the factors that lead to the model's outcome. Figure 3 shows the essential elements of each category's images. The network identifies the most significant lesion area, demonstrating the efficacy of our proposed methodology.

Wang et al. [11] utilized Id-Net and Gr-Net were utilized to identify ROP and assess its severity. They developed an Id-Net that had a sensitivity and specificity of 84.9%

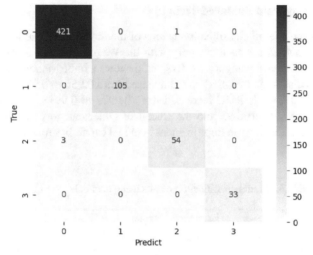

Fig. 2. Confusion matrix calculated based on SE-ResNet50 after using weight sampler.

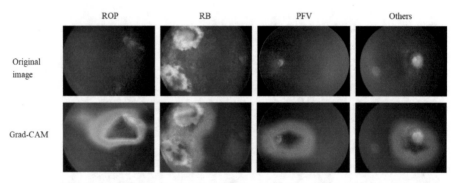

Fig. 3. Grad-CAM visualization of images with four different diseases.

and 96.9% for identifying ROP. The I-ROP computer system, designed by J. Peter Campbell et al.[21] to diagnose diseases based on the features of arteries and veins, has a 95% accuracy rate. Zhang et al. [13] developed DLA-RB model and validated using 36623 pictures of 713 patients, and it achieved an AUC of 0.9982. Our proposed model outperforms previous methods with an AUC of 0.9998 and an accuracy of 99.2%. We select a smaller data set and our model can recognize a wider variety of disorders. Several diseases can be identified in the images of the same patient in practical applications, enhancing screening capabilities.

This study still has some limitations: (1) The number of images in our dataset is limited, which may affect the performance of the model; (2) The fundus images in our study are collected from a single center and from single ethnicity, which may have the less data diversity affecting the generalization ability of algorithms; In the future, we will collect larger data sets and formulate new methods verifying the performance.

4 Conclusions

We present a four-class classification system based on Se-Resnet50 to detect retinal diseases in infants. The proposed methodology performs well with fewer or more illness types and is very simple, reliable, and efficient even with a small data set. It may help physicians to see the intermediate process and provide them with additional tools for making decisions. Using this method for the initial screening of eye issues in infants and newborn children can reduce the risk of vision loss or possibly blindness.

References

1. Blencowe, H., Lawn, J.E., Vazquez, T., Fielder, A., Gilbert, C.: Preterm-associated visual impairment and estimates of retinopathy of prematurity at regional and global levels for 2010. Pediatr Res. **74**(Suppl 1), 35–49 (2013)
2. Tong, Y., Lu, W., Deng, Q., et al.: Automated identification of retinopathy of prematurity by image-based deep learning. Eye Vis. **7**(1), 1–12 (2020)
3. He, J., Baxter, S.L., Xu, J., et al.: The practical implementation of artificial intelligence technologies in medicine. Nat. Med. **25**(1), 30–36 (2019)
4. Ting, D.S.W., Pasquale, L.R., Peng, L., et al.: Artificial intelligence and deep learning in ophthalmology. Br. J. Ophthalmol. **103**(2), 167–175 (2019)
5. Ongsulee, P.: Artificial intelligence, machine learning and deep learning. In: 2017 15th International Conference on ICT and Knowledge Engineering (ICT&KE), pp. 1–6. IEEE (2017)
6. Ting, D.S.W., et al.: Deep learning in ophthalmology: the technical and clinical considerations.Prog Retin Eye Res. 72, 100759 (2019)
7. Li, Z., Xu, M., Yang, X., Han, Y.: Multi-Label fundus image classification using attention mechanisms and feature fusion. Micromachines (Basel). **13**(6), 947 (2022). https://doi.org/10.3390/mi13060947.PMID:35744561;PMCID:PMC9230753
8. Mateen, M., Wen, J., Nasrullah, Song, S., Huang, Z.: Fundus image classification using VGG-19 architecture with PCA and SVD. Symmetry 11, 1 (2019). https://doi.org/10.3390/sym110 10001
9. Alyoubi, W.L., Abulkhair, M.F., Shalash, W.M.: Diabetic retinopathy fundus image classification and lesions localization system using deep learning. Sensors **21**, 3704 (2021). https://doi.org/10.3390/s21113704
10. Brown, J.M., Campbell, J.P., Beers, A., et al.: Automated diagnosis of plus disease in retinopathy of prematurity using deep convolutional neural networks. JAMA Ophthalmol. **136**(7), 803–810 (2018)
11. Wang, J., Ju, R., Chen, Y., et al.: Automated retinopathy of prematurity screening using deep neural networks. EBioMedicine **35**, 361–368 (2018)
12. Durai, C., Jebaseeli, T.J., Alelyani, S., et al.: Early prediction and diagnosis of retinoblastoma using deep learning techniques. arXiv preprint arXiv:2103.07622 (2021)
13. Zhang, R., Dong, L., Li, R., et al.: Automatic retinoblastoma screening and surveillance using deep learning. medRxiv (2022)
14. Li, X., Xia, C., Li, X., et al.: Identifying diabetes from conjunctival images using a novel hierarchical multi-task network. Sci. Rep. **12**(1), 1–9 (2022)
15. He K, Zhang X, Ren S, et al. Deep residual learning for image recognition[C]//Proceedings of the IEEE conference on computer vision and pattern recognition. 2016: 770–778
16. Hu, J., Shen, L., Sun, G.: Squeeze-and-excitation networks. In: Proceedings of the IEEE Conference on Computer Vision and Pattern Recognition, pp. 7132–7141 (2018)

17. Zhao, X., Li, K., Li, Y., et al.: Identification method of vegetable diseases based on transfer learning and attention mechanism. Comput. Electron. Agric. **193**, 106703 (2022)
18. Bonela, A.A., He, Z., Norman, T., et al.: Development and validation of the alcoholic beverage identification deep learning algorithm version 2 for quantifying alcohol exposure in electronic images. Alcoholism: Clin. Experimental Res. **46**(10), 1837–1845 (2022)
19. Yin, C., Zhu, Y., Fei, J., et al.: A deep learning approach for intrusion detection using recurrent neural networks. IEEE Access **5**, 21954–21961 (2017)
20. Selvaraju, R.R., Cogswell, M., Das, A., et al.: Grad-CAM: visual explanations from deep networks via gradient-based localization. In: Proceedings of the IEEE International Conference on Computer Vision, pp. 618–626 (2017)
21. Ataer-Cansizoglu, E., Bolon-Canedo, V., Campbell, J.P., et al.: Computer-based image analysis for plus disease diagnosis in retinopathy of prematurity: performance of the "i-ROP" system and image features associated with expert diagnosis. Transl. Vis. Sci. Technol. **4**(6), 5 (2015)

Predicting Stroke-Associated Pneumonia from Intracerebral Hemorrhage Based on Deep Learning Methods

Guangtong Yang[1(✉)], Min Xu[2], Lulu Gai[1], Wei Chen[3], Jin Ma[4], Xu Qiao[1], Hongfeng Shi[2], and Yongmei Hu[1]

[1] School of Control Science and Engineering, Shandong University, 250061 Jinan, China
`guangtongyang@mail.sdu.edu.cn, qiaoxu@sdu.edu.cn`
[2] Neurointensive Care Unit, Shengli Oilfield Central Hospital, Dongying, Shandong 257034, China
[3] Department of Radiology, Shandong First Medical University and Shandong Academy of Medical Sciences, 271000 Taian, China
[4] School of Economics, Shandong Normal University, 250358 Jinan, China

Abstract. Stroke-associated pneumonia (SAP) is a very common complication in patients with intracerebral hemorrhage (ICH), which makes the nursing challenging and increases the patients risk of poor health. Most previously proposed SAP recognition methods are based on clinical data, which sometimes are time-consuming for collecting. In this paper, deep learning models using 3D-CNNs and 3D-ViTs networks were used in order to diagnose SAP rapidly. In addition, we performed image registration to integrate the spatial information to enhance the model. We have collected brain CT images of 244 patients to use in the SAP recognition studies, the experimental results demonstrate our deep learning models outperformed the previous methods achieving an AUC value of 0.8. And image registration also plays a key role in improving performance.

Keywords: Intracerebral hemorrhage · Pneumonia classification · Deep learning

1 Introduction

Patients who have intracerebral hemorrhage (ICH) frequently develop stroke-associated pneumonia (SAP), which extends the length of hospital stay and makes nursing more challenging [1]. In addition, pneumonia has been found to increase the risk of several non-pneumonia-related medical complications, such as deep vein thrombosis, gastrointestinal bleeding, and atrial fibrillation [2].

Earlier studies use clinical data from patients for SAP prediction and risk grading [3]. Based on the multivariable logistic regression method, Ruijun Ji et al. [4] developed the ICH-APS model, which was divided into the ICH-APS-A model without hematoma and the ICH-APS-B model with hematoma volume.

G. Yang and M. Xu—contributed equally.

The area under the receiver operating characteristic curve (AUC) was used as the evaluation index. The insignificant variables in the model were removed using a stepwise backward estimation method by building a model from demographic data, stroke risk factors, and past medical history, and finally, a scoring system for SAP was obtained achieving better experimental results (AUC = 0.76). In addition, Jing Yang et al. [5] took fasting blood glucose and c-reactive protein into consideration, constructing the ICH-LR2S2 model based on logical regression, and obtained good performance (AUC = 0.75). However, as collecting the clinical data from patients is time-consuming and complicated, novel strategies are required to predict SAP.

Nowadays, deep learning-based method has become the most advanced technology. Convolutional neural networks (CNNs) provide advancements for computer vision [6], CNNs has been widely used in medical imaging for various task including registration, diagnosis and prognosis [7]. In addition, the Vision Transformer (ViT) [8] has demonstrated excellent potential in image classification, and has been proved to be superior to CNNs for the ImageNet classification task [8], which is a famous benchmark image classification dataset. Gai et al. [9] effectively implemented 3D-ViTs to medical images using the idea of transfer learning, achieving better results in comparison to 3D-CNNs. As a result, we present SAP predicting frameworks based on deep learning, including Efficient-Net [12] of 3D-CNNs and DeiT_S [16] of 3D-ViTs.

In this study, we present an end-to-end pipeline for predicting SAP in ICH patients. Our proposed models only require CT scans as input and could rapidly generate classified results. This is potentially useful for saving doctors' time and effort on collecting clinical data. Due to the clear presentation of the brain structure by MRI, we also utilized a registration method to match CT and MRI, so that the model can learn the spatial characteristics of ICH, which further improved the classification accuracy.

2   Materials and Methods

2.1   Patients

Our dataset consists of 244 brain CT images from the neurointensive care unit of Shengli Oilfield Central hospital. We classified the severity of pneumonia to mild, moderate and severe based on the corresponding chest CT scans [10]. All chest CT images were independently reviewed by two radiologists with over 10 years of experience who were blinded to clinical and laboratory findings. There are 19 cases of severe pneumonia, 47 cases of moderate pneumonia, 77 cases of mild pneumonia, and 101 cases of non-pneumonia. In summary, there are 143 SAP patients in our dataset, accounting for 58.6% of the total samples. There are 66 cases of moderate or above, accounting for 27% of the total samples.

The CT images are used for further research after obtaining informed consent from the local Ethics Committee. No is Q/ZXYY–ZY–YWB–LL202243.

2.2   MRI Atlas for Registration

We use normal human brain MRI images as reference image for registration, which from the OASIS project [11], these images clearly present the brain structures, as shown in Fig. 1.

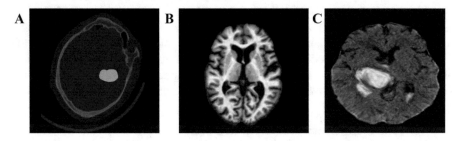

Fig. 1. Example images of the dataset used for this paper. (A) Brain CT and its ICH region is highlighted. (B) Brain MRI utilized as reference for registration. (C) The brain CT scan after registration.

2.3   Predicting SAP Based on Deep Learning Network

Our deep learning-based methods can be divided into two ways to conduct prediction, the EfficientNet model representing 3D-CNNs and the DeiT-S model representing 3D-ViTs. The CTs are provided as input to the models after performing some specific preprocessing, including transformations such as random values of horizontal and vertical flip, blur, anisotropic and affine. In addition, according to the doctor's recommendation, we conduct experiments on the prediction of SAP above mild level, because it is considered to be treated with endotracheal intubation.

3D-CNNs. The CTs are provided to the network after preprocessing. EfficientNet_B0 includes 9 stages, stage 1 contains $Conv3 \times 3$, stage from 2 to 8 are $MBConv$ layers with different kernel size, and stage 9 includes full connection layer. EfficientNet uses Neural Architecture Search (NAS) technology to search the reasonable configuration of three parameters, namely, the resolution of image input, the depth of the network, and the width of the channel [12]. The target of EfficientNet is to maximize the accuracy under the given resource limitations, which can be formulated as an optimization problem:

$$\max_{d,w,r} ACCURACY\left(N\left(D,W,R\right)\right)$$
$$s.t. N\left(d,w,r\right) = \odot_{i=1...s} F_l^{d \cdot L_i}\left(X_{\left(r \cdot H_i, r \cdot W_i, w \cdot C_i\right)}\right)$$
$$Memmory\left(N\right) \leq target_memmory$$
$$FLOPS\left(N\right) \leq target\_flops$$

(1)

where w, d, r are coefficients for scaling network width, depth, and resolution; F_i, L_i, H_i, W_i, C_i are predefined parameters in baseline network. We resized the CTs to $224 \times 224 \times 16$.

3D-ViTs. Figure 2 shows the structure of ViTs, which mainly includes Linear Projection, Transformer Encoder, and MLP Head. Linear Projection is responsible for mapping the input patches to tokens and add positional embedding. Transformer Encoder is based on the self-attention mechanism, Multi-Head Attention is mined for features after the input vector is normalized. The MLP Head is mainly responsible for the output of classification results. GAI et al. [9] have proved that it is feasible to apply ViTs to 3D medical images. Inspired by this, using ViTs on our dataset may obtain a better performance than 3D-CNNs. For ViTs, 3D medical images should to be divided into patches in size of $16 \times 16 \times 16$, and every patch should embed the spatial information into tokens. In the experiment, we used transfer learning with pre-trained weights.

2.4 Registration Between CT and MRI

Due to the differences between CT scans and the MRI atlas, preprocessing operations were required: skull-stripped and resizing CTs to the same size of MRI atlas. As the skull is not present in the MRI image, removing it enhances the accuracy of registration. It is possible to remove the skull and its external tissues from CTs by using thresholding and treating the internal tissues as regions of maximum connectivity as the skull has substantially higher Hu values than other body parts. Then resize the size of CTs to $x = 160$, $y = 192$, and $z = 224$.

We transform the image by applying rigid and non-rigid registration [13]. We use rigid transformation to translate and rotate the original image without changing its size and internal curve as the moving images and fixed images have different origins and orientations. Then we apply non-rigid transformation using 'bspline' method to exactly match CTs to the MRI atlas. In the process, the CTs is the moving image $I_m (v)$ and the MRI atlas is the fixed image $I_f (v)$,

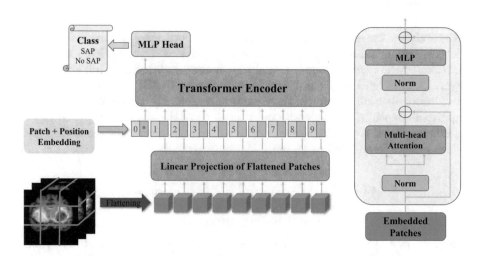

Fig. 2. Overview of the proposed 3D-ViTs for predicting SAP.

where v is voxels of image; the moving image iterated continuously in order to find a most suitable transform $T(v)$, aiming to minimize the mutual information between two images.

$$\min_{x=3} MI\left(T\left(I_m(v), I_f(v)\right)\right) \tag{2}$$

where, $x = 3$ means image is 3D type. We used a multi-resolution strategy to create a resolution pyramid. To find the optimum outcome, a maximum number of iterations for each layer is performed.

$$T = T_{rigid} + T_{nonreigid} \tag{3}$$

We use mutual information (MI) as our evaluation metric for each iteration. MI is a measure of the amount of information that a random variable (image intensity in one image) tells another random variable (image brightness of another image) [14]. Therefore, it is very suitable for multimodal image pairs and single-mode images. The moving image with the highest processor score is obtained as our output image.

3 Results

Table 1 shows the results of SAP prediction. Evaluation indexes include AUC, accuracy, sensitivity, and precision score. Sensitivity, also called recall, represents the proportion of all positive cases that are predicted as positive. It should be noted that we only report experimental results of ICH-APS-A [4] and ICH-LI2S2 [5] model as we are unabled to obtain all the clinical data used by these. Moreover, their experiments lack the ability to predict SAP above mild level, hence we do not show the values in Table 2. And two tables also include the results using our previously proposed radiomics model. The ViT-based Deit_S model achieves the best model performance in predicting the occurrence of SAP (AUC = 0.8), and is further improved after registration achieving an AUC value of 0.85. The registration process also enhances CNNs-based frameworks' performance in terms of accuracy, sensitivity, and precision.

Table 1. Experiment results for predicting SAP.

Method	Model	AUC	Accuracy	Sensitivity	Precision
ICH-APS-A	Logistic regression	0.76	-	-	-
ICH-LR2S2	Logistic regression	0.75	-	-	-
Radiomics	Logistic regression	0.74	0.75	**0.79**	0.65
3D-CNNs	EfficientNet_B0	0.76	0.69	0.68	0.68
	EfficientNet_B0+Registration	**0.85**	**0.74**	0.68	**0.79**
3D-ViTs	Deit_S	0.8	0.69	0.64	0.73
	Deit_S+Registration	0.85	0.74	0.76	0.76

Table 2 shows the results for predicting SAP above mild level. All evaluation for EfficientNet increase if the registered images are used as model input (AUC = 0.83), while three of evaluation for DeiT have improved (AUC = 0.82), in exception for accuracy.

Table 2. Experiment results for predicting SAP above mild level.

Method	Model	AUC	Accuracy	Sensitivity	Precision
Radiomics	Logistic regression	0.77	0.72	0.54	**0.88**
3D-CNNs	EfficientNet_B0	0.77	0.56	0.62	0.74
	EfficientNet_B0+Registration	**0.83**	**0.76**	0.75	0.75
3D-ViTs	Deit_S	0.8	0.74	0.64	0.73
	Deit_S+Registration	0.82	0.67	**0.76**	0.76

4   Discussion

Our work demonstrates that the use of imaging data for SAP prediction is an effective approach that outperforms previous studies based on clinical data in terms of availability and model performance.

The experimental results on the test set demonstrate that after data registration processing, the performance of both CNNs-based and ViTs-based models is enhanced. This section discusses why the registration method improves model performance even when using a simple network. Our original data are brain CT scans. After being admitted to the hospital, patients with ICH usually undergo a CT imaging test, which allows medical professionals to quickly determine the size, shape and scope of hematoma and the compression of surrounding brain tissues. In CT scan, hematoma, cerebrospinal fluid and brain parenchyma can be easily recognized because of their different Hu values, but more complex brain structure cannot be easily recognized [15]. After having cerebral hemorrhage, the degree of pulmonary infection may be affected directly or indirectly depending on the location of the hemorrhage and the affected brain regions. For example, if the hematoma affects the basal ganglia, the patient may have difficulty swallowing or consciousness, which is a risk factor for SAP. Although brain MRI images can reveal specific brain anatomical regions, it is not often used to diagnose ICH due to its high clinical cost. Therefore, we proposed registering CTs to the brain MRI template to take advantage of both CT and MRI to increase the accuracy of the network. ViTs can visualize the salience diagram of the self-attention mechanism, which we can use to determine the key attention of our ViTs both before and after registration. The attention maps for the final Deit_S module are visualized in Fig. 3, with brighter areas denoting higher response output of the model. Before registration, the model learns the outline of the edge of the brain, but there is no obvious difference inside of the brain except the bleeding area,

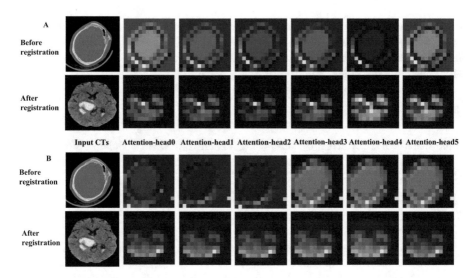

Fig. 3. Attention maps generated using the final module of Deit-S. (A) Predicting SAP. (B) Predicting SAP above mild level.

indicating that the model could not learn the details of brain structure. After the registration precedure, the multiple attention regions with different colors are displayed in the brain image (Fig. 3), demonstrating how the model not only learns the characteristics of cerebrospinal fluid, brain parenchyma, hematoma, left and right brain, and other regions, but also enhance them with different attention, which improves the effectivenss of the model for classification task. The proportion of the brain in the whole image also increases after the registration procedure. The model acceptance domain expanded along with the increase in key information area, and now features can be learned more in-depth. The improvement in model performance could possibly from the increased contrast between the hematoma and the brain tissue after the skull is removed.

The study has the following limitations: it is a retrospective study using samples from a single center. In order to advance our work and finally make it relevant in a clinical context, more data and external validation are required. The segmentation of bleeding areas can be added through the multi-task learning model, which may further improve model performance and automation. In addition, the various types of extracted features are expected to be shared in subsequent work.

5   Conclusion

This paper constructed a risk model based on deep learning methods for feature extraction and prediction of SAP. According to clinical practice, we also presented a prediction for SAP above mild level. In two classification tasks, the experimental results demonstrate that deep learning network-based models outperform other methods. Image registration is applied to the CTs to further improve performance of the model. The SAP prediction model based on deep learning techniques can also achieve end-to-end result output and reduce the time needed for clinical availability.

Funding

This work was supported by Shandong Provincial Natural Science Foundation (Grant No. ZR202103030517) and National Natural Science Foundation of China (Grant No. U1806202 and 82071148).

References

1. Hannawi, Y., Hannawi, B., Rao, C.P.V., et al.: Stroke-associated pneumonia: major advances and obstacles. Cerebrovascular diseases **35**(5), 430–443 (2013)
2. Smith, C.J., Kishore, A.K., Vail, A., et al.: Diagnosis of stroke-associated pneumonia: recommendations from the pneumonia in stroke consensus group. Stroke **46**(8), 2335–2340 (2015)
3. Sui, R., Zhang, L.: Risk factors of stroke-associated pneumonia in Chinese patients. Neurological Res. **33**(5), 508–513 (2011)
4. Ji, R., Shen, H., Pan, Y., et al.: Risk score to predict hospital-acquired pneumonia after spontaneous intracerebral hemorrhage[J]. Stroke **45**(9), 2620–2628 (2014)
5. Yan, J., Zhai, W., Li, Z., et al.: ICH-LR2S2: a new risk score for predicting stroke-associated pneumonia from spontaneous intracerebral hemorrhage. J. Transl. Med. **20**(1), 1–10 (2022)
6. Alzubaidi, L., Zhang, J., Humaidi, A.J., et al.: Review of deep learning: concepts, CNN architectures, challenges, applications, future directions. J. Big Data **8**(1), 1–74 (2021)
7. Kattenborn, T., Leitloff, J., Schiefer, F., et al.: Review on Convolutional Neural Networks (CNN) in vegetation remote sensing. ISPRS J. Photogrammetry Remote Sens. **173**, 24–49 (2021)
8. Dosovitskiy, A., Beyer, L., Kolesnikov, A., et al.: An image is worth 16x16 words: Transformers for image recognition at scale. arXiv preprint arXiv:2010.11929 (2020)
9. Gai, L., Chen, W., Gao, R., et al.: Using vision transformers in 3-D medical image classifications. In: 2022 IEEE International Conference on Image Processing (ICIP), pp. 696–700. IEEE (2022)
10. Zapata-Arriaza, E., Moniche, F., Blanca, P.G., et al.: External validation of the ISAN, A2DS2, and AIS-APS scores for predicting stroke-associated pneumonia. J. Stroke Cerebrovasc Dis. **27**(3), 673–676 (2018)
11. Daniel, S, Marcus, et al.: Open Access Series of Imaging Studies (OASIS): cross-sectional MRI data in young, middle aged, nondemented, and demented older adults. J. Cognitive Neuroscience (2007)
12. Tan, M., Le, Q.: Efficientnet: rethinking model scaling for convolutional neural networks. In: International Conference on Machine Learning, pp. 6105–6114. PMLR (2019)
13. Zitova, B., Flusser, J.: Image registration methods: a survey. Image Vision Comput. **21**(11), 977–1000 (2003)

14. Batina, L., Gierlichs, B., Prouff, E., et al.: Mutual information analysis: a comprehensive study. J. Cryptology **24**(2), 269–291 (2011)
15. Gillebert, C.R., Humphreys, G.W., Mantini, D.: Automated delineation of stroke lesions using brain CT images. NeuroImage Clin. **4**, 540–548 (2014)
16. Touvron, H., Cord, M., Douze, M., et al.: Training data-efficient image transformers & distillation through attention. In: International Conference on Machine Learning, pp. 10347–10357. PMLR (2021)

An Efficient Dual-Pooling Channel Attention Module for Weakly-Supervised Liver Lesion Classification on CT Images

Duong Linh Phung[1], Yinhao Li[1], Rahul Kumar Jain[1], Lanfen Lin[2(✉)],
Hongjie Hu[3(✉)], and Yen-Wei Chen[1(✉)]

[1] College of Information Science and Engineering, Ritsumeikan University, Kyoto, Shiga, Japan
chen@is.ritsumei.ac.jp
[2] College of Computer Science and Technology, Zhejiang University, Hangzhou, China
llf@zju.edu.cn
[3] Department of Radiology Sir Run Run Shaw, Zhejiang University, Hangzhou, China
hongjiehu@zju.edu.cn

Abstract. The classification of liver lesions on computed tomography (CT) images is vital for early liver cancer diagnosis. To aid physicians, several methods have been proposed to perform that task automatically. These methods mostly use regions of interest (ROIs) that are manually or automatically selected from liver CT slices as training and testing data. However, the manual selection of ROIs requires a lot of time and effort from experienced physicians making the number of available fully labeled datasets limited. When it comes to automatic ROIs selection using segmentation methods, some incorrect mask predictions that might occur can affect the quality of the selected ROIs causing the model for the final task to be trained improperly. In this paper, we explore the potential of using the whole liver CT slice in combination with the lesion type label for weakly-supervised lesion classification. We exploit the ability of attention mechanisms to lead convolutional neural networks (CNNs) to focus on important regions in the input image. Then, we propose a lightweight attention module modified from the Efficient Channel Attention (Eca) module, called Efficient Dual-Pooling Channel Attention (EDPca). Our experimental results show that attention mechanisms can significantly boost the performance of CNNs for the task of weakly-supervised liver lesion classification, bringing the results closer to that of the supervised task. Besides, our proposed module achieves better classification results than the other channel attention ones. Moreover, the combination of it and the spatial attention module from CBAM module outperforms other methods.

Keywords: liver lesion classification · weakly-supervised · CNN · attention · multi-phase CT images

1   Introduction

Liver cancer is one of the major causes of cancer deaths worldwide. Early detection of liver lesions is vital to prevent its progression, and CT scans are commonly used for diagnosis. However, the interpretation of CT scans requires physicians to be well-trained and experienced. To aid physicians, many computer-aided diagnoses (CAD) systems have been developed for automatic classification of liver lesions on CT images.

Commonly, CAD systems have two main stages: detection of regions of interest (ROIs) and construction of a classifier using the selected ROIs. The first stage can be done by experienced physicians or by using automatic segmentation tools. However, the state-of-the-art method for liver tumor segmentation [1] only achieves a dice metric score less than 0.75. Many studies have suggested using the machine learning approach to carry out the second stage. Low-level features (i.e., density, texture etc.) extracted from selected ROIs are used for classification in several studies [2, 3]. Mid-level features (i.e., bag of visual words) have also been utilized for the same task [4]. High-level features extracted by deep convolution neural networks (DCNNs) have also shown their strong potential for multiple classification tasks, including liver lesions classification on CT images [5, 6]. While these approaches have good performances, their success is heavily dependent on the selection of ROIs (the tumors), which is time-consuming and labor-intensive for experienced radiologists to do manually or not so accurate to be done automatically.

The above problem suggests using the whole liver slice for classification instead. The reason behind it is that we can use segmentation tools to automatically cut out the entire liver from CT scans. It will be easier than tumor segmentation as the liver does not vary much in size and shape, and the contour of the liver is normally clearer than that of the tumors through all CT phases. Moreover, by using liver segmentation we can lower the risk of losing some parts of the tumors inside it, which is the major problem of tumor segmentation. That approach may be data-efficient but the noises from non-ROI areas may negatively impact the performance of the classifier. That causes another challenge that is how to lead DCNNs to focus more on the task-relevant areas and ignore the irrelevant ones, and attention mechanisms appear to be a good solution to tackle it. They work by assigning weights to different regions of the input image, allowing the network to dynamically focus on the most relevant features for the target task while suppressing the impact of non-relevant information.

Several channel and spatial attention modules have been proposed for the classification of natural images. Squeeze-and-Excitation (SE) module [7] uses fully connected layers following a global average pooling operation to learn to reweight the channels. The Efficient channel attention module (Eca) [8] later replaces the fully connected layers in the SE module with a lightweight 1D convolution layer to make the learned weights become more direct from the channels. In addition to an SE module combining both global average and max pooling, Convolution Block Attention Module (CBAM) [9] further inserts a spatial attention module based on a 2D convolution operation to reweight the spatial positions of the feature map. When it comes to classifying lesions of the liver on CT images, Chen [10] utilized a Dual-self-attention module to enhance the long-range dependencies within the feature map extracted by a Dilated Residual Network (DRN) and obtained a 6.07% accuracy gain compared with no attention network. In their later work [11], they used convolution long-short-term memory (ConvLSTM) layers to extract spatial-temporal information of the different phases from the ROI predicted by a well-trained Dual-Attention DRN and the accuracy gain is 2.04% compared with the method in [10]. In [12], Xi et al. also use the attention approach for weakly-supervised skin lesion classification. They proposed a distinct region proposal module (DRPM) which combines both channel and spatial attention to guide the network to focus on the lesion areas and achieved an average AUC of 93.2%.

In this paper, we explore the ability of attention mechanisms to enhance the classification of a DRN by refining its extracted high-resolution feature map. Then, inspired by the lightweight Eca module, we modify it to propose a new Efficient Dual-Pooling channel attention (EDPca) module, that uses both Global Average and Max Pooling operations to further improve the attention weight calculation.

Our main contributions in this paper are as follows: (1) we have investigated and compared the performances of multiple existing attention modules for the task of weakly-supervised liver lesion classification on CT images; (2) our proposed EDPca module achieves better accuracy gain compared to other channel attention modules and the combination of it and the spatial attention module from CBAM module outperforms other methods; (3) our experimental results show that attention mechanisms can significantly boost the performances of CNNs for the mentioned task, bringing the results closer to that of the ROI-level liver lesion classification.

2 Methods

Our overall framework for weakly-supervised liver lesion classification on CT images is shown in Fig. 1. It consists of four main components: (1) the DRN backbone to extract high-resolution feature maps from the input CT liver slice; (2) the attention module to enhance the features and areas within the feature maps; (3) the classifier to predict the type of lesion existing in the input image; (4) the localization branch using Gradient-weighted Class Activation Mapping (Grad-CAM) algorithm.

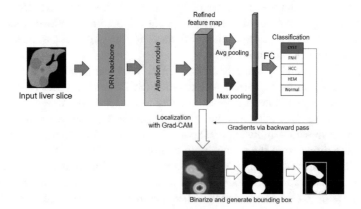

Fig. 1. The overall framework

2.1 Revisiting Efficient Channel Attention (Eca) Module

Given an input feature map $X \in \mathbb{R}^{C \times W \times H}$, Eca module (Fig. 2a) first performs a Global Average Pooling (GAP) operation like in Squeeze-and-Excitation (SE) module (Fig. 2b) to obtain channel descriptors of shape $\mathbb{R}^{C \times 1 \times 1}$. Then a lightweight 1D convolution followed by a Sigmoid function is used to replace the fully connected (FC) layers in SE module. By doing so, the number of additional parameters will be ignorable and the learned weights will become more direct from the channel descriptors as there is no intermediate layers.

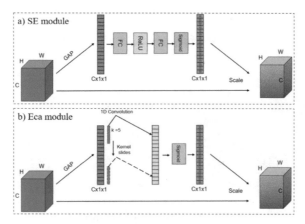

Fig. 2. SE and Eca modules

Finally, Eca module multiplies the learned weights with the input feature map to adjust the importance of each channel. The equations below show the process of weight calculation in Eca module.

$$z_{Eca} = \frac{1}{W \times H} \sum_{i=1}^{W} \sum_{j=1}^{H} X(i, j) \tag{1}$$

$$attention_{Eca} = \sigma(C1D_k(z_{Eca})) \tag{2}$$

where z_{Eca} is the channel descriptors tensor, σ is a Sigmoid function and $C1D_k$ is a 1D convolution with kernel size of k.

2.2 The Proposed Efficient Dual-Pooling Channel Attention Module

In SE and Eca modules, they both have the first stage as the Global Average Pooling (GAP) operation, which outputs a single average value of the whole channel for each channel. The major drawback of it is the loss of spatial information of the whole channel. With that in mind, our key idea is to add more channel information to the attention weights calculation, in addition with the use of GAP operation. That is our motivation to combine the use of both GAP and Global Max Pooling (GMP) as the first stage of our proposed EDPca module (Fig. 3).

For the first stage, it performs both GAP and GMP operations to obtain two $\mathbb{R}^{C\times 1\times 1}$ tensors and then concatenate them to form a tensor of size $\mathbb{R}^{C\times 2\times 1}$. Here, each channel will have two different descriptors from GAP and GMP operations, allowing more channel information to be utilized for the computation of the weights, making them more accurate. In the next stage, we apply a lightweight 1D convolution layer with the kernel size of k to learn the weights. Finally, a Sigmoid function will be applied to normalized the weights. The whole process can be summarized as follows:

$$z_{GAP} = \frac{1}{W \times H} \sum_{i=1}^{W} \sum_{j=1}^{H} X(i,j); \ z_{GMP} = Max(X); \ z_{EDPca} = [z_{GAP}, z_{GMP}]$$
(3)

$$attention_{EDPca} = \sigma(C1D_k(z_{EDPca}))$$
(4)

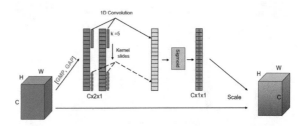

Fig. 3. The proposed EDPca module

Where $[z_{GAP}, z_{GMP}]$ is the concatenation of the output of the two pooling operations with the shape of $\mathbb{R}^{C\times 2\times 1}$, σ represents a Sigmoid function and $C1D_k$ is a 1D convolution layer with the kernel size of k and the shape of the kernel weights is of $\mathbb{R}^{k\times 2}$.

2.3 The Combination of Our EDPca Module with CBAM'S Spatial Attention Module

We propose to combine our EDPca module with the spatial attention module from the CBAM module. Thus, the network will be more flexible in the process of choosing what (channel) and where (position) to pay more attention to. The spatial attention module from CBAM module (CBAM_s) can be described as in Fig. 4.

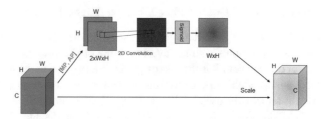

Fig. 4. The spatial attention module from the CBAM module

At first, an average and max pooling operation (AP and MP) is applied for each position $X(i, j)$ of the input feature map $X \in \mathbb{R}^{C \times W \times H}$ to get two spatial representations of size $\mathbb{R}^{1 \times W \times H}$. Next, they are concatenated to form a tensor of size $\mathbb{R}^{2 \times W \times H}$ and then a 2D convolution layer with the kernel size of k × k is applied to learn the weights. The final step is to normalize the learned weights using a Sigmoid function and spatial-wise multiply them with the input feature map to perform spatially reweighting.

To use this module in conjunction with our EDPca module, we follow the same strategy in the CBAM module, that is placing the spatial attention module after the channel attention module as in Fig. 5.

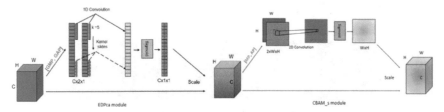

Fig. 5. The combination of our proposed EDPca and CBAM_s module

2.4 Configuration Details of Attention Modules

In our work, we set the parameters of attention modules based on the DRN backbone network. Specifically, we use a DRN with 26 layers and the shape of the output feature map is $\mathbb{R}^{512 \times 28 \times 28}$. For SE module, we use the same reduction ratio of 16 as in the original work. When it comes to the kernel size of the 1D convolution operation of the Eca and EDPca modules, we follow the formular suggested in [8]: $k = \psi(C) = \left| \frac{\log_2(C)}{\gamma} + \frac{b}{\gamma} \right|_{odd}$, where C is the channel dimension and $|t|_{odd}$ is the nearest odd number of t. Given the values of C, γ, and b as 512, 2, and 1 respectively, the kernel size k will be 5. Finally, for the CBAM module, we also set its channel attention (CBAM_c) module's reduction ratio to 16 like in SE module. We use a 2D convolution kernel of size 7 × 7 for the CBAM_s module as suggested in the original work.

3 Experimental Results

3.1 Dataset and Implementation Details

In this study, we conduct our experiments on an in-house multi-phase CT liver lesion dataset (MPCT-FLLs) [13] with 4 types of lesion namely Cyst, Focal Nodular Hyperplasia (FNH), Hepatocellular Carcinoma (HCC), and Hemangioma (HEM), which were collected by Sir Run Run Shaw Hospital, Zhejiang University, China. The dataset has a total of 106 patient cases, each case is provided with a lesion type and tumor masks for all slices in NC, ART, and PV phases. We utilize an iterative probabilistic atlas model [14] to perform liver segmentation on original abdomen CT scans. The results are checked by experienced radiologists to ensure their accuracy. We also extract liver slices that have no tumors from some of the above cases and use them as the Normal class. The ROI for each Normal slice is considered as the largest rectangle inside the liver. In order to utilize the three phases of each slice, we stack them together (the center of each tumor is at the same position for the three phases) to form an RGB-like 2D image and resize it to the size of 224×224 for training and testing our models. We also make sure that there is no patient case overlapping between the training and testing set. Some sample images can be seen in Fig. 6 and the data distribution is shown in Table 1. For the weakly-supervised classification task, we use whole-liver images similar to the ones in Fig. 6 combing with their class labels. On the other hand, we generate bounding boxes covering the tumor masks and use them as the ground truth for the localization task only.

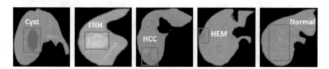

Fig. 6. Sample images from the dataset used in this study

Table 1. Data distribution of the dataset: *number of slices (number of cases)*. The number of cases of the Normal class (marked with *) is not counted in the Total column as they are extracted from the other four classes.

Class	Cyst	FNH	HCC	HEM	Normal	**Total**
Training set	142 (28)	66 (13)	146 (16)	102 (17)	106 (*47)	**562 (74)**
Test set	54 (9)	23 (7)	51 (7)	36 (9)	25 (*14)	**189 (32)**

Our models are built with Pytorch deep learning framework and the experiments are done using a NVIDIA GeForce GTX 980 Ti device with 6 GB of memory. We use Adam as the optimizer for training, and the other hyperparameters are set as follows: weight decay is 0.0001, initial learning rate is 0.0001, training epoch is 150 and a decay of 0.1 after every 50 epochs, batch size is 8 and we use pre-trained weights on ImageNet dataset to initialize the DRN backbone weights. For data augmentation, we use vertical, horizontal flipping and image rotation ($15°$).

Our models are evaluated using classification accuracy and localization accuracy. Classification accuracy depicts how good the attention modules are in leading the network to focus more on discriminative features of each lesion type. On the other hand, the localization accuracy shows how the attention modules force the network to give more weight to the ROIs in the input image. Classification or localization accuracy for each class is the ratio of the number of correct classified or localized slices of that class over the total number of slices of that class. Classification or localization total accuracy is the ratio of the number of correct classified or localized slices of the whole test set over the total number of slices of the whole test set.

3.2 Classification Results

The classification results of the DRN backbone using different attention modules are shown in Table 2. It can be clearly seen that for the task of weakly-supervised classification, attention modules can significantly improve the performance of the network without attention (at least 1.59% total accuracy gain for the case of SE module). In terms of channel attention, our proposed EDPca module improved from Eca module obtains higher amount of total accuracy gain than the others (3.18%) while having just a small amount of additional parameters (only 10 parameters). Moreover, the combination of our EDPca module and the CBAM_s module outperforms all other methods, having the smallest gap with the results of the supervised task (4.24%).

Table 2. Classification results using different attention modules. (c) means channel attention, (c,s) means channel and spatial attention

Task	Backbone	Attention module	Classification accuracy					
			Cyst	FNH	HCC	HEM	Normal	Total
Supervised classification	ResNet 18	×	1.0	0.8261	0.7843	0.9167	1.0	0.9048
Weakly-supervised classification	DRN 26	×	0.9074	0.7826	0.7451	0.7500	0.9200	0.8201
		SE [7] (c)	0.9259	0.7826	0.8039	0.7500	0.8800	0.8360
		Eca [8] (c)	**0.9815**	0.7391	0.7843	0.7222	0.9200	0.8413
		CBAM_c [9] (c)	0.9630	0.6087	0.8235	**0.8056**	0.9200	0.8466
		Channel self-attention [10] (c)	0.9444	**0.9565**	0.8235	0.6389	0.8400	0.8413
		EDPca (**Ours**) (c)	0.9630	0.7391	0.8039	0.7778	0.9200	0.8519
		CBAM [9] (c,s)	**0.9815**	0.7826	0.8039	**0.8056**	0.8400	0.8571
		Dual self-attention [10] (c,s)	**0.9815**	0.6957	**0.8431**	0.7222	0.9600	0.8571
		EDPca (**Ours**) + CBAM_s (c,s)	0.9630	0.7391	**0.8431**	0.7222	**1.0**	**0.8624**

3.3 Localization Results

In this study, for each testing image having the actual label other than Normal, we use Gradient-weighted Class Activation Maps (Grad-CAM) for the predicted class to do the task of weakly-supervised localization. We upsample the Grad-CAM to the same size with the input image (224 × 224) and binarize it with a threshold of 25% of the max intensity. Then, we generate a bounding box that covers all activated pixels (Fig. 7) and use an IoU threshold of 0.3 with the ground truth for evaluation.

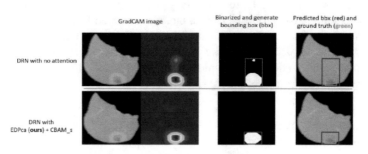

Fig. 7. An example of localization with GradCAM for class Cyst

Finally, the localization accuracy for a class will be the number of slices having the tumors correctly localized over the total number of slices of that class. We present the comparison of localization performance of different attention modules using Grad-CAM in Table 3. The experimental results show that, compared with using the backbone only, almost all attention modules can boost the localization accuracy. The combination of our proposed EDPca module and the CBAM_s module achieves the highest total classification accuracy but it is just ranked second among the modules that have the best overall localization performance (1.83% lower than the best one). That can be explained as when a network is good at classification, it will mainly focus on the parts of the ROI that is most discriminative, and not every part of the ROI is beneficial for classification, causing the predicted localization bounding boxes to not cover the whole ROI and thus having lower localization accuracy.

Table 3. Localization accuracy comparison of different attention modules. (c) means channel attention, (c,s) means channel and spatial attention

Task	Backbone	Attention module	Localization accuracy				
			Cyst	FNH	HCC	HEM	Total
Weakly-supervised localization	DRN 26	×	0.6481	0.6087	0.7647	0.6944	0.6890
		SE [7] (c)	0.6852	0.4783	0.7255	0.8056	0.6951
		Eca [8] (c)	**0.7037**	**0.9130**	0.8039	**0.8611**	**0.7988**
		CBAM_c [9] (c)	0.6852	0.4783	0.8235	0.8333	0.7317

(continued)

Table 3. (*continued*)

Task	Backbone	Attention module	Localization accuracy				
			Cyst	FNH	HCC	HEM	Total
		Channel self-attention [10] (c)	0.6111	0.8261	0.5490	0.5833	0.6159
		EDPca (**Ours**) (c)	0.6481	0.7391	0.8431	0.8333	0.7622
		CBAM [9] (c,s)	**0.7037**	0.8261	0.7255	0.6944	0.7256
		Dual self-attention [10] (c,s)	0.6667	0.6957	**0.8627**	0.6944	0.7378
		EDPca (**Ours**) + CBAM_s (c,s)	**0.7037**	0.7391	**0.8627**	0.8056	0.7805

4 Conclusions

In this paper, we propose an Efficient Dual-Pooling Channel Attention module that is very lightweight and integrate it to a Dilated ResNet backbone to improve the results of the weakly-supervised liver lesion classification on CT images task. Our EDPca module outperforms other channel attention modules and when combine it with the spatial attention module from CBAM module we achieve the highest total classification. Although it is only ranked second in terms of boosting the overall localization accuracy, the performance gap between it and the best module is not so considerable.

Acknowledgement. This research was supported in part by the Grant-in Aid for Scientific Research from the Japanese Ministry for Education, Science, Culture and Sports (MEXT) under the Grant No. 21H03470, 20KK0234 and No. 20K21821.

References

1. Li, X., Chen, H., Qi, X., Dou, Q., Fu, C.-W., Heng, P.-A.: H-DenseUNet: hybrid densely connected UNet for liver and tumor segmentation From CT volumes. IEEE Trans. Med. Imaging **37**, 2663–2674 (2018)
2. Roy, S., Chi, Y., Liu, J., Venkatesh, S.K., Brown, M.S.: Three-dimensional spatiotemporal features for fast content-based retrieval of focal liver lesions. IEEE Trans. Biomed. Eng. **61**, 2768–2778 (2014)
3. Xu, Y., et al.: Combined density, texture and shape features of multi-phase contrast-enhanced CT images for CBIR of focal liver lesions: a preliminary study. In: Chen, Y.-W., Toro, C., Tanaka, S., Howlett, R.J., Jain, L.C. (eds.) Innovation in Medicine and Healthcare 2015. SIST, vol. 45, pp. 215–224. Springer, Cham (2016). https://doi.org/10.1007/978-3-319-23024-5_20

4. Yang, W., Lu, Z., Yu, M., Huang, M., Feng, Q., Chen, W.: Content-based retrieval of focal liver lesions using bag-of-visual-words representations of single- and multiphase contrast-enhanced CT images. J. Digit. Imaging **25**, 708–719 (2012)

5. Yasaka, K., Akai, H., Abe, O., Kiryu, S.: Deep learning with convolutional neural network for differentiation of liver masses at dynamic contrast-enhanced CT: a preliminary study. Radiology **286**, 887–896 (2018)

6. Liang, D., et al.: Combining convolutional and recurrent neural networks for classification of focal liver lesions in multi-phase CT images. In: Frangi, A.F., Schnabel, J.A., Davatzikos, C., Alberola-López, C., Fichtinger, G. (eds.) MICCAI 2018. LNCS, vol. 11071, pp. 666–675. Springer, Cham (2018). https://doi.org/10.1007/978-3-030-00934-2_74

7. Hu, J., Shen, L., Sun, G.: Squeeze-and-excitation networks. CoRR, abs/1709.01507 (2017)

8. Wang, Q., Wu, B., Zhu, P., Li, P., Zuo, W., Hu, Q.: ECA-net: efficient channel attention for deep convolutional neural networks. CoRR, abs/1910.03151 (2019)

9. Woo, S., Park, J., Lee, J.-Y., Kweon, I.S.: CBAM: convolutional block attention module. CoRR, abs/1807.06521 (2018)

10. Chen, X., et al.: A dual-attention dilated residual network for liver lesion classification and localization on CT images. In: 2019 IEEE International Conference on Image Processing (ICIP) (2019)

11. Chen, X., et al.: A cascade attention network for liver lesion classification in weakly-labeled multi-phase CT images. In: Wang, Q., et al. (eds.) DART/MIL3ID -2019. LNCS, vol. 11795, pp. 129–138. Springer, Cham (2019). https://doi.org/10.1007/978-3-030-33391-1_15

12. Xue, X., Kamata, S.-I., Luo, D.: Skin lesion classification using weakly-supervised fine-grained method. In: 2020 25th International Conference on Pattern Recognition (ICPR) 2021

13. Xu, Y., et al.: PA-ResSeg: a phase attention residual network for liver tumor segmentation from multiphase CT images. Med. Phys. **48**, 3752–3766 (2021)

14. Dong, C., et al.: Segmentation of liver and spleen based on computational anatomy models. Comput. Biol. Med. **67**, 146–160 (2015)

Diffusion Models for Realistic CT Image Generation

Maialen Stephens Txurio[1,2,3(✉)], Karen López-Linares Román[1,2],
Andrés Marcos-Carrión[4], Pilar Castellote-Huguet[4],
José M. Santabárbara-Gómez[4], Iván Macía Oliver[1],
and Miguel A. González Ballester[3,5]

[1] Vicomtech, Basque Research and Technology Alliance,
Donostia-San Sebastian, Spain
mstephens@vicomtech.org
[2] Biodonostia Health Research Institute, Donostia-San Sebastian, Spain
[3] BCN Medtech, Department of Information and Communication Technologies,
Universitat Pompeu Fabra, Barcelona, Spain
[4] Biomedical Engineering Unit, Ascires Biomedical Group, Valencia, Spain
[5] ICREA, Barcelona, Spain

Abstract. Generative networks, such as GANs, have been applied to
the medical image domain, where they have demonstrated their ability
to synthesize realistic-looking images. However, training these models is
hard, as they show multiple challenges like mode collapse or vanishing
gradients. Recently, diffusion probabilistic models have revealed to outperform GANs in the context of natural images. However, only a few
early works have attempted their use in medical images. Hence, in this
work we aim at evaluating the potential of diffusion models to generate
realistic CT images. We make use of the Frechet Inception Distance to
quantitatively evaluate the trained model at different epochs, as a metric
to provide information about the fidelity of the synthetic samples, dis-
playing a clear convergence of the value in the advance of the training
process. We quantitative and qualitatively show to successfully achieve
coherent and precise CT images, compared to real images.

Keywords: CT synthesis · Diffusion probabilistic model · Image
generation · Medical imaging · Deep learning

1 Introduction

Medical imaging is fundamental in healthcare, with an increasing role in the
diagnosis and follow-up of diseases. It also plays a major role in the development of new therapeutics during clinical trials, where quantitative image-based
biomarkers help to detect diseases and estimate the patient's response to different
drugs [1]. For a fair and comprehensive evaluation, collecting sets of heterogeneous images, including rare clinical cases, is needed. However, it is tedious and
time consuming to recruit large enough cohorts to achieve statistical power and
to develop robust algorithms for imaging biomarker extraction. Furthermore,

© The Author(s), under exclusive license to Springer Nature Singapore Pte Ltd. 2023
Y.-W. Chen et al. (Eds.): KES InMed 2023, SIST 357, pp. 335–344, 2023.
https://doi.org/10.1007/978-981-99-3311-2_30

data privacy and security concerns prevent access to and/or reuse of valuable research data. Hence, generating synthetic images is thought to be a good alternative to overcome the difficulty of selecting representative and diverse cohorts for biomedical research and development.

Lately, deep learning based generative networks have demonstrated their potential to provide realistic and high quality images. To date, GANs [2] are leading the generative models and have been widely explored and applied, surpassing state-of-the-art results. However, GANs are usually challenging to train as they suffer from mode collapse, which leads to the synthetic data not sufficiently covering the whole distribution, and thus generating poor variety of images. Recently, diffusion models have emerged as an alternative generative approach, reporting better results than GANs [3]. Nevertheless, there are very few works that have explored the use of diffusion models for medical image synthesis.

The aim of this study is to prove the ability of diffusion models to generate realistic Computed Tomography (CT) images, to the best of our knowledge, for the first time in the literature. We qualitative and quantitatively evaluate the generated samples demonstrating the potential of these networks to further be used to generate different image modalities, contributing to the medical image generation approaches proposed in the literature.

2   State of the Art

GANs have emerged as a powerful tool for image generation tasks. Researchers have successfully employed GANs and their extensions to generate some medical image modalities like T1-weighted brain MRI [4], MRI prostate lesions [5], CT lung cancer nodules [6] and liver lesion ROIs [7], retinal images [8] or skin lesions [9]. They have also shown the capability to solve domain adaptation, reconstruction and classification tasks as addressed in [10]. Despite the achieved results, GANs still suffer from multiple issues which make the training process difficult, such as convergence, vanishing gradients or mode collapse.

Recent research has shown that diffusion probabilistic models outperform state-of-the-art results obtained by GANs with regard to natural images [3]. Diffusion models are a type of likelihood-based models that are trained to reverse a diffusion process that consists on gradually adding noise to the data in the opposite direction of sampling until the image is wiped out [11]. The main advantages of these models compared to GANs are the distribution coverage, stationary training objective and easy scalability. The promising results obtained with natural images suggest that these models could be useful to improve medical image generation for virtual cohort generation or data augmentation. Still, very few works use diffusion models in the medical imaging domain. Two very recent works report the generation of synthetic magnetic resonance data for the first time [12–14]. Other examples include the use of diffusion models for localization and semantic segmentation [15–17], score-based reconstruction [18], under-sampled medical image reconstruction [19,20], anomaly detection [21] and image translation [22]. According to [23], no previous work has applied diffusion models to solve the CT image generation problem, yet, a recent study employs a modified diffusion model architecture that works on the latent space to generate CT images [24]. However, the latent space generated by the diffusion model is subsequently passed to a VQ-GAN [25] that decodes the input into a synthetic CT. Thus, the work in [24] does not prove the ability of diffusion models on their own to generate high quality synthetic CT images from random noise. Given the benefits of diffusion models, in this study we propose generating CT scans using pure diffusion models, quantitatively and qualitatively validating the synthetic CT images.

3   Methods

3.1   Dataset

The employed images are chest-abdomen-pelvis CTs that have been provided and by Ascires Biomedical Group, obtained from scanners of different manufacturers. In total, we work with 559 CTs from healthy subjects (Table 1).

Table 1. Summary of the employed CT images to train and evaluate the developed diffusion model.

	Train		Test	
	Female	Male	Female	Male
20-40 years	71	77	18	19
40-65 years	76	76	19	19
> 65 years	74	73	19	19
Total	**447**		**112**	

To train the diffusion model, we firstly transform image intensities to Hounsfield Units (HU). We then modify the image intensities by a window/level transformation according to the target values for abdominal CTs (window = 40 HU, level = 400 HU) in order to remove the histogram differences identified in the whole dataset. Finally, we resize the images to $128 \times 128 \times 128$ to reduce computational costs and normalize the intensity values between 0 and 1. As we later train a 2D network, we split the 3D volumes into slices resulting in 57216 and 14336 CT images of size 128×128 for training and testing, respectively.

3.2   Diffusion Models and Training

Hereby, we generate CT images employing diffusion probabilistic models. Inspired by non-equilibrium thermodynamics, the process consists in defining a generative Markov chain able to learn the reverse of a diffusion process that progressively adds random Gaussian noise to real data until the signal is lost, resulting in a sequence of variables in which the state of one variable depends only on the previous one [26].

Thus, given input training data, we firstly define a gradual noising process by randomly adding Gaussian noise during $t \in T$ timesteps with a variance of $\beta_t \in (0, 1)$. The diffusion model is then trained to repeatedly predict slightly denoised x_{t-1} given x_t, starting from x_T. As the model samples during several time steps until producing the denoised image, these models provide more training stability than GANs. The optimized loss function during training is defined in Eq. 1, which is the mean-squared error between the real and the predicted noise.

$$L = E_{t \sim [1,T], x_0 \sim q(x_0), \epsilon \sim \mathcal{N}(0,I)} \left[\| \epsilon - \epsilon_\theta (x_t, t) \|^2 \right] \tag{1}$$

where $\epsilon_\theta (x_t, t)$ is the noise prediction at time t, ϵ is the true noise, T is the number of diffusion steps and $q (x_0)$ is the initial noise Gaussian distribution.

As an imaging generative model, we use the approach and improvements proposed in [3], which synthesizes high quality natural images using diffusion models. As the backbone, we use BigGAN [27] residual blocks for upsampling and downsampling the activations, attention at resolutions 32, 16 and 8, adaptive group normalization, 64 base channels, and 2 residual blocks per resolution. We define the hyperparameters experimentally, selecting the ones providing highest quality images. We set 1000 diffusion steps, a linear noise shedule and a batch size of 2 to reduce the computational cost. We train the network using PyTorch [28] on a NVIDIA Tesla V100 (32 GB) during 7K iterations with the Adam optimizer with a constant learning rate of 1e–04.

3.3   Evaluation Metrics

We evaluate the trained diffusion model with the *Frechet Inception Distance* (FID) first proposed by [29] and detailed in Eq. 2 and widely applied to quantitatively assess generative networks. FID commonly uses the Inception-V3 network [30] pretrained on the ImageNet dataset [31]. We firstly feed the network with the real and generated samples, from where we extract the mean and covariance of the activations of the final block for both sets, and later compute the *Frechet distance* between them. The FID is believed to better capture the human perception, fidelity and diversity by measuring the distance between the distributions of the latent space. Despite the Inception network being pretrained with natural images, the study [10] demonstrates that the FID is a reliable metric for medical images as it improves when the generated sample quality increases. Furthermore, [32] shows that a pretrained Inception model is more appropriate than a randomly initialized model for synthetic medical image quality evaluation. We also estimate the sFID [33] which uses spatial features instead of standard pooled features to account for the spatial relationships and consistent high-level structures.

$$\text{FID} = \| \mu_r - \mu_g \|^2 + \text{Tr} \left(\Sigma_r + \Sigma_g - 2 (\Sigma_r \Sigma_g)^{1/2} \right) \tag{2}$$

where μ_r and μ_g are the feature-wise mean of the real and generated images, Tr refers to the trace linear algebra operation, and Σ_r and Σ_g denote the covariance matrix for the real and generated images.

In addition, for the model returning the best FID and sFID values, we calculate the precision and recall metrics. The precision allows quantifying fidelity and the recall captures diversity [34].

4   Results

Once the network is trained, our objective is to test the ability of the model to generate realistic CT images that resemble structures seen in real CT scans. Thus, we quantitatively evaluate the model in different stages of the training process estimating the previously described FID and relating it to the visual quality improvements of the generated samples. We also calculate the aforementioned metrics for the best FID value obtained to support the fidelity of the synthetic CTs.

We firstly analyze the trained diffusion model behaviour over time by estimating the FID and sFID curves for the first 4000 iterations. In order to improve computational efficiency, we generate 100 synthetic samples per each 100 iterations and compare them with 100 real CT slices based on the FID. For this step, from the real 112 testing CT volumes, we randomly select one slice per each CT image in order to cover the whole variety of slices present in the dataset. We observe from Fig. 1 that both the FID and the sFID decrease the during training process, which indicates the diffusion model convergence and hints at an improvement of the generated CT image quality and the representation of the main structures.

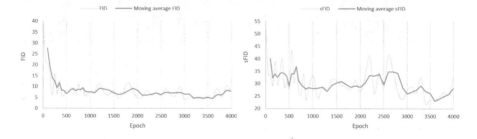

Fig. 1. FID (left) and sFID (right) values together with their corresponding moving average with a period of 3, comparing synthetic CT samples with the real test CT slices. The values are estimated on the first 4000 models obtained during the training process of the diffusion model. The curves suggest the quality of the images improves over time.

To further confirm the reliability of these metrics to guide the diffusion model convergence using CT images, we compare the FID value of models saved at different epochs with the visual qualitative appearance of the generated samples. Figure 2 demonstrates that a lower FID involves a more realistic synthetic sample generation. We can notice in Fig. 1 that at the beginning the FID falls abruptly and decreases more slowly after epoch 500. Figure 2 visually confirms that the high initial decrease of FID value implies a substantial improvement of the image quality. Likewise, the gentle improvement of the value shows slight detail refinements of the generated CT samples, in which the coherence of the spatial placement and shape of the organs improves to precisely resemble real images.

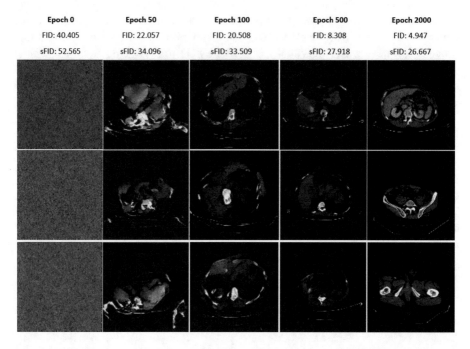

Fig. 2. Visual results of sampling three different synthetic images employing models trained for different epochs. We can observe that the FID metric clearly indicates image quality, as the value reduces according to the representation quality of the generated synthetic images. The same happens for the sFID metric, which decreases when the spatial consistency improves.

The model providing the best FID value is the model at epoch 3600. Hence, we generate up to 1000 synthetic samples and compare them to 1000 real CT images from the testing set for a thorough model evaluation. The obtained FID and sFID scores are 4.002 and 23.32, respectively. Figure 3 displays qualitative results of the generated samples in epoch 3600. The generated synthetic images show well defined structures and precise spatial integrity, when compared to real CT images. These results suggest that the trained diffusion model is capable of generating realistic CT images.

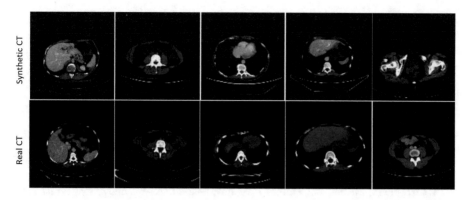

Fig. 3. Generated CT samples employing the diffusion model trained for 3600 epochs, and compared to non-paired real CT images.

5   Conclusions

This study aimed at evaluating the ability of diffusion models to generate realistic CT images, as a promising data augmentation technique to enhance the development of forthcoming deep learning approaches. Diffusion models have recently shown to surpass the results of the well-known GANs, which have been the best models for image generation tasks in recent years. Therefore, this work explored the use of diffusion models, mainly employed for natural image generation, to synthesize CT images.

We have proved to successfully generate realistic images by training a diffusion probabilistic model, qualitatively and quantitatively comparing the generated samples with the real CT images. We have evaluated the models at different points of the training process to assess the convergence and the reliability of the FID and sFID as metrics to guide the precision of the process. We have seen that although the Inception network is trained with natural images, the FID is a trustworthy metric for our diffusion model as the decrease of the metric entails an improvement of the generated CT images. The FID curve also confirms the convergence property observed in the literature with natural images, again confirming that diffusion models are more robust than GANs. Moreover, we have qualitatively compared the generated CT samples with real images, proving that the synthetic images correctly resemble the organ structures and their spatial location.

As future work, we aim at further validating the potential of these generated images to reinforce different task-specific deep learning model training approaches. Furthermore, we would like to include class conditional restrictions to guide the diffusion models, for example to generate pathological organ images. Finally, the extension to 3D will also be addressed in future work.

6   Compliance with Ethical Standards

Approval for this study was granted by the Drug Research Ethics Committee of the Hospital Clínic in Barcelona.

References

1. Miller, C.G., Krasnow, J., Schwartz, L.H. (eds.): Medical Imaging in Clinical Trials. Springer, London (2014). https://doi.org/10.1007/978-1-84882-710-3
2. Goodfellow, I., et al.: Generative adversarial nets. Adv. Neural. Inf. Process. Syst. **27**, 2672–2680 (2014)
3. Dhariwal, P., Nichol, A.: Diffusion models beat GANs on image synthesis. Adv. Neural. Inf. Process. Syst. **34**, 8780–8794 (2021)
4. Bermudez, C., Plassard, A.J., Davis, L.T., Newton, A.T., Resnick, S.M., Landman, B.A.: Learning implicit brain MRI manifolds with deep learning. Med. Imag. 2018: Image Process. **104574**, 408–414 (2018)
5. Kitchen, A., Seah, J.: Deep generative adversarial neural networks for realistic prostate lesion MRI synthesis. arXiv preprint arXiv:1708.00129 (2017)
6. Chuquicusma, M.J., Hussein, S., Burt, J., Bagci, U.: How to fool radiologists with generative adversarial networks? A visual turing test for lung cancer diagnosis. In: 2018 IEEE 15th International Symposium on Biomedical Imaging, pp. 240–244 (2018)
7. Frid-Adar, M., Diamant, I., Klang, E., Amitai, M., Goldberger, J., Greenspan, H.: GAN-based synthetic medical image augmentation for increased CNN performance in liver lesion classification. Neurocomputing **321**, 321–331 (2018)
8. Guibas, J.T., Virdi, T.S., Li, P.S.: Synthetic medical images from dual generative adversarial networks. arXiv preprint arXiv:1709.01872 (2017)
9. Baur, C., Albarqouni, S., Navab, N.: MelanoGANs: high resolution skin lesion synthesis with GANs. arXiv preprint arXiv:1804.04338 (2018)
10. Skandarani, Y., Jodoin, P.M., Lalande, A.: GANs for medical image synthesis: an empirical study. arXiv preprint arXiv:2105.05318 (2021)
11. Ho, J., Jain, A., Abbeel, P.: Denoising diffusion probabilistic models. Adv. Neural. Inf. Process. Syst. **33**, 6840–6851 (2020)
12. Dorjsembe, Z., Odonchimed, S., Xiao, F.: Three-dimensional medical image synthesis with denoising diffusion probabilistic models. Medical Imaging with Deep Learning (2022)
13. Kim, B., Ye, J.C.: Diffusion deformable model for 4D temporal medical image generation. In: International Conference on Medical Image Computing and Computer-Assisted Intervention, pp. 539–548 (2022)
14. Pinaya, W.H., et al.: Brain imaging generation with latent diffusion models. In: Mukhopadhyay, A., Oksuz, I., Engelhardt, S., Zhu, D., Yuan, Y. (eds) Deep Generative Models. DGM4MICCAI 2022. Lecture Notes in Computer Science, vol. 13609, pp. 117–126. Springer, Cham (2022). https://doi.org/10.1007/978-3-031-18576-2_12
15. Wolleb, J., Sandkühler, R., Bieder, F., Valmaggia, P., Cattin, P.C.: Diffusion Models for Implicit Image Segmentation Ensembles. In: International Conference on Medical Imaging with Deep Learning, pp. 1336–1348 (2022)
16. Pinaya, W.H., et al.: Fast unsupervised brain anomaly detection and segmentation with diffusion models. Medical Image Computing and Computer Assisted Intervention, pp. 705–714 (2022)

17. Sanchez, P., Kascenas, A., Liu, X., O'Neil, A.Q., Tsaftaris, S.A.: What is Healthy? Generative counterfactual diffusion for lesion localization. In: Mukhopadhyay, A., Oksuz, I., Engelhardt, S., Zhu, D., Yuan, Y. (eds) Deep Generative Models. DGM4MICCAI 2022. Lecture Notes in Computer Science, vol. 13609, pp. 34–44. Springer, Cham (2022). https://doi.org/10.1007/978-3-031-18576-2_4

18. Chung, H., Ye, J.C.: Score-based diffusion models for accelerated MRI. Med. Image Anal. **80**, 102479 (2022)

19. Xie, Y., Li, Q.: Measurement-conditioned denoising diffusion probabilistic model for under-sampled medical image reconstruction. Medical Image Computing and Computer Assisted Intervention–MICCAI 2022: 25th International Conference, Singapore, 18–22 September 2022, Proceedings, Part VI, pp. 655–664 (2022)

20. Peng, C., Guo, P., Zhou, S.K., Patel, V.M., Chellappa, R.: Measurement-conditioned denoising diffusion probabilistic model for under-sampled medical image reconstruction. Medical Image Computing and Computer Assisted Intervention–MICCAI 2022: 25th International Conference, Singapore, 18–22 September 2022, Proceedings, Part VI, pp. 623–633 (2022)

21. Wolleb, J., Bieder, F., Sandkühler, R., Cattin, P.C.: Diffusion models for medical anomaly detection. In: Wang, L., Dou, Q., Fletcher, P.T., Speidel, S., Li, S. (eds.) Medical Image Computing and Computer Assisted Intervention – MICCAI 2022. MICCAI 2022. Lecture Notes in Computer Science, vol. 13438. Springer, Cham (2022). https://doi.org/10.1007/978-3-031-16452-1_4

22. Özbey, M., et al.: Unsupervised medical image translation with adversarial diffusion models. arXiv preprint arXiv:2207.08208 (2022)

23. Kazerouni, A., et al.: Diffusion models for medical image analysis: a comprehensive survey. arXiv preprint arXiv:2211.07804 (2022)

24. Khader, F., et al.: Medical diffusion–denoising diffusion probabilistic models for 3D medical image generation. arXiv preprint arXiv:2211.03364 (2022)

25. Esser, P., Rombach, R., Ommer, B.: Taming transformers for high-resolution image synthesis. In: IEEE/CVF Conference on Computer Vision and Pattern Recognition, pp. 12873–12883 (2021)

26. Sohl-Dickstein, J., Weiss, E., Maheswaranathan, N., Ganguli, S.: Deep unsupervised learning using nonequilibrium thermodynamics. In: International Conference on Machine Learning, pp. 2256–2265 (2015)

27. Brock, A., Donahue, J., & Simonyan, K.: Large scale GAN training for high fidelity natural image synthesis. In: International Conference on Learning Representations (2018)

28. Paszke, A., et al.: PyTorch: an imperative style, high-performance deep learning library. Advances in Neural Information Processing Systems, vol. 33 (2019)

29. Heusel, M., Ramsauer, H., Unterthiner, T., Nessler, B., Hochreiter, S.: GANs trained by a two time-scale update rule converge to a local Nash equilibrium. Advances in Neural Information Processing Systems, vol. 30 (2019)

30. Szegedy, C., Vanhoucke, V., Ioffe, S., Shlens, J., Wojna, Z.: Rethinking the inception architecture for computer vision. In: Proceedings of the IEEE Conference on Computer Vision and Pattern Recognition, pp. 2818–2826 (2016)

31. Deng, J., Dong, W., Socher, R., Li, L.J., Li, K., Fei-Fei, L.: ImageNet: a large-scale hierarchical image database. 2009 IEEE Conference on Computer Vision and Pattern Recognition, pp. 248–255 (2009)

32. O'Reilly, J. A., Asadi, F.: Pre-trained vs random weights for calculating Fréchet inception distance in medical imaging. In: 2021 13th Biomedical Engineering International Conference (BMEiCON), pp. 1–4 (2021)

33. Nash, C., Menick, J., Dieleman, S., Battaglia, P.W.: Generating images with sparse representations. In: International Conference on Machine Learning, pp. 7958–7968 (2021)
34. Kynkäänniemi, T., Karras, T., Laine, S., Lehtinen, J., Aila, T.: Improved precision and recall metric for assessing generative models. Advances in Neural Information Processing Systems, vol. 32 (2019)

Unsupervised Data Drift Detection Using Convolutional Autoencoders: A Breast Cancer Imaging Scenario

Javier Bóbeda[1(✉)], María Jesús García-González[1],
Laura Valeria Pérez-Herrera[1], and Karen López-Linares[1,2]

[1] Vicomtech Foundation, Basque Research and Technology Alliance (BRTA), San Sebastian, Spain
`jbobeda@vicomtech.org`
[2] Biodonostia Health Research Institute, San Sebastian, Spain

Abstract. Imaging AI models are starting to reach real clinical settings, where model drift can happen due to diverse factors. That is why model monitoring must be set up in order to prevent model degradation over time. In this context, we test and propose a data drift detection solution based on unsupervised deep learning for a breast cancer imaging setting. A convolutional autoencoder is trained on a baseline set of expected images and controlled drifts are introduced in the data in order to test if a set of metrics extracted from the reconstructions and the latent space are able to distinguish them. We prove that this is a valid tool that manages to detect subtle differences even within these complex kind of images.

Keywords: data drift detection · deep learning · convolutional autoencoder · medical imaging · breast cancer

1 Introduction

The number of commercial Artificial Intelligence (AI)-based medical image analysis applications, lead by deep learning-based approaches, is notably increasing in the last years [1]. However, there is still some reticence for its broad adoption in healthcare. This is due to several reasons related to data access, integration with current workflows or trust, among others. One of the big topics under discussion is how to ensure the expected functioning of deployed AI applications.

It is largely known that the performance of deployed AI models degrades with time because of variations in the assumptions made during the algorithm development phase. This phenomenon is called model drift and depending on the source causing the variation, it can be subdivided in different categories: concept, label and data drift. Concept drift happens when the relation between the data and the labels changes. Label drift, when the distribution in the labels varies. Finally, data drift occurs when data changes in some unexpected manner with respect to the set used to develop the model. Even if a proper commercial model should be trained with a large, heterogeneous dataset that encompasses

Y.-W. Chen et al. (Eds.): KES InMed 2023, SIST 357, pp. 345–354, 2023.
https://doi.org/10.1007/978-981-99-3311-2_31

the variability of the data in the real setting, there are still potential variations in the population, imaging protocols, imaging infrastructures and so on that may not be anticipated and may prevent the model to work as expected. This study focuses on addressing data drift detection for models deployed at healthcare facilities.

Different tools have emerged in the last years to tackle data drift detection. Good examples of open-source toolkits are Evidently AI [2] and Deepchecks [3]. However, both of them use only tabular features and lack the ability to directly analyze the image itself to detect drifts due to complex features that cannot be manually pre-computed. For that, different techniques based on dimensionality reduction using deep learning have been proposed in the literature [4], including convolutional autoencoders (CAE) and domain classifiers. In that same study, autoencoders are reported to be the best-performing methods for this task. A CAE is a type of convolutional neural network that is able to compress the information present in the image to a latent space with lower dimensionality while learning important image features in the process, and reconstruct it back. The original and reconstructed images can be compared and a reconstruction error can be computed, which should increase for images drifted in any perceivable way from the set used during training. Although this technique has been proven useful in the computer vision domain [4–6], to the best of our knowledge there is only one recent pre-print focused on the medical imaging field [8]. Specifically, the work aims at detecting drifts that may occur with a deployed model that classifies chest X-ray images of different diseases. Authors show that a combination of features extracted from DICOM metadata, classification model predicted probabilities and a latent representation produced by a variational autoencoder (VAE) allow to accurately detect data drifts. They use the latent representation instead of the reconstruction metrics to determine if there is a drift, stating that the latent space can more easily be checked for distributional shifts. Within their experiments, they present one in which the detector only relies on VAE features.

In this work, we aim to go deeper into the idea of using autoencoders for data drift detection. We investigate the potential of using not only the latent space but also the reconstructions to detect drifts. The latent space is a compressed space and we believe that some important information could be lost if we do not analyze the complete reconstructions. We also want to increase the evidence that the image content alone can be trusted to detect drift, as there are situations in which it is not feasible to use DICOM metadata (i.e. digital pathology images). We run several experiments simulating a variety of potential drifts using public datasets from two imaging modalities used for breast cancer detection and diagnosis: mammography and digital pathology (whole slide images-WSI). As per our current understanding, this is the first time the method is tested with these imaging modalities.

2   Methods

This section presents the general idea behind the technique and how we plan to validate its performance. Afterwards, details on the experiments, data, metrics and training process are described.

2.1   Data Drift Detector

We implement our data drift detector based on the CAE architecture shown in Fig. 1. It is composed of an encoding and a decoding path. The encoding path has 3 convolutional layers with a stride of 2 to reduce image resolution and extract image features, projecting them into a lower dimensional space, the so-called latent space or bottleneck. The decoding path is made of 3 transposed convolutional layers that allow reconstructing the original image from the compressed version in the bottleneck. This process is guided by a reconstruction loss that compares the input and output images.

The latent space can be understood as a compressed version of the most important properties of the images in the training set, which organizes them in a coordinate system where the ones with similar properties lie closer to each other than the ones with different characteristics. Intuitively, when images somehow different from the ones used for training pass through the autoencoder, the features generated by the encoder path lie far from the previously learnt latent space and the quality of the reconstruction provided by the decoder path decreases. We try to get profit of this idea to automatically detect changes in new data with respect to the one used during training.

It is important to note that these data drifts need to be detected from a set of images, and not from a single study. The reasoning behind this is that in the medical domain it is very difficult to distinguish when a subtle change in an image is due to some unexpected drift or if it comes from the intrinsic high variability of the data. When the change is global and a group of images present it, it is more easily perceivable and it can be affirmed with greater statistical significance that a drift has occurred. We can measure this with statistical tests specifically designed to detect differences between distributions.

In order to test the performance of this method under different potential drift scenarios we design a set of experiments, all of them with the same skeleton. A dataset is selected to serve as the source data a deployed model could have been trained on. We extract 70% of its samples to create a **baseline training set** used to train the CAE. The remaining 30% constitute the **baseline test set**, with images extracted from the same source than the baseline train set, but unseen by the model during training. A third set, called the **target test set**, is created with images different from the baseline sets in some form. We reconstruct these three sets with the CAE and calculate our metrics for each one of them, obtaining three distributions per metric. The baseline and target test set distributions are then compared to the baseline train set. An experiment is considered successful if we find deviations for the target test set distribution but not for the baseline test set. The complete experiment architecture is represented in Fig. 1.

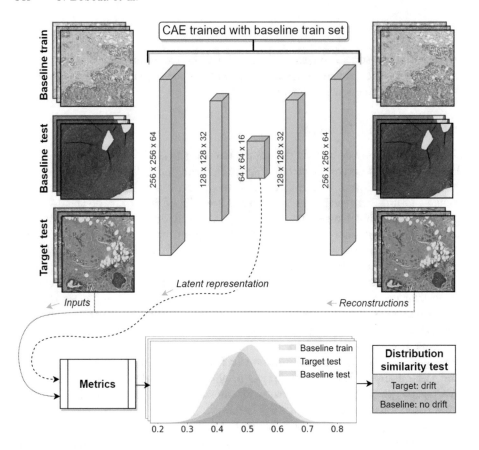

Fig. 1. Proposed data drift detection approach. The CAE is composed of convolutional layers forming the encoder and decoder branches (pink blocks) and the latent space (blue block). The printed block dimensions correspond to an input size of $512 \times 512 \times 3$, used for pathology images, but they can be extrapolated to any other input size. The CAE generates reconstructions and latent representations for the different sets. Then, metric distributions are computed and statistically compared.

2.2 Experiments

We carry out 4 experiments to evaluate the drift detector. The specifics of the data used for each of them is explained in Sect. 2.3.

1 - Dataset Drift. In a general scenario, we simulate how a model trained on a dataset of a certain image modality starts receiving images from a different dataset. Drifts here could appear from a range of differences. For example, the selected population or the equipment and acquisition parameters used.

2 - Acquisition Drift. Equivalent images of the same body part taken with different equipment can have similar characteristics to the human eye but completely trick a model if it is not prepared for them. Examples of this problem are using MRI from different manufacturers or digital and digitized film mammography at the same time. We simulate how a model trained with images taken with certain equipment, starts receiving equivalent images acquired with a different machine.

3 - Sample Drift. This experiment aims at simulating a sample selection failure. A model trained to detect breast cancer starts receiving images with apparently similar visual characteristics but from lung cancer tissue.

4 - Pre-processing Drift. The goal is to detect drifts due to unnoticed variations in the image pre-processing pipeline, i.e. a model trained on images with certain transformations starts receiving ones pre-processed in a slightly different way.

2.3   Datasets

The data under analysis is further explained and the final number of samples per experiment is displayed in Table 1.

Mammography Datasets. We employ two publicly available mammography datasets: Breast Cancer Digital Repository (BCDR) and INBreast [9,10]. BCDR contains 1164 digital mammography studies and 1686 digitized film mammograms, while INBreast contains 410 digital ones. Both datasets contain images taken in different contexts and with different machines. We use these datasets to perform experiments 1 and 2.

Digital Pathology Datasets. We use 3 collections extracted from The Cancer Genome Atlas (TCGA) Imaging Archive: Breast Invasive Carcinoma (BRCA), Lung Adenocarcinoma (LUAD) and Lung Squamous Cell Carcinoma (LUSC) [11–13]. We filter the data to get only the slides that have been used for cancer diagnosis, yielding a total of 576 breast samples and 373 lung samples. These images are taken by digitally scanning a microscope slide of tainted tissue and saved in SVS format. With these files, the image information can be accessed at different resolution levels. In order to perform experiment 3, we use the breast and lung tissue images, using the resolution level whose size is closer to $\frac{1}{4}$ of the size of the maximum resolution in x and y dimensions. For experiment 4, we use the three collections and pre-process them as above but with $\frac{1}{4}$ and $\frac{1}{6}$ size reductions for the baseline (train and test) and target sets, respectively. We extract 16 patches that contain tissue from each image, filtering out non informative patches. These patches are the ones we use as the input of our models.

Table 1. Number of samples per experiment and set.

	Set		
Experiment	Baseline train	Baseline test	Target test
1	815	349	410
2	815	349	1686
3	6448	2768	5968
4	10624	4560	12952

2.4   Metrics

We propose three metrics to assess differences between our sets of data: mean squared error (MSE), structural similarity (SSIM) and latent space distance (LATD). MSE and SSIM provide different ways of measuring the similarity between two images and are computed according to Eqs. 1 and 2, respectively. While MSE calculates the error between pairwise pixels for the two images, SSIM looks for similarities within groups of pixels using a windowing approach.

$$MSE(X,Y) = \frac{1}{n} \sum_{i=1}^{n} (X_i - Y_i)^2 \qquad (1)$$

$$SSIM(x,y) = \frac{(2\mu_x\mu_y + c_1)(2\sigma_{xy} + c_2)}{(\mu_x^2 + \mu_y^2 + c_1)(\sigma_x^2 + \sigma_y^2 + c_2)} \qquad (2)$$

with X and Y being the two images to compare, n the number of pixels in an image, x and y windows of same size of the given images, μ_x the pixel sample mean of x, μ_y the pixel sample mean of y, σ_x^2 the variance of x, σ_y^2 the variance of y, σ_{xy} the covariance of x and y, $c_1 = (k_1L)^2, c_2 = (k_2L)^2$ two variables to stabilize the division with weak denominator, L the dynamic range of the pixel-values (typically this is $2^{\#bits\ per\ pixel} - 1$), $k_1 = 0.01$ and $k_2 = 0.03$ by default.

LATD explores differences on the latent space representations of the images instead of the actual pixel values. It is computed as follows: first, every image representation gets flattened; then, using only the baseline representations we perform a principal component analysis (PCA), which computes a linear transformation of the feature space such that the greatest variance of the transformed data comes to lie on the first coordinate (first principal component), the second greatest variance in the second one, and so on; the resulting PCA transformation is applied to the whole set of representations, keeping the first 50 principal components; then, the mean for these 50 features of the baseline PCA representations is computed, giving us an approximate center of their representations in the PCA coordinate system; finally, the euclidean distance to this center is computed for every PCA representation of our three different sets of data.

For the experiments using WSIs, it is important to note that we average the results obtained for each patch or tile, as we have 16 patches per image.

Finally, to measure distribution shifts of variables compared to a reference sample, we use a **two-sample Kolmogorov-Smirnov (K-S) test**. It is appropriate for continuous numerical data and is non-parametric, which implies that it does not assume any specific distribution on the data under testing. It provides a p-value of the null hypothesis that the two distributions are equal. We determine a threshold of 0.005 on this p-value to find non-similar distributions.

2.5 Training Details

The trainings have been run in a Nvidia A40 GPU (48GB) using Tensorflow 2.8.0. A **mean squared error loss** between the original and reconstructed images has been minimized. The rest of the parameters used to train the CAE when using each image modality are summarized in Table 2. It must be noted that experiments have been carried out to try and reduce the latent space size with a final flattening and dense layers, trying to obtain a one dimensional vector of features. Anyhow, they have not been successful. This fact matches results in other articles dealing with autoencoders and medical imaging with complex features [15]. Having a spatial 3-dimensional bottleneck instead of a 1-dimensional representation allows for geometrical information to be preserved and leads to better reconstructions.

Table 2. Convolutional Autoencoder hyper-parameters.

	Mammography	Pathology
Learning rate	0.0001	=
Max epochs	300	=
Batch size	16	=
Strides per layer	2	=
Kernel size	5	=
Activation function	ReLu	=
Input size	$512 \times 1024 \times 1$	$512 \times 512 \times 3$
Latent space size	$64 \times 128 \times 16$	$64 \times 64 \times 16$

3 Results

To evaluate the ability of the CAE to compress and recreate the images under test, we display example model reconstructions per experiment in Fig. 2. Afterwards, drift detection results per experiment and metric are commented using Fig. 3.

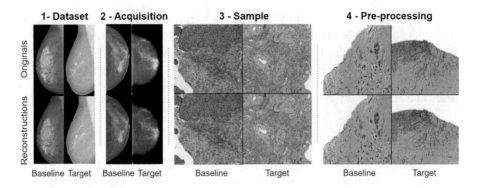

Fig. 2. Sample originals and reconstructions per experiment and test set

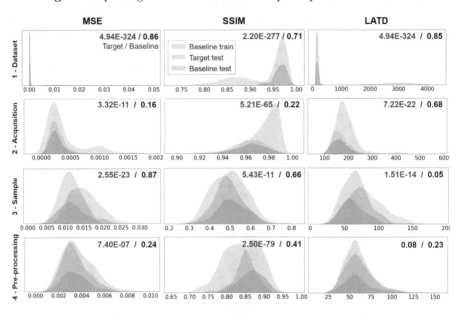

Fig. 3. Drift detection results. Rows correspond to experiments and columns to our three metrics. K-S p-values are provided for each case in the upper-right corner, comparing the similarity of the target (left) and baseline (right) test sets with the baseline train set. Red color marks out values under our detection threshold of 0.005.

The CAE correct performance has been assessed by visual inspection of the reconstructions and by checking that the baseline train set MSEs are always below 0.01 error. Even for the target set, originals and reconstructions do not present big perceivable differences to the human eye. Thus, a quantitative similarity test must be performed to evaluate their reconstruction quality.

In Fig. 3 we observe how the target test set is recognized as drifted for every experiment at least by two metrics, while the baseline test set is never marked out. This coincides with the expected behavior. MSE and SSIM, being the metrics extracted from the reconstructions, capture the drifted set in every scenario, while LATD fails to do so in some cases. For every case, p-values are lower for MSE or SSIM than for LATD. This translates to the notion that we extract more discriminative power from the reconstruction quality metrics than from the latent space.

In experiment 1 the target set distribution is almost completely separated apart from the other, leading to very low K-S test p-values. Experiment 3 is the one that presents less discriminative power, with a minimum p-value between all metrics of 2.55E-23, which is still satisfactory.

4 Conclusions

We have proved that the CAE data drift detector is a valid technique for the imaging modalities used in breast cancer: mammography and pathology. The models are able to learn the intricacies of the data and the metrics detect the drifted sets without providing false positives. We also prove that for our use case, analyzing reconstruction metrics is necessary to catch every drift scenario and that in general their p-values are lower than for LATD. This contradicts the idea presented in [8] that the latent space can more easily be checked for distributional shifts. Still, a future experiment should use a bigger sample size, aiming for lower latent space dimensions to corroborate if it is better to use the latent space or the reconstruction for drift detection.

Further steps on this topic include investigation more complex dimensionality reduction architectures, as variational autoencoders or generative adversarial networks (GANs). Additionally, the proposed experiments should be expanded to different modalities and drift scenarios.

Our experiments suggest that the simplest form of an autoencoder seems to be enough to capture data drift coming from different sources and can be applied to control the live cycle of deployed AI models. Still, we recommend that the performance of the method is specifically evaluated for different imaging modalities and use cases. The decisions on architecture and hyperparameters made in this study have been optimized only for our choice of image modalities and thus, they could be suboptimal for other scenarios.

Regarding the application of this technique in a real setting, it would imply training the autoencoders with the same training sets that the models they will monitor. When new data reaches the main model, it must pass through the CAE as well and the obtained metrics must be stored in a database alongside the ones retrieved from the baseline set. When a representative number of new samples is collected, the distribution comparison tests can be performed comparing new and baseline data. This process can be repeated with a given time frequency, using a windowing approach partitioning the new data in time windows. In this way, a drift metric over time could be obtained.

References

1. van Leeuwen, K.G., Schalekamp, S., Rutten, M.J.C.M., van Ginneken, B., de Rooij, M.: Artificial intelligence in radiology: 100 commercially available products and their scientific evidence. Eur. Radiol. **31**(6), 3797–3804 (2021). https://doi.org/10.1007/s00330-021-07892-z
2. Evidently AI. https://www.evidentlyai.com/
3. Deepchecks. https://deepchecks.com/
4. Rabanser, S., Günnemann, S., Lipton, Z.C.: Failing loudly: an empirical study of methods for detecting dataset shift. In: Proceedings of the 33rd International Conference on Neural Information Processing Systems, Article 125, pp. 1396-1408 (2019). arXiv:1810.11953
5. Lohdefink, J., et al.: Self-supervised domain mismatch estimation for autonomous perception. In: IEEE/CVF CVPRW, pp. 1359-1368 (2020). https://doi.org/10.1109/CVPRW50498.2020.00175
6. Suprem, A., Arulraj, J., Pu, C., Ferreira, J.: ODIN: automated drift detection and recovery in video analytics. arXiv e-prints (2020). https://doi.org/10.48550/arXiv.2009.05440
7. Yan, W., et al.: The domain shift problem of medical image segmentation and vendor-adaptation by Unet-GAN. In: Shen, D., et al. (eds.) MICCAI 2019. LNCS, vol. 11765, pp. 623–631. Springer, Cham (2019). https://doi.org/10.1007/978-3-030-32245-8_69
8. Soin, A., et al.: CheXstray: real-time multi-modal data concordance for drift detection in medical imaging AI. arXiv preprint (2022). arXiv:2202.02833
9. Arevalo, J., González, F.A., Ramos-Pollán, R., Oliveira, J.L., Guevara, M.A.: Representation learning for mammography mass lesion classification with convolutional neural networks. Comput. Methods Programs Biomed. **127**, 248–257 (2016). https://doi.org/10.1016/j.cmpb.2015.12.014
10. Moreira, I.C., Amaral, I., Domingues, I., Cardoso, A., Cardoso, M.J., Cardoso, J.S.: INbreast: toward a full-field digital mammographic database. Acad. Radiol. **19**(2), 236–248 (2012). https://doi.org/10.1016/j.acra.2011.09.014
11. Lingle, W., et al.: The cancer genome atlas breast invasive carcinoma collection (TCGA-BRCA) (Version 3) [Data set]. Cancer Imag. Arch. (2016). https://doi.org/10.7937/K9/TCIA.2016.AB2NAZRP
12. Albertina, B., et al.: Radiology data from the cancer genome atlas lung adenocarcinoma [TCGA-LUAD] collection. Cancer Imag. Arch. (2016). https://doi.org/10.7937/K9/TCIA.2016.JGNIHEP5
13. Kirk, S., et al.: The cancer genome atlas lung squamous cell carcinoma collection (TCGA-LUSC) (Version 4) [Data set]. Cancer Imag. Arch. (2016). https://doi.org/10.7937/K9/TCIA.2016.TYGKKFMQ
14. García-González, M.J., et al.: CADIA: a success story in breast cancer diagnosis with digital pathology and AI image analysis. Applications of Medical Artificial Intelligence. AMAI 2022. Lecture Notes in Computer Science, vol. 13540. Springer, Cham (2022) https://doi.org/10.1007/978-3-031-17721-7_9
15. Baur, C., Denner, S., Wiestler, B., Navab, N., Albarqouni, S.: Autoencoders for unsupervised anomaly segmentation in brain MR images: a comparative study. Med. Image Anal. **69**, 101952 (2021). ISSN 1361–8415 (2021). https://doi.org/10.1016/j.media.2020.101952

Deep Learning-Based Assessment of Histological Grading in Breast Cancer Whole Slide Images

María Jesús García-González[1,5(✉)], Karen López-Linares Román[1,2],
Esther Albertín Marco[3], Iván Lalaguna[3], Javier García Navas[4],
Maria Blanca Cimadevila Álvarez[4], Ana Calvo Pérez[4],
and Valery Naranjo Ornedo[5]

[1] Vicomtech, Basque Research and Technology Alliance, San Sebastián, Spain
mjgarcia@vicomtech.org
[2] Biodonostia Health Research Institute, San Sebastián, Spain
[3] Instrumentación y Componentes SA, Inycom, Zaragoza, Spain
[4] Servicio Gallego de Salud, Galicia, Spain
[5] Universitat Politècnica de València, València, Spain

Abstract. Histological grading of breast cancer samples is critical for determining a patient's prognosis. Automatic grading of pathological cancer images promotes early diagnosis of the disease, as it is a long and tedious task for health professionals. In this paper, we propose an algorithm capable of predicting each component of the histological grade in Hematoxylin and eosin (H&E)-stained Whole-Slide Images (WSIs) of breast cancer. First, the WSI is split into tiles, and a classifier predicts the grade of both tubular formation and nuclear pleomorphism. Experiments are carried out with a proprietary database of 1,374 breast biopsy DICOM WSIs and evaluated on an independent test set of 120 images. Our model allows us to accurately classify the constitutive components of the histological grade both for all tumour samples and only-invasive samples.

Keywords: Digital pathology · breast cancer · histologic grade · deep learning

1 Introduction

According to the World Health Organisation (WHO), 2.3 million women were diagnosed with breast cancer in 2020, causing 685,000 deaths globally. Considering the 5-year relative survival rate, breast cancer is the world's most prevalent type of cancer [1].

To successfully control and manage the disease, the standardization of robust prognostic factors, both clinical and pathological, is critical to aid in patient decision-making and selecting suitable treatment options. In routine clinical practice, lymph node status, tumour size, and histological grade are used as prognostic factors. An expert pathologist's analysis of a hematoxylin and eosin

© The Author(s), under exclusive license to Springer Nature Singapore Pte Ltd. 2023
Y.-W. Chen et al. (Eds.): KES InMed 2023, SIST 357, pp. 355–364, 2023.
https://doi.org/10.1007/978-981-99-3311-2_32

(H&E)-stained biopsy is the current standard for determining all three factors. Focusing on the histological grade, several international health entities such as WHO, AJCC, EU, and UK RCPath recommend following the Nottingham Grading System (NGS) for its evaluation. NGS indicates the "degree of resemblance" of tumour cells to healthy tissue cells, and it is composed of three individual features [2]:

- Tubular formation. It relates to the percentage of tumour cells that forms tubular structures:
  - Grade 1 means more than 75% of cells are in tubule formation.
  - In grade 2, between 10 and 75% of cells form tubular structures.
  - A score of 3 is used when less than 10% of cells form tubules.
- Nuclear pleomorphism. It scores from 1 to 3 the degree of nuclear atypia.
  - Grade 1 is assigned when nuclei are only slightly enlarged and have minor variations in size, shape and chromatic pattern.
  - In grade 2, nuclei are enlarged and may be variable in shape.
  - Grade 3 is used for samples with markedly enlarged vesicular nuclei with often prominent nucleoli and a general variation in size and shape.
- Mitotic count. It is calculated as the number of mitoses per 10 high-power fields in the most mitotic active region in the tumour. It considers the number of mitoses and the specific microscope field diameter.

Lately, Digital Pathology (DP) is becoming more widespread and is revolutionizing histological features analysis. Although there are numerous definitions of this term, they all have in common the digitization of physical specimens, obtaining *Whole Slide Images (WSIs)*, and their use within the pathology workflow by substituting or complementing the physical samples for several tasks.

Many studies have evaluated the performance of using WSIs instead of physical samples observed under the microscope, demonstrating their non-inferiority in primary diagnosis [3]. Furthermore, DP opens up new opportunities such as telepathology or the development of artificial intelligence-driven digital pathology methods, which are accurate, unbiased and consistent [4]. Moreover, in 2017 the FDA approved pathology specimen scans, boosting their use and implementation in clinical routines [5].

Regarding breast cancer histological grading using WSIs, some interesting approaches have been proposed in the literature. In [6], they develop three deep-learning models to assess breast biopsy samples. First, they build a model able to segment the invasive component for the tumour in the sample and use the predicted region to feed three classifiers, one per each component of the NGS. Finally, they train a deep learning model to predict the patient's prognosis. In [7], they also exploit invasive breast biopsy samples to build a model that predicts the final histological grade for each input WSI. However, they do not consider grade II and use their trained model to reassign the grade II samples to the other classes.

In this work, we propose an AI-driven digital framework to support the histological grading of images from breast cancer biopsy samples by automatically predicting the individual components, i.e. tubular formation degree and nuclear pleomorphism, at a tile level. We discard the mitotic count assessment because it is predicted by counting individual mitoses of ten regions of the tumour. We train and evaluate our proposed methodology with an extensive and real-world proprietary database of H&E-stained WSIs derived from different hospitals, which includes samples with variations in staining and degradation due to the time they have been stored before being scanned, proving that our algorithm is robust against this source of bias. We run experiments considering all tumor types or only invasive carcinoma samples, as in [6].

Section 2.1 and Sect. 2.2 describe the input data and the preprocessing applied, respectively. The training procedure and the experimental setup followed during model development are described in Sect. 2.3. Finally, we present and discuss the results in Sect. 3 and provide some conclusions in Sect. 4.

2   Materials and Methods

In the following subsections, we describe our proposed method and database. Shortly, we begin with the extraction of tiles from the WSI's, considering the input expert annotations, and it's preprocessing. Then, a deep learning classifier outputs the tubular formation and the nuclear pleomorphism grades for each tile. Finally, a reconstruction step generates an image with the grade overlaid, showing the most relevant areas of the tumour and it's characteristics. Figure 1 depicts an scheme of the whole method.

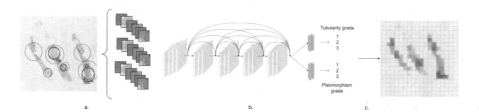

Fig. 1. Layout of the proposed method. a - tile extraction and labelling from expert annotations, b - deep learning architecture, and c - model outputs and reassembling the original image.

2.1   Input Data

This study uses retrospective and anonymized data collected from various Galician Healthcare System hospitals during the development of the CADIA project [8]. The database comprises 1,925 breast biopsy samples stained with H&E and scanned with a maximum resolution of 40x with the VENTANA DP 200 slide scanner, resulting in RGB WSIs. These samples are distributed into many histological types. As the histological grade is only given in association with a tumor, all benign samples were discarded, giving as a result a database with 1,374 tumor samples.

Each sample in the database is linked to a unique patient and is stored following the typical WSI structure -a pyramid of resolutions-, resulting in multiple DICOM instances. The instances are composed of a large number of tiles, mosaicking the original image.

To generate the training database, it is essential to capture pathologists' knowledge associated with a breast cancer diagnosis to use it as ground truth during model training and validation. For this reason, gathering values for tubularity and pleomorphism grades from pathologists was required; clinicians were asked to contour representative tumour regions of each histological type of breast cancer in the WSI and annotate the tubular and pleomorphism grades for each region. Each study was annotated by three pathologists in order to filter out some annotation mistakes and single-annotator biases. It is important to note that each annotator selected regions according to preference. In Fig. 2, an example of the annotations is shown.

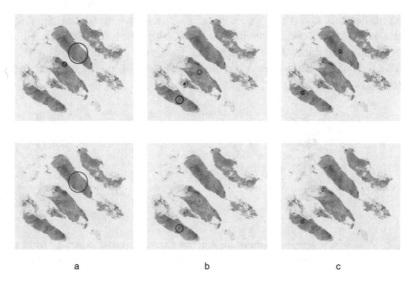

a   b   c

Fig. 2. Example of an annotation. top: tubular formation annotation, bottom: nuclear pleomorphism annotation. a) annotator 1, b) annotator 2, c) annotator 3. Green: grade I, yellow: grade II, red: grade III.

2.2 Tile Extraction and Preprocessing

In order to transform the pathologists' manual annotations into training samples, the next process is followed:

- According to expert pathologists' feedback, we select the second level of magnification of the pyramid of resolutions.

– Obtain the pixel coordinates at the selected level of resolution from the manual annotations.
– Retrieve the corresponding tiles with a shape of 1024×1024 pixels.
– Filter the background tiles (tiles with no tissue). To perform this step, we use the mean of all tiles in the database and check if the mean of the tile is higher than the mean to ignore it.
– Label the tiles with the aggregated information of the three annotators using majority voting. If there is no agreement, the higher annotated grade is selected.

We construct a second training database by filtering out only invasive samples and annotations because some experiments make predictions only with these samples.

The total number of training, validation and test images (tiles) used for our experiments after applying the described methodology is displayed in Table 1.

Table 1. Data distribution into training, validation and test data splits for all the grades. a - All tumor samples database, b - filtered dataset with only invasive samples.

Split	Grade	All tumors		Only IC	
		Tubularity	Pleomorphism	Tubularity	Pleomorphism
	I	24887	15660	3812	4670
Train	II	15037	67459	11646	28961
	III	57420	14225	23331	5236
	I	150	201	102	118
Validation	II	93	798	604	1070
	III	870	114	508	32
	I	2589	1962	412	541
Test	II	1340	6323	1073	3103
	III	5724	1368	2334	181

2.3   Deep Learning Architecture and Training Approach

We base all our experiments in a deep learning architecture, which has two independent classifiers, one for each component of the histological grade, but which share the feature extractor. We use a Densenet-121 [9] initialised with Imagenet weights as a feature extractor and add some new dense layers to classify the extracted features into the contemplated classes.

To make a prediction, the model processes all tiles that make up a WSI and performs the tubular and pleomorphism grading for each input tile. A heatmap is then constructed for each grade by reassembling the WSI, highlighting areas of interest in the image.

In order to train our model, we divide the database into training, validation, and test splits at the patient level. The test set counts with 10% of the samples, which were retrieved considering the hospital they came from; 8 examples for each hospital define the test set, equaling 120. The remaining 1,254 examples comprised the train set for all the models.

As the number of tiles in each class of the training dataset is unbalanced and could lead to a bias towards the majority class, we re-sample the dataset during training to ensure that each class has the same probability of being seen by the network on each epoch. To avoid the side effects of having multiple hospitals supplying samples, such as differences in the staining, we apply multiple forms of colour augmentations during training. The samples are randomly modified in hue, saturation and contrast, as well as random rotations and flip to avoid overfitting. We also normalize the images following the z-score equation, using the mean and standard deviation of the training database.

Regarding training hyperparameters, we use a batch size of 4, a learning rate of $1e-5$ and the Adam optimizer. The loss function used to optimize the parameters is the categorical cross-entropy for all the outputs and the one-hot encoding of the real class. All the experiments are executed on a single NVIDIA Tesla V100 SXM2 GPU Accelerator 32 GB, and the code is implemented in python 3.6 and Tensorflow 2.8.1.

2.4 Experimental Setup

From previous literature, we have extracted two main ideas, which lead us to define the following two experiments:

- Experiment 1: Grade-II samples should be analyzed independently because they might be subdivided into grade-I-like and grade-III-like samples. To test this hypothesis, we develop two models: 1) a model to predict grade I, grade II and grade III samples, and 2) a model to predict only grades I and III.
- Experiment 2: previous works only predict the histological grade in Invasive Carcinoma samples. To analyze this decision's influence on model performance, we train a model able to grade only invasive samples.

3   Results

This section summarizes the results obtained for the described experiments. The following statistical measurements are computed for the predicted outputs per class: sensibility (recall, True Positive Rate-TPR), specificity (True Negative Rate-TNR), and mean accuracy. We will also plot the confusion matrix for each experiment. In addition, we plot an example of the WSI reassembled with the model predictions overlayed.

3.1   Experiment 1

This section summarizes the results achieved with the database containing all tumour types.

We have developed a first model to predict grades I, II and III for all samples. The first column in Tables 2 and 3 shows the model performance for each grade evaluated on the test split. The first column of Fig. 3 (a) and (b) contains the confusion matrix for tubularity and pleomorphism, respectively. As observed, grade-II results corroborate the idea that these samples introduce noise in the optimal characterization of the grading problem.

As explained in Sect. 2.4 and based on model 1 results, we have developed a second model which only predicts grades I and III. The middle column in Tables 2 and 3 summarizes the achieved performance for each grade evaluated on the test split. The middle column of Figs. 3 (a) and (b) contain the confusion matrices for each component of the histologic grade. Comparing grades I and III results with the previous experiment performance, we can conclude that a vast improvement in model performance for these classes is achieved, supporting the idea that grade-II samples should be assessed independently.

Table 2. Results predicting the tubular formation grade in the test set in terms of sensibility and specificity for all experiment and classes.

	Exp. 1 - model 1			*Exp. 1 - model 2*		*Exp. 2*	
	Grade I	*Grade II*	*Grade III*	*Grade I*	*Grade III*	*Grade I*	*Grade III*
Sensibility	0.77	0.36	0.80	0.73	0.80	0.78	0.83
Specificity	0.94	0.89	0.68	0.80	0.73	0.83	0.78
Accuracy		0.75			0.78		0.82

Table 3. Results predicting the nuclear pleomorphism grade in the test set in terms of sensibility and specificity for all experiment and classes.

	Exp. 1 - model 1			*Exp. 1 - model 2*		*Exp. 2*	
	Grade I	*Grade II*	*Grade III*	*Grade I*	*Grade III*	*Grade I*	*Grade III*
Sensibility	0.73	0.26	0.80	0.73	0.93	0.91	0.94
Specificity	0.78	0.92	0.57	0.93	0.73	0.94	0.91
Accuracy		0.79			0.88		0.94

3.2   Experiment 2

This section summarizes the results achieved only by predicting grades I and III for the invasive samples. We have filtered the samples in the database, training, validating and testing the model with the data distribution shown in Table 1, only the IC column.

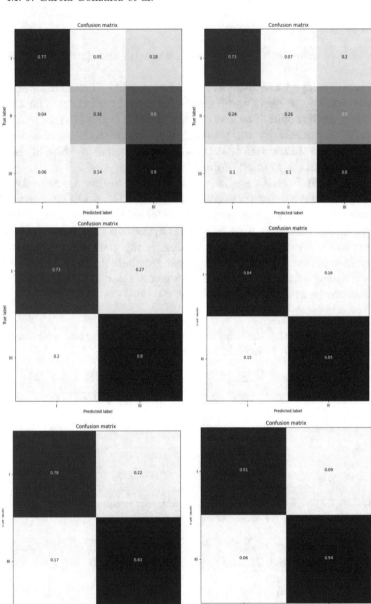

Fig. 3. Tubular formation (a) and nuclear pleomorphism (b) confusion matrices for experiment 1.

The last column in Tables 2 and 3 contains the quantitative evaluation of the model performance; in the last column of Figs. 3 (a) and (b) the confusion matrices for the prediction of the tubularity and nuclear pleomorphism grades are displayed. Analyzing the results for this experiment, only predicting the histological grade in invasive samples seems to simplify the problem, improving the performance of the model.

In Fig. 4, we depict an example of the reassembling of a WSI with the model's predictions overlayed.

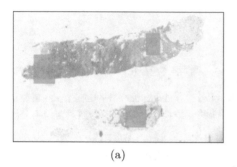 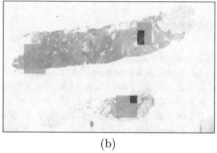

(a)   (b)

Fig. 4. Example of model's predictions overlayed in the reassembled WSI. Green: grade I, red: grade III. a) Tubular formation predictions, b) nuclear pleomorphism predictions.

4   Conclusions and Future Perspectives

In this paper, we introduced a deep learning-based approach for automatically grading WSIs in different histological grades.

We have demonstrated that our developed system can accurately grade all tumours in the database, not only focusing on the invasive samples. This makes our model clinically more interesting as compared to other state-of-the-art works, giving insights into the degree of differentiation for all tumour samples.

Another strength of the proposed approach is that the model independently predicts the constitutive components of the histological grade. This fact, combined with the WSI reassembling overlayed with the grades, acts as model interpretability, which raises the clinician's trust in the decisions automatically made.

One of the main drawbacks of the approximation is that all tissue samples of the database were scanned with the same device, so its performance on digital samples from other scanners should be checked. Also, we do not predict the mitotic count component of the histological grade.

In conclusion, this approach results in an accurate and potential solution for breast cancer histological grading that can support pathologists' daily work. In future work, we will expand the model robustness by enlarging the database with samples for other scanners.

Acknowledgements. The authors do not declare any conflict of interest. This work has been partially funded by FEDER "Una manera de hacer Europa". This research has been done within the project CADIA - Sistema de Deteccion de Diversas Patologias Basado en el Analisis de Imagen con Inteligencia Artificial (DG-SER1-19-003) under the Codigo100 Public Procurement and Innovation Programme by the Galician Health Service - Servizo Galego de Saude (SERGAS) co-funded by the European Regional Development Fund (ERDF).

We would like to acknowledge the work done by the pathologists at Ferrol, Lugo, Ourense, Pontevedra, Santiago, and Vigo health service areas from the Galician Health System.

References

1. World Health Organization (WHO): Breast Cancer (2021). https://www.who.int/news-room/fact-sheets/detail/breast-cancer
2. Rakha, E.A., Reis-Filho, J.S., Baehner, F., et al.: Breast cancer prognostic classification in the molecular era: the role of histological grade. Breast Cancer Res. **12**, 207 (2010). https://doi.org/10.1186/bcr2607
3. Mukhopadhyay, S., et al.: Whole slide imaging versus microscopy for primary diagnosis in surgical pathology: a multicenter blinded randomized noninferiority study of 1992 cases (pivotal study). Am. J. Surg. Pathol. **42**(1) (2018). ISSN 0147-5185. https://journals.lww.com/ajsp/Fulltext/2018/01000/Whole_Slide_Imaging_Versus_Microscopy_for_Primary.6.aspx
4. Baxi, V., Edwards, R., Montalto, M., et al.: Digital pathology and artificial intelligence in translational medicine and clinical practice. Mod. Pathol. **35**, 23–32 (2022). https://doi.org/10.1038/s41379-021-00919-2
5. Food and Drug Administration: FDA allows marketing of first whole slide imaging system for digital pathology (2017). https://www.fda.gov/news-events/press-announcements/fda-allows-marketing-first-whole-slide-imaging-system-digital-pathology
6. Jaroensri, R., Wulczyn, E., Hegde, N., et al.: Deep learning models for histologic grading of breast cancer and association with disease prognosis. NPJ Breast Cancer **8**, 113 (2022). https://doi.org/10.1038/s41523-022-00478-y
7. Wang, Y., et al.: Improved breast cancer histological grading using deep learning. Ann. Oncol. **33**(1), 89–98 (2022). https://doi.org/10.1016/j.annonc.2021.09.007
8. Garcia-Gonzalez, M.J., et al.: CADIA: a success story in breast cancer diagnosis with digital pathology and AI image analysis. In: Wu, S., Shabestari, B., Xing, L. (eds.) AMAI 2022. LNCS, vol. 13540, pp. 79–87. Springer, Cham (2022). https://doi.org/10.1007/978-3-031-17721-7_9
9. Huang, G., Liu, Z., Maaten, L., Weinberger, K.: Densely connected convolutional. Networks (2016). https://doi.org/10.48550/ARXIV.1608.06993

Sample Viability Assessment from H&E Whole Slide Images for Lung Cancer Molecular Testing

Laura Valeria Perez-Herrera[1][(✉)], María Jesús García-González[1],
Ruth Román Lladó[2], Cristina Aguado[2], Josep Castellvi[2], Sonia Rodriguez[2],
Erika Aldeguer[2], María Teresa Torrijos[3], and Karen Lopez-Linares[1]

[1] Fundación Centro de Tecnologías de Interacción Visual y Comunicaciones Vicomtech, Donostia-San Sebastian, Spain
lvperez@vicomtech.org
[2] Pangaea Oncology SA, Barcelona, Spain
[3] Instrumentación y Componentes SA Inycom, Zaragoza, Spain

Abstract. Molecular testing has become an essential tool in precision oncology as targeted therapies have shown to increase the survival rate of patients. However, for molecular test results to be reliable, some requirements must be met, such as the presence of a minimum percentage of tumor cells in a minimum area of the sample. Currently, this analysis is performed by viewing the histopathological slides under the microscope and manually quantifying and highlighting the areas with the highest tumor cellularity. This results in low reproducibility and high subjectivity. To address these problems, we propose a deep learning framework to assist pathologists in the evaluation of the viability of a sample for molecular testing. The developed approach highlights viable sample regions, as well as areas that require further processing. To this aim, we implement a 3-step methodology to analyze Whole Slide Images (WSI): 1) stain normalization of WSI tiles, 2) classification of tiles by a cascade approach, 3) heatmap generation to determine the area of the WSI to perform molecular testing. Moreover, we use three lung cancer subtypes and compare the performance when the models are trained separately for each type or jointly. We achieve a F1-score of **0.63** at tile-level, while at the WSI-level the F1-scores were **0.71** and **0.96**.

1 Introduction

Lung cancer is the second most common cancer worldwide, with more than 2.2 million new cases diagnosed in 2020 [1]. There are two main types of lung cancer: non-small cell (NSCLC) and small-cell carcinoma (SCLC). 80% to 85% of lung cancers are NSCLC and its main subtypes are adenocarcinoma and squamous cell carcinoma.

The gold standard for diagnosing lung cancer is to perform a biopsy, in which a small amount of tissue is removed for microscopic examination by a pathologist.

Y.-W. Chen et al. (Eds.): KES InMed 2023, SIST 357, pp. 365–374, 2023.
https://doi.org/10.1007/978-981-99-3311-2_33

Then, several tests, such as molecular tests, can be performed to characterize the tumor and its prognosis, and make treatment decisions.

Precision oncology uses information about a tumor's genes or proteins to better diagnose and treat a patient. It has shown to contribute to improved treatment outcomes and quality of life for patients. Whenever molecular testing is requested, pathologists need to determine whether a sample contains sufficient tumor tissue for testing. The viability of the sample depends on different factors: the percentage of tumor cells, the area in which this percentage is found, the sensitivity of the test to be performed and the platform used. For instance, to perform next generation sequencing (NGS) the requirement ranges from 10 to 25 percent of tumor cells on an area of more than $4\,mm^2$ or more than 25% on a smaller area. However, there are many cases where this is not met and areas with more than 10% may be considered too.

If the estimate of tumor cellularity (TC) is below the analytical sensitivity of the assay, the sample should be discarded, as otherwise the test could be run with the risk of obtaining a false result, resulting in an incorrect treatment selection. On the other hand, if quality and quantity requirements are met, it is important to locate the area from which tissue should be extracted to increase the reliability and accuracy of the results.

The ability of deep learning (DL) to perform repetitive tasks with human-like or better performance makes it a great tool for assisting clinicians in the interpretation of medical images. Some of the tasks that can be performed by DL to assist in the workflow of pathologists is the quantification of TC, as currently, this quantification is too time-consuming and prone to high inter- and intra-observer variability [2]. In [3], authors observed that the first analysis of TC performed by the pathologists often resulted in an overestimation of the percentage of tumor nuclei but that it could be reduced after providing an adequate training and feedback. Similarly, [4] conducted an analysis to determine the reliability of the estimated percentages of tumor cells and observed that 38% of samples were considered eligible for testing when in fact there was an insufficient percentage of tumor cells (less than 20%). This overestimation, found in pathologists' quantification in both studies, is considered particularly serious as it could lead to false results and, consequently, misdiagnosis.

To the best of our knowledge, there is only one work addressing the problem of TC quantification for molecular testing in lung cancer [5]. The work implemented a tumor segmentation network and a nuclear counting algorithm only for adenocarcinoma samples, which was then used to adjust the scores determined by pathologists. They demonstrated that by incorporating AI, pathologists modified their initial estimate in 87% of the samples and achieved a more precise score.

Based on the relevance of an accurate assessment of TC for the performance of molecular tests, the aim of this paper is to present our ongoing work about the implementation of a system to determine if a sample is viable for testing, providing the area with the highest TC from which molecular tests should be performed to obtain a reliable result. The remainder of this paper is organized as follows. Section 2 presents the dataset used to develop our method. The proposed approach is explained in Sect. 3. Next, section 4 presents the obtained results and an interpretation of them. Finally, Sect. 5 summarizes the conclusions.

2 Dataset

The data for this work consists of 65 H&E-stained tissue samples collected retrospectively from Pangaea; a company focused on precision oncology. The samples were already diagnosed with lung cancer and manually scored with respect to the percentage of tumor cells in the whole sample and the maximum percentage in a manually delineated area. Samples were selected considering these percentages to have variability in the dataset. In addition, only samples with less than two years were included in the study to ensure degradation of staining was not present.

The slides were scanned using an Aperio CS2 Scanner, generating the WSIs in .svs format. According to pathologists' feedback, it is enough for TC quantification to work with a magnification of 10x, where a WSI tile corresponds to an area of $1mm^2$ and has a total of 1024×1024 pixels.

2.1 Annotation Approach

Regarding image labelling, a tile-by-tile annotation approach was followed. First, all the tiles from the WSI were extracted and the ones with no tissue were discarded. The resulting tiles, saved in .png format, were presented to annotators.

Focusing on the tissue area, annotators assigned a numeric value to each tile from 0 to 100%. The annotation included each type of tissue category (tumor, stroma, inflammation, and necrosis) adding up to a total of 100%. This way, a pathologist, and an experienced molecular biologist responsible for pathological anatomy within Pangaea annotated a total of 4,466 tiles, divided as shown in Table 1.

Table 1. Number of patients and tiles by type of carcinoma, including mean ± std of percentage of tumor cells for WSIs and for region with maximum tumor tissue.

Type	# Pat	# Tiles	Mean %	Max %
Adenocarcinoma	15	2016	31.67±18.77	48.57±15.05
Squamous	20	1465	45.75±23.51	56.00±21.07
Small-cell	30	985	65.16±21.73	72.16±18.82

Finally, as the goal of this work is to determine if a sample is viable for testing, indicating the area, tiles were grouped according to TC into *no tumor* (0), *non-viable* (from 1-10 percent), *probably viable* (from 11 to 25 percent) and *viable* (more than 25 percent) for algorithm development, as suggested by pathologists.

3   Methodology

To predict if a sample is viable for testing, highlighting the area from which the tissue should be extracted, we implement a three-step methodology: 1) stain normalization; 2) DL-based classification of TC in the groups mentioned in 2, following a cascade approach; and 3) WSI viability determination with TC heatmap generation. Steps 1 and 2 were performed at tile level and are shown in Fig. 1.

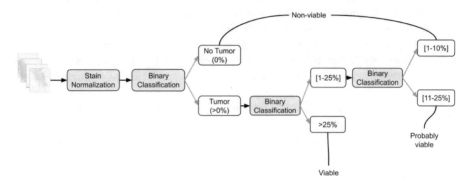

Fig. 1. Overview of the cascade approach to assess viable samples for molecular testing and rule out inadequate ones.

3.1   Stain Normalization

The first step of the workflow corresponds to tile resizing to $512 \times 512 \times 3$ pixels and stain normalization following the methodology proposed in [6]. This step is considered essential since pathology images present variations in stain intensities that greatly influence the performance of DL models. These variations come from different sources such as the slide preparation and storage. Examples of the normalization results are shown in Fig. 2. After that, z-score normalization (subtracting the mean and dividing by the standard deviation) is applied. The mean and standard deviation are computed with the training set for each model in the cascade, considering only the specific type of carcinoma or all types.

3.2   Tile-level Classification of TC

For this step, a cascade approach composed by three models is implemented, as shown in Fig. 1. The first model classifies tiles as tumor or no tumor. Then, a second model predicts whether the tile has less or more than 25% of TC. Finally, a third model stratifies tiles with less than 25% into 1-10% or 11-25%. In addition, we tried to determine whether performance would improve with more samples (all carcinoma types together for training) or by focusing on one carcinoma type

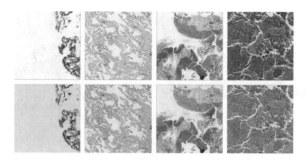

Fig. 2. First row: original tiles. Second row: tiles after normalization.

at a time. For all classification models we use a VGG16 architecture pretrained on ImageNet, without the last fully-connected layers.

Furthermore, based on the work of [7] we implement a simplified deep supervision (adding supervision only on one hidden layer). Thus, in the selected hidden layer, a classification is made from its output to add supervision and the loss of such supervision is combined with the final loss. The main advantage of this method is that it simultaneously minimizes the classification error while making the learning process of hidden layers direct and transparent. Moreover, it results in faster convergence of the network and acts as a feature regularization (allowing to obtain more discriminative and robust features).

The classification block consists of six layers. The first layer corresponds to a global average pooling, which is followed by two dense layers (varying number of units), each with a dropout layer of 0.2, and a final classification by a dense layer with 2 units and softmax as activation function. The activation function of the previous dense layers is a relu and a $l2$ kernel regularizer is used to decrease the risk of over-fitting. This classification block is added after both the selected hidden layer and the last layer from VGG16. The architecture is shown in Fig. 3.

The training and validation sets are split by tiles. For the test set, 4 separate patients for each carcinoma type are selected to avoid overly optimistic results and to ensure the presence of all classes. All models are trained with a learning rate of 1e-6 with Adam optimizer and categorical cross-entropy. Furthermore, to avoid overfitting, we use online data augmentations (random rotations, vertical and horizontal flipping) and we use early stopping if the validation loss stops decreasing after 30 epochs. All models are implemented with the Keras and Tensorflow frameworks on a NVIDIA GeForce RTX 2080 Ti with 12 GB.

3.3   Sample Viability Assessment and Testing Area Selection from TC Heatmap

As the goal is to determine if a sample is viable for molecular testing, a post processing of the output of the tile-level cascade classifiers is performed, which includes the generation of a WSI heatmap of TC and determination of the region

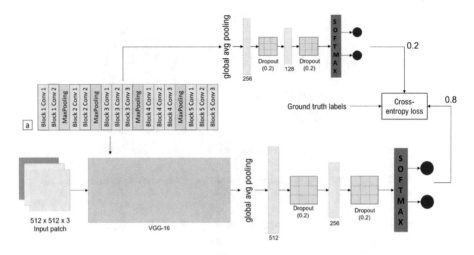

Fig. 3. Network architecture for classification of tumor percentage, a) shows VGG16 architecture. Loss from the selected hidden layer is added with less weight (0.2) than loss from the last layer of VGG16 (0.8).

of interest (ROI) with maximum TC meeting the requirements for molecular testing.

As each tile represents an area of $1mm^2$, but $4mm^2$ are usually needed for testing, a tile-grouping algorithm is proposed to generate the heatmap and extract the ROI. First, we predict TC for each tile using the cascade classifiers and assemble a WSI heatmap with those predictions. From there, we estimate whether there is an area with more than 4 adjacent tiles (corresponding to the minimum area for molecular testing) with more than 25% TC. If this criterion is met, a ROI is created surrounding all the tiles that fit this ROI (which may include other adjacent tiles with different TC percentages). The median value in the ROI is computed and this result is assigned to the entire ROI to assess whether it is a valid region to extract tissue for testing.

Conversely, if there are no 4 neighboring tiles with 25% TC, we search for the 11-25% tiles to add to the 25% area and perform the above steps to create the ROI and analyze it. Finally, the last possibility is to consider that there are no 25% tiles and select tiles only with 11-25% TC. Hence, the output of our approach is a heatmap of TC from the WSI and the viable area for testing. An example of the process for defining the ROI is shown in Fig. 4.

To evaluate the proposed approach we compared our results with the maximum percentage of tumor specified in the pathologists' report from when the sample was first analyzed and with the tile-level annotations with the same post processing.

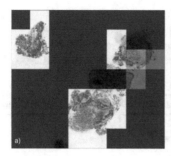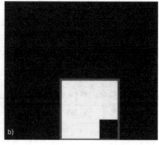

Fig. 4. Overview of the ROI definition determining if a sample is viable for testing. The WSI with the overlay heatmap is shown in a), areas with more than 25% are highlighted with white. The area with more tumor percentage is shown in b) with the yellow region corresponding to tiles with more than 25% and the red rectangle is the final ROI from which tissue should be removed for testing.

4   Results

We evaluate the performance of our proposed approach in two ways: 1) evaluation of cascade classifiers for tile-lever TC quantification, and 2) evaluation of whole sample feasibility for molecular testing.

Results for the whole cascade approach at tile-level are shown in Table 2. The best results for adeno- and small-cell carcinomas were obtained with the models trained with all tumor subtypes. However, for squamous carcinoma there were highly increased with the specialized network (trained only with its own samples).

Based on these results, it was considered that the model performed best when trained with only its samples for the specific case where there were enough samples for learning and especially if the distribution was similar across all sets. Tissue samples contain a wide variety of cells and not only tumor cells. Thus, in a sample there are nuclei corresponding to tumor cells but also to non-tumorous or normal tissue components, which may induce the model to predict a percentage of tumor cellularity different from the real one. In our problem, the annotations included inflamed cells, necrosis, and stroma.

Generally, in the presence of stromal cells the model tended to predict less TC than that observed in a tile. And in the presence of more inflamed cells the model predicted more TC. This affected adenocarcinoma and small-cell more, as their test sets had more samples with more inflammation and less stroma compared to training and validation. Thus, they benefited when squamous carcinoma was added to training, as the distribution was more similar.

Looking at the results of each step of the cascade approach, it was observed that the most difficult prediction was found in the last step. The first classifier divides tiles as tumor or no tumor, being the F1-scores **0.80**, **0.77** and **0.82** for adeno-, squamous and small-cell carcinoma, respectively. In the second model, trained to distinguish between tiles with more or less than 25% of TC, we obtain

Table 2. Evaluation of performance on the test sets obtained from *cascade approach* at tile-level. Models were trained with all carcinomas (*), adenocarcinoma samples (A), squamous carcinoma (SQ) or small-cell carcinoma (SC). Metrics are computed considering the number of examples per class. Best results on each type of carcinoma are highlighted.

Model	Test	Specificity	Sensitivity	Precision	F1-score
*	*	0.81	0.61	0.60	0.61
*	**A**	**0.78**	**0.65**	**0.63**	**0.63**
*	SQ	0.86	0.47	0.52	0.49
*	**SC**	**0.78**	**0.65**	**0.63**	**0.63**
A	A	0.72	0.59	0.61	0.59
SQ	**SQ**	**0.83**	**0.64**	**0.62**	**0.62**
SC	SC	0.80	0.58	0.66	0.61

F1-scores of **0.74**, **0.78** and **0.73**. Finally, the third classifier provides F1-scores of **0.59**, **0.74** and **0.45**. The best results of this third model were obtained with squamous carcinoma and the worst with the small-cell subtype.

Results at WSI-level (sample viability) are shown in Fig. 5 and Table 3. It can be observed that our proposed approach achieved a similar F1-score to that of the pathologists' report when compared to the tile-level annotations. Furthermore, when comparing our results with those of the report, we only misclassified one sample. However, in the entire dataset (considering the pathologists' report) there were only four samples corresponding to the *probably viable* class and none in the *unviable* class. Therefore, the performance of the model in these classes could not be properly evaluated. Finally, since at the tile-level the model performed well with no tumor cells, it is believed that non-viable samples would be correctly detected. Some examples of the prediction at WSI-level are shown in Fig. 6.

Table 3. Evaluation of performance on the test set obtained from comparison between the results of the proposed methodology using the tile-level annotations (TL-A), the ones from the pathologists' report (PR) and the proposed approach (PA).

	Specificity	Sensitivity	Precision	F1-score
PR vs TL-A	1	0.83	0.69	0.76
PA vs TL-A	0.90	0.75	0.68	0.71
PA vs PR	0.92	0.92	1	0.96

It was observed that the main problem with the model arose when distinguishing between 1-10% and 11-25% tiles. There were two reasons for this. Firstly, there were fewer examples for these classes and secondly, there is likely

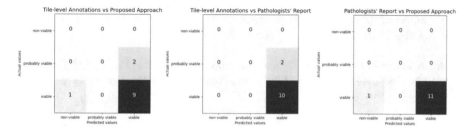

Fig. 5. Confusion matrix for viability assessment. Comparison between tile-level annotations, pathologists' report and the predictions made by the proposed approach.

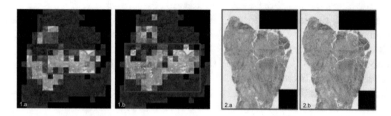

Fig. 6. 1.a and 2.a show the model predictions, while 1.b and 2.b represent the heatmaps made from the tile-level annotations.

to be a lot of noise present in the annotations, as these ranges are very small and accurate estimation by pathologists is very complicated. In addition, it is common practice for more than two pathologists to annotate the images and reach a consensus. However, in our case this was not possible, as this is a costly and a time-consuming process. In fact, this variability can be confirmed by analyzing the results of the tile-level annotations and the pathologists' report, as there are differences between them that should not be present. Thus, it is believed that training the model with more reliable annotations or with techniques to address the problem of noisy labels, could improve the performance.

5   Conclusions

In this work, we evaluated whether DL algorithms could help pathologists select viable areas for analysis in a WSI to ensure compliance with quantitative requirements. Our results suggest that, although there is room for improvement, it is possible for DL algorithms to determine the percentage of tumor cells in a sample. Furthermore, it was observed that the use of more samples, even if they contained different morphologies, is beneficial to the model, especially if there is variability between the training, validation, and test sets. Thus, stratification should be performed with two objectives, to balance the percentage of tumor in all sets and to consider the distribution of other tissues present in the samples.

These are preliminary results of work in progress. Therefore, further analysis will be performed to evaluate the best approach to determine the most viable area. Some of the possible improvements could be to assign more weight to specific classes in the training of the model.

Acknowledgments. This work has been done within the PATHFLOW project, funded by the Spanish Ministry of Industry, Commerce and Tourism under grant AEI-010500-2021b-181.

References

1. Lung cancer statistics — world cancer research fund international. https://www.wcrf.org/cancer-trends/lung-cancer-statistics/
2. Holzinger, A., Goebel, R., Mengel, M., Müller, H. (eds.): Artificial Intelligence and Machine Learning for Digital Pathology. LNCS (LNAI), vol. 12090. Springer, Cham (2020). https://doi.org/10.1007/978-3-030-50402-1
3. Mikubo, M., et al.: Calculating the tumor nuclei content for comprehensive cancer panel testing. J. Thoracic Oncol. **15**, 130–137 (2020)
4. Smits, A.J., et al.: The estimation of tumor cell percentage for molecular testing by pathologists is not accurate. Mod. Pathol. **27**, 168–174 (2014)
5. Sakamoto, T., et al.: Collaborative workflow between pathologists and deep learning for evaluation of tumor cellularity in lung adenocarcinoma. Histopathology **81**, 758–769 (2022)
6. Vahadane, A., et al.: Structure-preserving color normalization and sparse stain separation for histological images. IEEE Trans. Med. Imag. **35**, 1962–1971 (2016)
7. Lee, C.Y., et al.: Deeply-supervised nets. J. Mach. Learn. Res. **38**, 1962–1971 (2015)

Lobar Emphysema Quantification on Chest X-Rays Using a Generative Adversarial Regressor

Mónica Iturrioz Campo[1,2], Javier Pascau[2], and Raúl San José Estépar[1](✉)

[1] Applied Chest Imaging Laboratory, Brigham and Women's Hospital, Boston, MA, USA
rsanjose@bwh.harvard.edu
[2] Dept. de Bioingeniería e Ingeniería Aeroespacial, Universidad Carlos III de Madrid, Madrid, Spain

Abstract. Emphysema quantification and localization is a key factor determining COPD treatment, as the efficacy of each procedure varies with the burden of disease and its distribution; emphysema quantification is done on CT imaging, despite chest X-rays (CXR) being the preferred, and more clinically available, tool for diagnosis and management of COPD patients. We present a method to quantify lobar emphysema using digitally reconstructed radiographs (DRR) obtained from CT scans, based on a Sim-GAN regressor network which aims to both refine the DRR to make them look more realistic and calculate the emphysema percentage of each lobe for any given subject. The developed model was able to improve X-ray-based emphysema diagnosis, correctly understanding the volumetric distribution of each lung region, with a mean absolute error of 4.46 and an accuracy of 87.97% for an emphysema definition of $\geq 10\%$, with a mean sensitivity of 81.61%. CXR-based Upper vs. Lower lobe predominant classification had an accuracy of 66% and 67% for the left and right lung, respectively. These results could open the door to further explore the role of X-ray for patient selection for therapeutic treatment of emphysema using lung volume reduction techniques.

Keywords: X-ray · Emphysema quantification · CNN · Sim-GAN · Biomarker regression · COPD

1 Introduction

Emphysema is a condition of the lung characterized by the damage and destruction of the lung tissue, without any obvious scarring. Along with chronic bronchitis, it is one of the components of Chronic Obstructive Pulmonary Disease (COPD), which was the 3rd leading cause of death worldwide as of 2019, being responsible for over 3 million deaths that year [1]. COPD has no cure and treatment is merely palliative, whether in the form of surgery, medication and/or respiratory rehabilitation. The recommended treatment for severe emphysema is to undergo Lung Volume Reduction Surgery (LVRS), which consists of resecting and removing the most affected parts of the lung. In recent years, a new approach has been developed, Bronchoscopic Lung Volume Reduction (BLVR),

© The Author(s), under exclusive license to Springer Nature Singapore Pte Ltd. 2023
Y.-W. Chen et al. (Eds.): KES InMed 2023, SIST 357, pp. 375–384, 2023.
https://doi.org/10.1007/978-981-99-3311-2_34

which consists of deflating the most affected area of the lung through the placement of an endobronchial valve. This procedure yields similar results to LVRS, with the advantage of being less invasive as it is done endoscopically [2]. The main drawback, however, is the patient selection, as this procedure is only recommended to patients with localized severe emphysema, which calls for both localization and quantification of the condition, which can only be done using quantitative CT imaging to define the amount of emphysema per lobe and their distribution. Despite the availability of CT, chest X-Rays (CXR) continues to be the most readily available imaging modality for the management of chronic subjects.

To bridge the gap between emphysema quantification in CT and CXR, Digitally Reconstructed Radiographs (DRRs) can be a useful tool. On our previous work we developed a method to quantify emphysema on X-rays, as they are routinely used to diagnose chest diseases given that they are fast and cheap when compared with CT scans. Through the design and use of a CNN we proved that it is possible to obtain an accurate emphysema percentage of any given patient using an antero-posterior chest DRR [3]. Other authors have similarly explored the use of DRRs to quantify total lung volumes [4]. We aim to advance these works in two different areas: first, we want to improve the generative model in order to create more realistic DRRs; second, we want to expand our regressor model to include the spatial distribution of emphysema along with the percentage score. Our goal is to build a regressor model with an integrated generative adversarial network (GAN) that will take in DRRs, refine them to make them look more realistic, and output the emphysema percentage distribution throughout the lung lobes to develop a tool to assess the quantitative distribution of emphysema on X-rays.

2 Material and Methods

2.1 Emphysema Scoring

The emphysema scores were calculated on 4,095 inspiratory CT scans of the phase 2 of the COPDGene cohort [5], using the LAA% approach. First, we segmented the lungs, along with their lobes, using the approach provided in the Chest Imaging Platform (www. chestimagingplatform.org). LAA% was computed as the percentage of lung voxels below -950HU. A total of 8 scores were generated per scan: the total score, the score of each individual lung (left vs. right), and of each individual lobe.

2.2 X-ray Generation

We generated DRRs from the CT scans to create a database of X-ray images with corresponding emphysema scores in a two-step process. First, we created an initial approximation of the projection based on the parallel projection model using our previous proposed approximation [3]. We optimized β (the boosting of X-ray absorption through the tissues) using an anthropomorphic phantom scanned on both a CT and a CXR, setting it to 0.9982. All CT scans were resampled to 512x512x600 (ensuring no distortion of the volumes through stretching) and processed to remove the CT table and outside air using Otsu thresholding and applying hole filling to the largest component. Both antero-posterior (AP) and lateral (LAT) views were generated for each subject. We then applied a CNN-based generative model, G(x), to alter the appearance of our projections to make them look more realistic. The generator was trained in an adversarial structure with both DRRs and real X-rays, forcing it to learn the characteristics present in real X-ray images to apply them to DRRs to make them look more realistic. The generative model is further explained in Sect. 2.4.

2.3 Dataset

We made use of 3 different databases: COPDGene phase 2, NIH ChestX-ray14 and the National Lung Screening Trial (NLST) cohort (Fig. 1).

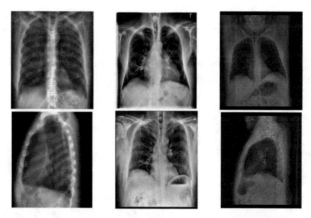

Fig. 1. Sample DRRs (left), real X-rays (NIH ChestX-ray14) (middle) and scouts (NLST) (right).

The COPDGene portion of our data consists of 4,095 subjects with their respective emphysema scores. Analyzing the distribution of scores of our data, we observed that it was severely skewed to the right, with roughly 75% of the scores being below 5%. To overcome this problem, we decided to perform weighted data augmentation on the dataset to balance the score distribution. We divided our data in 4 groups depending on the emphysema severity (no emphysema, mild, moderate and severe), augmented the largest group by a factor of 2, and then adjusted this value for the 3 remaining groups so that each group would have the same number of images as the first one. The transformations included small rotations of the CT volume around the z-axis (up to $\pm 10°$), changes of the β coefficient (from 0.9 to 1.8), small rotations of the X-ray projection (up to $\pm 5°$), small vertical shifts and small horizontal shifts (up to ± 30 pixels). We selected 1,124 subjects for training and, by means of weighted data augmentation, we generated 15,000 DRR samples (both AP and LAT), and used the remaining 2,971 subjects for testing (with no data augmentation).

The NIH ChestX-ray14 database contains 112,120 real AP X-rays that have been manually tagged with 14 different thoracic diseases, including emphysema. We retrieved those images that were either classified as *"no findings"* or *"emphysema"*, excluding all other 13 conditions and those subjects that were labeled with more diseases than just emphysema. Using this criterion, we ended up with a set of 1,000 AP NIH real X-ray images. We tagged them as having emphysema or not, to later use them in the Sim-GAN training portion of our proposed regression network.

Lastly, the NLST cohort is composed of 17,147 low dose CT scans, out of which 8,222 have both AP and LAT scouts, as well as the associated regional emphysema score extracted from CT as mentioned above.

Both NIH and NLST images were resampled to match the DRR dimensions (512x600). We then equalized the histograms of all three datasets using CLAHE [6] to improve contrast and enhance small details in the lungs and normalized their intensities.

2.4   Network

We built a regression model composed of two sequential networks: a Sim-GAN and a regressor. Sim-GANs (Simulated Generative Adversarial Networks) are composed of two competing CNNs, a refiner and a discriminator, and their goal is to take an artificially generated image and alter its appearance to give it a more realistic look without changing the information represented in the original image [7] (Fig. 2).

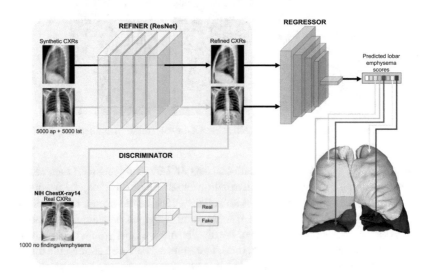

Fig. 2. Architecture of the Sim-GAN emphysema regressor.

The refiner (a 4-block ResNet) of our network takes as input the COPDGene DRR (a pair of AP and LAT images) and it outputs a more realistic depiction of them. The inputs of the discriminator (a simple classifier CNN) are a subset of the real NIH X-ray images and the refined AP projections, and its outputs are binary labels representing whether an image is thought to be real or not. The regressor network (a CNN composed of a concatenating layer, followed by 2 blocks of 3 Conv2D followed by a MaxPool2D, and a block of 5 Dense layers) takes the output of the generator (a pair of images, AP and LAT) as input, and it outputs a vector of 8 values, each one representing the emphysema score of each of the already defined lung regions. We used a regularized Mean Squared

Error loss function to train the regressor, which also takes into consideration the Mean Absolute Error following MSE +0.05*MAE.

Due to time and computational restraints, we selected 4,500 DRR samples (both AP and LAT) for training, another 500 to use for validation, and all 1,000 real X-rays for the discriminator. The 2 networks (Sim-GAN and regressor) were independently pre-trained for a few epochs, and then trained simultaneously to ensure that the refined images were adequate to predict the emphysema scores. Once the training was completed, we took a separate set of 10,000 DRRs and ran them through the refiner, to then use them to retrain the regressor network on its own (9,000 for training and 1,000 for validation).

3   Results

We selected 2,971 COPDGene subjects that had not been used for training nor validation to test the performance of our regressor. These images were first run through the refiner, and then through the regressor to get the emphysema predictions for each subject. This set was not augmented, and so the distribution of scores is heavily unbalanced, with most subjects in the 0–5% range.

3.1   GAN DRR Visual Performance

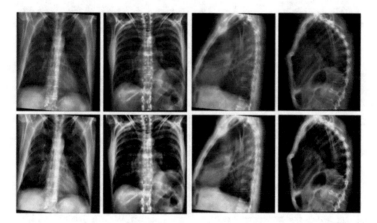

Fig. 3. Synthetic (top) and refined (bottom) AP and LAT DRRs.

To assess the effectiveness of the refiner network, we evaluated the discriminative ability of our trained discriminator on both the pre-refinement and post-refinement digital reconstructed radiographs (DRRs). The pre-refinement DRRs had an average probability of being classified as "artificial" of 0.99 ± 0.007, while the refined DRRs had an average probability of 0.98 ± 0.011 ($p < 0.001$). Visually comparing the images, the refined DRRs showed a decrease in contrast in bright areas, such as the central thorax where the heart overlaps the spinal cord, and an increase in contrast between the lungs and their surrounding structures. These changes resulted in a more realistic appearance.

Interestingly, these changes were observed in both lateral and anterior-posterior projections, even though only the latter was used in the discriminator. This suggests that our Sim-GAN was able to effectively identify the distinguishing features that separate real projections from DRRs, regardless of the input image structure (Fig. 3).

3.2   CXR Lobar Emphysema Validation

The performance of the regressor portion of our model was assessed using the Relative Error (RE) between emphysema scores stratified by four emphysema severity groups (as described in Sect. 3): no emphysema, mild, moderate and severe (Fig. 4).

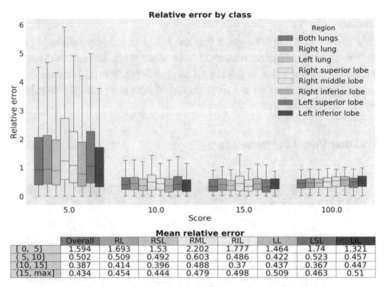

	Overall	RL	RSL	RML	RIL	LL	LSL	LIL
[0, 5]	1.594	1.693	1.53	2.202	1.777	1.464	1.74	1.321
(5, 10]	0.502	0.509	0.492	0.603	0.486	0.422	0.523	0.457
(10, 15]	0.387	0.414	0.396	0.488	0.37	0.437	0.367	0.447
(15, max]	0.434	0.454	0.444	0.479	0.498	0.509	0.463	0.51

Fig. 4. Boxplot of the relative error of the predicted scores on artificial X-rays, organized by emphysema severity (no emphysema (5.0), mild (10.0), moderate (15.0) and severe (100.0)) and lung region (color).

The distribution of the RE across regions is quite homogeneous, which is a good indicator that our model has learned to discern the spatial distribution of emphysema throughout the lungs for a severity group. The no-emphysema group has highest mean RE, with values larger than 1 for all regions, meaning that the predicted scores differ at least by 1 time the actual value. If we consider that these scores are smaller than 5%, these large relative errors become relevant for scores higher than 3–4%, as a relative error of 1.5 could make a negative emphysema diagnosis into a positive one. The mean RE is mostly constant for all 3 remaining groups, with values roughly centered around 0.45 indicating their utility to monitor emphysema distribution in subjects with disease.

3.3   Validation of Emphysema Distribution Quantification

Upper/lower lobe ratio (U/L ratio) is a measurement used for characterization of emphysema, as heterogeneity is a relevant marker when considering treatment. We analyzed the ability of our model for localizing emphysema on those subjects with moderate to severe emphysema (>10%) by calculating the U/L ratio per lung and assessing whether each test case has upper (U/L > 1) or lower (U/L < 1) lobe predominant emphysema. By looking at the confusion matrix of each lung, we observe that our model overdiagnoses upper lobe dominant emphysema for both right and left lungs, with an accuracy of 66.38% and 67.23% respectively (Figs. 5 and 6).

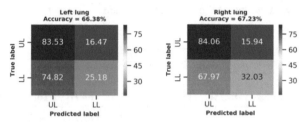

Fig. 5. Confusion matrix (normalized by row) of U/L lobe ratio > 1 and < 1 for mild to severe emphysema for each lung.

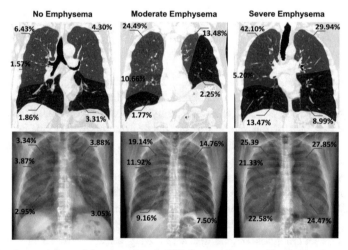

Fig. 6. Visual comparison of the ground truth CT lobar emphysema distribution (top row) and the predicted scores on the respective DRRs (bottom row) for three different emphysema severities: no emphysema (left), moderate (middle) and severe (right).

3.4 Emphysema Diagnostic Performance on CXR

Lastly, to further study the diagnostic ability of our regressor model (how well it can discern between sick and healthy subjects) we computed the AUC of several ROC curves establishing different emphysema thresholds for each lobe, as well as the overall score, and compared it to the AUC achieved in our previous work [3]. We can observe that by increasing the threshold (the pathological definition of emphysema) the performance of our model improves, which was expected given that more advanced emphysema stages present more noticeable alterations on X-ray images. If we look at the 10% threshold row (corresponding to moderate to severe emphysema), the mean sensitivity is 81.61% with an AUC of 87.97. Comparing the results to our previous model in which we solely estimated the total emphysema score with a simple CNN [3], we can see that the AUCs of our Sim-GAN model are comparable to those of the simpler model, which means that we have improved the diagnostic information including spatial distribution of emphysema without sacrificing accuracy of the overall performance (Table 1).

Table 1. AUC of our regressor for different diagnostic criteria for each lobe (RUL, RML, RLL, LUL, LLL) as well as the overall score (Total) and the AUCs of our previous work (Total 2018).

Emph Thres %	RUL	RML	RLL	LUL	LLL	Total	Total (2018)
≥ 5	82.58	79.24	84.48	82.93	83.96	84.99	85.91
≥ 10	**85.43**	**83.78**	**87.93**	**86.79**	**86.74**	**87.97**	**90.73**
≥ 20	88.84	85.67	91.47	90.26	89.56	91.57	-

3.5 External Validation in Scout Projections

To validate our model, we ran it on the 8,222 scouts from NLST dataset. Just like we did for the DRRs, we refined the scouts and then ran them through the regressor to get the emphysema scores. Making the same analysis as we did on the DRRs, we notice that the performance of our model on this dataset decreases. The mean RE of each lobe for all 4 emphysema severity categories shows a similar behavior on scouts as it does on DRRs, with a homogeneous distribution of the error across regions for a given emphysema severity, with the higher values on the no-emphysema group. The mean RE for this group ranges from 1.664 (for LIL) to 3.235 (for RIL), being higher on scouts than on DRRs by a mean factor of 1.4; however, the behavior is almost identical on both datasets for scores larger than 5%. The AUC of the ROC curves show that our model does have sufficient diagnosis capability, with the highest AUC (for severe emphysema) being 71.38.

4   Discussion and Conclusion

We designed a Sim-GAN-like regressor network with which we aimed to solve two problems at once: making artificially generated X-ray projections look more realistic, and accurately quantifying and locating emphysema distribution throughout the pulmonary lobes of a given subject.

The results of the refining stage of the model showed an improvement on the visual aspect of the artificially generated projections, increasing the brightness of the heart and reducing the values of the air inside the lungs, giving them a more realistic look. However, we can still discern between real and refined projections, as real X-rays show more details inside the lungs, given by the fact that X-rays have a higher spatial resolution than standard CTs.

Analyzing the regressor portion of the network, we observed that our model properly learned the hierarchical distribution of the scores across lobes and lungs; this is, the scores obtained for each lobule add up to make up the score for each individual lung when taking the volumes of each region into account, so even when the prediction is wrong, all 8 scores are coherent with themselves. The model was also capable of predicting emphysema scores on DRR with an accuracy of 84.99% when studying emphysema under the condition that a positive diagnosis is given when the subject has at least 5% of emphysematous tissue in the lungs. By increasing this threshold to a 10%, the performance of our model increases, having an AUC of 87.97%, an improvement over the observer-based X-ray visual diagnostic technique which has an accuracy of 77% for mild to moderate severity [8]. The regressor shows a fixed positive bias when predicting small emphysema scores, while it tends to underestimate large scores.

Using our model as a tool to describe the heterogeneity of moderate to severe emphysema throughout the lobes, we observed that the regressor has an accuracy of roughly 66.8% at predicting upper vs. lower lobe emphysema dominance, with a tendency of favoring emphysema on the upper lobe over the lower lobe. This is likely because the moderate to severe emphysema cases of our training set were composed roughly 70% of upper lobe dominant cases. Although far from optimal, these results are still optimistic given that lung fissures are difficult to locate on X-rays and visual detection of emphysema on X-rays relies on the expression of symptoms rather than on the detection of the affected tissue.

However, our model's performance decreased when we used it on scouts, especially when analyzing its diagnostic capability, obtaining worse results than those attained when performing visual interpretation of the images.

While it is true that CT scans have an easily implemented and fast method to accurately quantify and localize emphysema, the main advantage our model presents over LAA% is that our regressor works on X-ray images, which are more frequently used than CT scans on a clinical setting, given that X-rays are acquired faster, the radiation dose the patient receives is lower, and the cost of a performing a single X-ray is cheaper. In addition to that, X-rays are also part of the follow-up of COPD patients [9]. Our model offers a reliable tool for assessing emphysema severity on chest X-rays, and -although with a lower accuracy- it can also describe the heterogeneity of the spatial distribution of emphysema throughout the lobes (U/L ratio). This opens the doors for a potential use for screening patients to undergo lung volume reduction using endobronchial valve treatment [2]; furthermore, studies show that an emphysema-percentage-based system could be used for stratification of lung cancer risk, as emphysema has been identified as a mayor risk factor [10].

The model designed for this project has room for improvement; the worsening of the performance of our model when used on scouts as compared to its performance on DRR images might be due to the fact that scouts are very noisy when compared with DRRs, along with the fact that the scouts were not preprocessed to remove the CT table and sheets. Despite the domain change, our model still provided results with diagnostic value. We can rule out overfitting of the training data as a problem source, as when we tested the model on a set of images that it had never seen, the results were optimistic. To overcome this issue, we could find out whether the problem is with the aspect of the input images or with the model by training a Sim-GAN to refine scouts, and then run them through our regressor to see if the results improve. It could also be argued that there is a potential miscalibration in the output of our network which might be decreasing its performance, which could be solved by recalibrating the system. However, our next step should be to try our regressor on a large collection of real X-rays with emphysema scoring, to test whether our results can be extrapolated to a real-life scenario.

Acknowledgments. This work was partially funded by the National Institutes of Health NHLBI award R01HL149877 and 5R21LM013670.

References

1. World Health Organization: The top 10 causes of death (2019), 2020. https://www.who.int/news-room/fact-sheets/detail/the-top-10-causes-of-death. Accessed Nov. 08, 2022
2. Hartman, J.E., Vanfleteren, L.E.G.W., van Rikxoort, E.M., Klooster, K., Slebos, D.J.: Endobronchial valves for severe emphysema. European Respiratory Rev. **28**(152), Jun 2019. https://doi.org/10.1183/16000617.0121-2018
3. Campo, M.I., Pascau, J., Estepar, R.S.J.: Emphysema quantification on simulated X-rays through deep learning techniques. In: Proceedings - International Symposium on Biomedical Imaging, May 2018, vol. 2018-April, pp. 273–276. https://doi.org/10.1109/ISBI.2018.8363572
4. Sogancioglu, E., Murphy, K., Scholten, E., Boulogne, L.H., Prokop, M., van Ginneken, B.: Automated estimation of total lung volume using chest radiographs and deep learning. Med. Phys. **49**(7), 4466–4477 (2022). https://doi.org/10.1002/mp.15655
5. Regan, E.A., et al.: Genetic Epidemiology of COPD (COPDGene) Study Design. COPD: Journal of Chronic Obstructive Pulmonary Disease, vol. 7, no. 1, pp. 32–43, Feb. 2011, doi: https://doi.org/10.3109/15412550903499522
6. Pizer, S.M., Johnston, R.E., Ericksen, J.P., Yankaskas, B.C., Muller, K.E.: Contrast-Limited Adaptive Histogram Equalization: Speed and Effectiveness (1990)
7. Shrivastava, A., Pfister, T., Tuzel, O., Susskind, J., Wang, W., Webb, R.: Learning from simulated and unsupervised images through adversarial training. In: Proceedings - 30th IEEE Conference on Computer Vision and Pattern Recognition, CVPR 2017, 2017, vol. 2017-Janua, pp. 2242–2251. https://doi.org/10.1109/CVPR.2017.241
8. Reid, L., Millard, F.J.: Correlation between radiological diagnosis and structural lung changes in emphysema. Clin. Radiol. **15**(4), 307–311 (1964). https://doi.org/10.1016/S0009-9260(64)80002-7
9. Miniati, M., et al.: Value of chest radiography in phenotyping chronic obstructive pulmonary disease. Eur. Respir. J. **31**(3), 509–514 (2008). https://doi.org/10.1183/09031936.00095607
10. Li, Y., et al.: Effect of emphysema on lung cancer risk in smokers: a computed tomography-based assessment. Cancer Prev. Res. **4**(1), 43–50 (2011). https://doi.org/10.1158/1940-6207.CAPR-10-0151

Thorax-Net: A Full Thoracic Chest X-Ray Segmentation Approach

Maria Rollan-Martinez-Herrera[1], Jagoba Zuluaga-Ayesta[1],
Francisco Martinez-Dubarbie[2,3], Marta Garrido-Barbero[4],
Ane Zubizarreta-Zamalloa[5], and Raul San José Estépar[1(✉)]

[1] Applied Chest Imaging Laboratory, Brigham and Womenś Hospital, Harvard
Medical School, Boston, MA, USA
rsanjose@bwh.harvard.edu
[2] Marqués de Valdecilla University Hospital, Santander, Cantabria, Spain
[3] Institute for Research "Marques de Valdecilla" (IDIVAL), University of Cantabria,
Santander, Cantabria, Spain
[4] Cruces University Hospital, Barakaldo, Bizkaia, Spain
[5] Basurto University Hospital, Bilbao, Bizkaia, Spain

Abstract. We propose a whole thorax segmentation approach in Chest
Radiographs based on a UNet architecture that captures useful information from the mediastinal region, which is often discarded in lung-based
segmentation. Our approach achieved excellent agreement with expert
readers, with 91% perfect segmentation and only 1% incorrect segmentations. When compared to lung-based segmentation, our thorax segmentation approach showed superior performance in preselection for a
diagnostic model, with higher validation and external validation areas
under the curve (AUCs). Our results suggest that thorax segmentation
may be a better preprocessing step for chest X-ray classification models.

Keywords: Thorax segmentation · CXR · UNet · Validation

1 Introduction

Chest X-ray (CXR) radiography is the most common and accessible medical
imaging technique [1]. It is commonly used as a first-line-of-care radiographic
test, even when more sophisticated tests are needed. Although CXR is mainly
used for detecting pulmonary pathology, it has utility beyond this purpose. Multiple thoracic pathologies with mediastinal manifestations can be detected by
this imaging technique, such as sarcoidosis, thymoma, lymphoma, cardiomegaly,
and ascending aortic aneurysm.

CXR segmentation is a preprocessing technique that provides semantic spatial context [2]. This can enable the extraction of features or enhance structures in a given anatomical area. It can also focus the attention of downstream
machine learning classification approaches on the area of interest for the pathology in question, thus eliminating anatomical and imaging confounders that could
hinder learning or induce uncontrolled learning biases.

© The Author(s), under exclusive license to Springer Nature Singapore Pte Ltd. 2023
Y.-W. Chen et al. (Eds.): KES InMed 2023, SIST 357, pp. 385–393, 2023.
https://doi.org/10.1007/978-981-99-3311-2_35

One of the main challenges for thoracic applications is the delineation of the lung regions that can show increased density in the presence of edema or pneumonia [3]. This specific task is difficult because these opacities often reach high intensity values that can be incorrectly interpreted as the lung limit. There are multiple segmentation works using neural networks focused on delineating the lung fields within chest radiographs. However, segmentation of the entire thorax, including lungs and the mediastinal region, has been largely unexplored. Full thorax segmentation is relevant since multiple extrapulmonary diseases can also be diagnosed based on chest radiography. In addition, lung-specific segmentation approaches ignore the fact that posterior lung segments are projected into the mediastinal portion of CXR, potentially excluding regions susceptible to disease as illustrated in Fig. 1. Therefore, segmentation of the pulmonary space alone obviates much useful information.

In this paper, we propose the implementation of a U-Net model for the segmentation of the entire thoracic space. We validate our segmentation results using a consensus-based approach with four clinicians. Finally, we compare the utility of our proposed thorax segmentation model with a lung-only segmentation model in focusing the attention of a classification model for pathology detection based on image masking. Our proposed model has the potential to provide more accurate and comprehensive information for thoracic disease diagnosis.

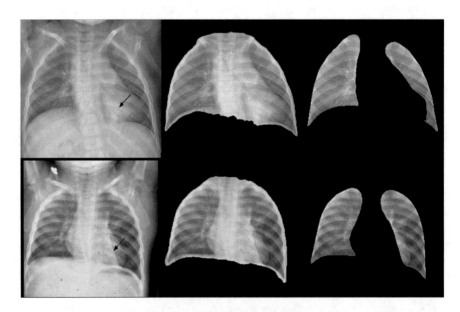

Fig. 1. Example of pathological cases where abnormal opacities are located within the anterior projection of the mediastinal region. The top image depicts a case of retrocardiac pneumonia, while the bottom image shows a case of retrocardiac atelectasis. Limiting a classification to the lung region in these cases would result in missing important diagnostic information.

2   Methods

2.1   Datasets

We utilized CXR images from four distinct data sources, namely the NIH Chest X-ray[1], JSRT dataset[2], Mongogomery County[3], Lung Segmentation from Chest-Xray dataset[4] and the Chest-Xray pneumonia[5]. These data sources were combined to create five separate datasets for our analyses:

- **General Dataset:** This dataset was used for training and testing the segmentation network. We randomly selected 500 images from the NIH Chest X-ray dataset. The median age of the subjects in this dataset was 48.5 years (interquartile range [IR] 34–58.25 years), and it included 206 (41%) females and 294 (59%) males. The dataset contained various radiographic findings, including Atelectasis, Cardiomegaly, Consolidation, Edema, Effusion, Emphysema, Fibrosis, Hernia, Infiltration, Mass, No Finding, Nodule, Pleural Thickening, Pneumonia, and Pneumothorax. The dataset was divided into training and testing sets in an 80:20 ratio.
- **Pathological Dataset:** We also used an independent set of 200 images randomly selected from the NIH Chest X-ray dataset with pathological findings.
- **Clinical Validation Dataset:** This dataset comprised 585 CXRs from three sources, including 200 randomly selected images from the NIH Chest X-ray dataset, 247 images from the JSRT dataset, and 138 images from the Montgomery County dataset. The median age of the subjects in this dataset was 51 years (IR 36.5–63 years), and it included 296 (51%) females and 288 (49%) males. Among the radiographs, 55% were normal.
- **Lung Segmentation Dataset:** This dataset has 21165 images already segmented. The dataset was divided into training and testing sets in an 80:20 ratio.
- **Classification Dataset:** This dataset was composed of 10,000 randomly selected images from the NIH dataset, with 5,000 having "no findings" and 5,000 having some findings, for training purposes. Additionally, 5,840 images from the Chest Xray Pneumonia dataset were used for external testing.

We used these datasets for various purposes, such as training and testing the segmentation and classification models, as well as validating our results against clinical scoring criteria.

2.2   Segmentation Ground-Truth

The thorax region in the General Dataset and the Pathological Dataset were manually segmented by a clinician with multi-year experinece reading CXR.

---

[1] https://www.kaggle.com/datasets/nih-chest-xrays/data.

[2] https://www.kaggle.com/datasets/raddar/nodules-in-chest-xrays-jsrt.

[3] https://www.kaggle.com/datasets/raddar/tuberculosis-chest-xrays-montgomery.

[4] https://kaggle.com/code/nikhilpandey360/lung-segmentation-from-chest-x-ray-dataset.

[5] https://www.kaggle.com/datasets/paultimothymooney/chest-xray-pneumonia.

2.3   Network Architecture

Our thorax segmentation model, called Thorax-net, was developed using the U-Net architecture [6] with a Dice coefficient loss function. Our U-Net has four downsample blocks, with two convolutions per level, with 64, 128, 264 and 512 channels respectevely; a bottleneck with 1024 channels, and four upsample blocks. To evaluate the effectiveness of our approach, we compared it to the encoder-decoder architecture proposed by Wufeng Liu et al. [4] (Efficientnet), which has five coding and decoding layers. The encoder was Efficientnet-b4, pre-trained on the Imagenet dataset. The decoder consisted of five blocks, each with a dropout layer, a two-dimensional convolution and padding layer, and two residual blocks with a LeakyReLU.

We trained both approaches ten times on the General Dataset's 400 training images, and then evaluated the resulting models on the General Dataset's test split (100 images) and the Pathologic Dataset (200 images). We performed data augmentation using spatial transformations (affine and elastic), blurring, and downsampling with the Albumentations library. We augmented the data with a factor of 2:1 to create a total of 1,200 training samples.

We compared the two approaches using the Dice coefficient, Euclidean Latent distance, accuracy, and area under the curve (AUC) metrics. The Euclidean latent distance was implemented in the following way using an autoencoder approach. First, a U-Net architecture was trained to generate a replica of the mask using the training dataset. The encoder portion of this trained U-Net was then extracted and utilized in the evaluation of a segmentation network's output. The encoder was applied to both the segmentation network's output and the corresponding ground truth mask. The output of the encoder was then compared to the ground truth using the absolute difference metric.

The network's output masks were post-processed to remove holes, and we retained the largest component for topological consistency. This post-processed result was used in our validation experiments.

2.4   Clinical Validation

The network results was visually validated by a group of four experts. Each expert assigned a score (1 to 3) to each segmentation. 1 was a perfect segmentation, 2 an acceptable segmentation but with some errors, and 3 an incorrect segmentation Fig. 2. The scores were unified using the Dawid-Skene method [5] to define a consensus score that was used a reference standard. Chi-squared test and pairwise post-hoc analysis were adjusted using Holm-method to assess difference between rating groups.

2.5   Impact of Segmentation in Classification Tasks

To further evaluate the clinical relevance of our full thorax segmentation approach, we compared it with a lung segmentation approach. To this end, we

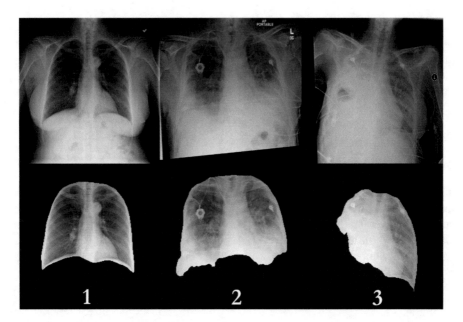

Fig. 2. Expert-based scoring for thorax segmentation evaluation. 1: perfect segmentation, 2: acceptable segmentation but with some errors, 3: incorrect segmentation.

trained a lung segmentation model using the same segmentation network architecture and the Thorax Segmentation Dataset. The trained lung segmentation model achieved a Dice coefficient of 0.988, an accuracy of 0.994, and an AUC of 0.992.

We trained two classification networks on the Classification Dataset to distinguish between normal and pathologic cases. These networks utilized different masking strategies based on either the full thorax or lung segmentation masks. The classification model was built on a pretrained Xception backbone network that was originally trained on ImageNet. To adapt gray-scale images, a 2D convolution of dimensions (1,1,3) was added as a preceding layer to the backbone. The backbone was then followed by a global max pooling and four dense layers. During training, the first half of the backbone was kept frozen while the second half was fine-tuned. Binary Crossentropy was used as the loss function with Adam optimizer and a learning rate of 10-4.

2.6   Reproducibility

To ensure the reproducibility of our work, we have made all the code and datasets generated during the replication of our results publicly available on the S3 bucket[6] and GitHub repository[7]. This includes the training and validation

---

[6] s3://cxr-thorax-segmentation.
[7] https://github.com/acil-bwh/CXRThoraxSegmentation.

datasets, data preprocessing steps, and the U-Net architecture used for thorax segmentation. We have also included detailed instructions and documentation to aid researchers in reproducing our results. We believe that sharing our code and data will not only help in validating our results, but also promote transparency and facilitate further research in the field of AI-driven CXR diagnosis.

3   Results

3.1   Segmentation Performance

The segmentation results of our method and the reference method in the testing datasets are shown in Table 1. The proposed model achieved best results in Dice coefficient over the test images in the General Dataset and the Pathological Dataset (0.96 and 0.97 respectively). Accuracy and AUC were 0.97 and 0.98 for the General Dataset and 0.98 and 0.98 for the Pathological Dataset respectively. For all the metrics, our method performance metric were superior ($p < 0.001$). Our approach also showed significance differences between the two different test datasets for all metrics, with better results in the Pathologic Dataset ($p = 0.02$).

Table 1. Results (mean and confidence interval) of the different approaches for the validation datasets using various metrics.

Method	Testing set	Eucl. Lat. Dist.	Accuracy	AUC	Dice coefficient
ThoraxNet	All	0.11 (0.10–0.12)	0.97 (0.97–0.97)	0.97 (0.97–0.97)	0.96 (0.960.97)
Efficientnet	All	0.18 (0.17–0.21)	0.95 (0.94–0.95)	0.95 (0.94–0.95)	0.93 (0.92–0.93)
ThoraxNet	General	0.11 (0.11–0.33)	0.97 (0.78–0.97)	0.97 (0.81–0.97)	0.96 (0.80–0.96)
Efficientnet	General	0.18 (0.17–0.22)	0.94 (0.93–0.95)	0.95 (0.94–0.95)	0.93 (0.91–0.94)
ThoraxNet	Pathologic	0.09 (0.09–0.33)	0.98 (0.78–0.98)	0.97 (0.81–0.98)	0.97 (0.80–0.97)
Efficientnet	Pathologic	0.18 (0.16–0.22)	0.95 (0.93–0.95)	0.95 (0.94–0.95)	0.93 (0.91–0.94)

In Fig. 3, we present a comparison of the performance of two segmentation methods, ThoraxNet and EfficientNet, in three different cases. Our findings indicate that ThoraxNet demonstrates superior performance in terms of accurately delineating the diaphragmatic arch and contouring the caudal mediastinal region.

3.2   Clinical Validation

The clinical validation showed good results (Table 2). There was a majority of evaluations with the highest score (91%) compared to 2 (8%) and 3 (1%). All the difference were significant ($p < 0.0001$).

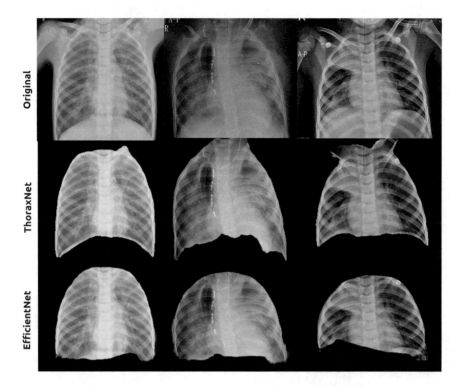

Fig. 3. Comparison between methods in three cases from the testing dataset.

3.3 Impact of Segmentation in Classification Problems

The thorax segmentation-based model classification was more stable across all the training experiment when evaluation over the testing split of the Classification Dataset Fig. 4. The classification model with thorax segmentation had a AUC of 0.8 (IC95% 0.79–0.81) while the lung segmentation-based model yielded a AUC of 0.72 (IC95% 0.7–0.734) on the external testing.

4   Discussion and Conclusions

In this study, we introduced and validated a U-Net architecture for thorax segmentation in CXR images, which outperformed a previously published method [4] in our validation datasets using multiple evaluation metrics.

To clinically validate our method, we assessed its performance against a consensus criteria between experts. Although the agreement between experts was reasonable, with a weighted Cohen's Kappa of 0.6, we employed a consensus score to define a reference using the Dawid-Skene method [5]. Overall, our results were promising, with 91% of masks evaluated as correct. However, the NIH dataset had the lowest percentage of correct masks (82%), which may be

Table 2. Proportion of testing images assigned to each evaluation score based on a consensus reading.

Evaluation label	Dataset	Frequency	N	Proportion (CI 95%)
1	TOTAL	534	585	91% (89%–93%)
2		46		8% (6%–10%)
3		5		1% (0%–2%)
1	JSRT	240	247	97% (94%–99%)
2		7		3% (1%–6%)
3		0		0% (0%–1%)
1	MONT	129	138	93% (88%; 97%)
2		9		7% (3%–12%)
3		0		0% (0%–3%)
1	NIH	165	200	82% (77%–87%)
2		30		15% (10%–21%)
3		5		2% (1%–6%)

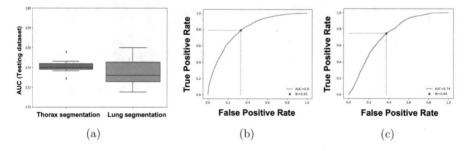

Fig. 4. (a) Testing AUC over the classification training. The box-plot shows the AUC results over the test split for all training, ten per each approach. ROC curve for the classification model using thorax-based (b) and lung-based (c) segmentations in the external testing dataset.

due to the higher variety of images with many non-pathological images being technically altered or having an underlying pathological thorax. In contrast, the Montgomery and JSRT datasets had more standardized images and their percentage of correct masks were 93% and 97%, respectively. Notably, the JSRT dataset, which had the highest number of pathological images, did not show differences in labels between non-pathological and pathological masks.

Moreover, we compared the utility of thorax segmentation and lung segmentation as part of a CXR masking preprocessing for a classification model to distinguish between normal and pathological CXR. Our hypothesis was that lung segmentation may overlook important information contained in the mediastinal area, as it focuses only on the primary lung fields. When comparing the results of the best model trained with thorax mask preprocessing and the best model trained with lung mask preprocessing over the validation dataset, we found that thorax segmentation was superior in the Classification Dataset validation folder (AUC 0.73 vs 0.72) but with no significant differences. However, with the External Classification Validation Dataset, the thorax segmentation preprocessing was significantly superior to the lung segmentation preprocessing (AUC 0.8 vs 0.74).

In conclusion, we presented a U-Net model for thorax segmentation in CXR, which was clinically validated by a consensus of human readers and achieved reliable results. Our model showed some limitations related to slightly inferior results in older subjects with preexisting pathologies. Our results suggested that thorax segmentation may be superior to lung segmentation as part of the preprocessing in AI-driven CXR diagnostic models.

Acknowledgments. This work has been funded by NIH awards R01HL149877 and 5R21LM013670, and a fellowship by Fundación Martín Escudero.

References

1. Mettler, F.A.: Essentials of Radiology, 3rd edn. Saunders Elsevier, Amsterdam (2013)
2. Mittal, A., Hooda, R., Sofat, S.: Lung field segmentation in chest radiographs: a historical review, current status, and expectations from deep learning. IET Image Process. **11**(11), 937–952 (2017)
3. Teixeira, L.O., Pereira, R.M., Bertolini, D., et al.: Impact of lung segmentation on the diagnosis and explanation of COVID-19 in chest x-ray images. Sensors **21**(21), 7116 (2021)
4. Liu, W., Luo, J., Yang, Y., Wang, W., Deng, J., Yu, L.: Automatic lung segmentation in chest x-ray images using improved U-net. Sci. Rep. **12**(1), 8649 (2022)
5. Dawid, A.P., Skene, A.M.: Maximum likelihood estimation of observer error-rates using the EM algorithm. J. R. Stat. Soc.: Ser. C: Appl. Stat. **28**(1), 20–28 (1979)
6. Ronneberger, O., Fischer, P., Brox, T.: U-net: convolutional networks for biomedical image segmentation. In: Navab, N., Hornegger, J., Wells, W.M., Frangi, A.F. (eds.) MICCAI 2015. LNCS, vol. 9351, pp. 234–241. Springer, Cham (2015). https://doi.org/10.1007/978-3-319-24574-4_28

Author Index

Y.-W. Chen et al. (Eds.): KES InMed 2023, SIST 357, pp. 395–396, 2023.
https://doi.org/10.1007/978-981-99-3311-2

Printed in the United States
by Baker & Taylor Publisher Services